Childhood Obesity: Contemporary Issues and Challenges

Childhood Obesity: Contemporary Issues and Challenges

Editor: Monica Slater

MURPHY & MOORE
www.murphy-moorepublishing.com

www.murphy-moorepublishing.com

MURPHY & MOORE

Cataloging-in-Publication Data

Childhood obesity : contemporary issues and challenges / edited by Monica Slater.
p. cm.
Includes bibliographical references and index.
ISBN 978-1-63987-778-2
1. Obesity in children. 2. Overweight children. 3. Metabolic disorders in children. 4. Children--Diseases. I. Slater, Monica.
RJ399.C6 C45 2023
618.923 98--dc23

Murphy & Moore Publishing
1 Rockefeller Plaza,
New York City,
NY 10020, USA

ISBN 978-1-63987-778-2

Contents

Preface

Over the recent decade, advancements and applications have progressed exponentially. This has led to the increased interest in this field and projects are being conducted to enhance knowledge. The main objective of this book is to present some of the critical challenges and provide insights into possible solutions. This book will answer the varied questions that arise in the field and also provide an increased scope for furthering studies.

Childhood obesity refers to a state in which a child's health or well-being is harmed by the presence of excess fat in the body. The methods to identify and evaluate body fat are problematic and due to this reason, BMI is frequently used to diagnose the presence and extent of obesity. The prevalence of obesity in children varies by gender and sex. The longer a child remains obese or overweight; the more likely it is that the child will grow up to be obese with all the associated morbidities. Children are exposed to a variety of social, nutritional and obesogenic environmental risks influencing their health throughout the life. Child obesity can be managed with physical activity and dietary changes. These play a significant role in ensuring a child's health and in maintaining the nutritional level, and diet patterns and quality. This book explores all the contemporary issues and challenges related to childhood obesity in the present day scenario. It strives to provide a fair idea about obesity in children and to help develop a better understanding of the latest advances in its clinical management. This book is appropriate for students seeking detailed information in this area as well as for experts.

I hope that this book, with its visionary approach, will be a valuable addition and will promote interest among readers. Each of the authors has provided their extraordinary competence in their specific fields by providing different perspectives as they come from diverse nations and regions. I thank them for their contributions.

Editor

Dietary Patterns and Risk of Obesity and Early Childhood Caries in Australian Toddlers

Lucinda K. Bell [1], Celeste Schammer [1], Gemma Devenish [2], Diep Ha [3], Murray W. Thomson [4], John A. Spencer [3], Loc G. Do [3], Jane A. Scott [2] and Rebecca K. Golley [1,*]

1 Caring Futures Institute, College of Nursing and Health Sciences, Flinders University, Adelaide 5001, Australia; lucy.bell@flinders.edu.au (L.K.B.); celesteschammer@gmail.com (C.S.)
2 School of Public Health, Curtin University, Perth 6102, Australia; gemma.devenish@curtin.edu.au (G.D.); jane.scott@curtin.edu.au (J.A.S.)
3 Australian Research Centre for Population Oral Health, School of Dentistry, The University of Adelaide, Adelaide 5000, Australia; diep.ha@adelaide.edu.au (D.H.); john.spencer@adelaide.edu.au (J.A.S.); loc.do@adelaide.edu.au (L.G.D.)
4 Division of Health Sciences, University of Otago, Dunedin 9016, New Zealand; murray.thomson@otago.ac.nz
* Correspondence: rebecca.golley@flinders.edu.au.

Abstract: We examined associations between dietary patterns at 12 months, characterised using multiple methodologies, and risk of obesity and early childhood caries (ECC) at 24–36 months. Participants were Australian toddlers (n = 1170) from the Study of Mothers' and Infants' Life Events affecting oral health (SMILE) birth cohort. Principal Components Analysis (PCA) and the Dietary Guideline Index for Children and Adolescents (DGI-CA) were applied to dietary intake data (1, 2 or 3-days) at 12 months, and regression analysis used to examine associations of dietary patterns with body mass index Z-score and presence of ECC at 24–36 months. Two dietary patterns were extracted using PCA: *family diet* and *cow's milk and discretionary combination*. The mean DGI-CA score was 56 ± 13 (out of a possible 100). No statistically significant or clinically meaningful associations were found between dietary pattern or DGI-CA scores, and BMI Z-scores or ECC (n = 680). Higher *cow's milk and discretionary combination* pattern scores were associated with higher energy and free sugars intakes, and higher *family diet* pattern scores and DGI-CA scores with lower free sugars intakes. The association between dietary patterns and intermediate outcomes of free sugars and energy intakes suggests that obesity and/or ECC may not yet have manifested, and thus longitudinal investigation beyond two years of age is warranted.

Keywords: dietary patterns; diet quality; obesity; dental caries; early childhood; toddlers; child (List three to ten pertinent keywords specific to the article; yet reasonably common within the subject discipline.)

---

1. Introduction

Childhood obesity and early childhood caries (ECC) are two highly prevalent conditions affecting children [1,2]. In Australia, 26% of children have overweight or obese [3] and 34% have ECC by five years of age [4]. Given the commonality of both these conditions in early childhood, and evidence of an association between the two [5], the case has been made that obesity prevention could be targeted within the dental remit [6,7]. The Common Risk Factor Approach (CRFA) seeks to target risk factors common between conditions [8], with potential efficiencies and benefits over utilizing an approach that is disease-specific [8]. Thus, adopting a collaborative approach to tackling both childhood obesity and ECC may be more effective than an individual condition approach.

Poor diet in early life is a major modifiable risk factor for both obesity and ECC. This is particularly true for high intakes and frequencies of free sugars [9–11]. For example, an Australian study of over 4000 children aged 4–8 years found that obesity and ECC were both associated with sugary drink consumption [12]. Given that the first years of life are a critical period when dietary behaviours and food preferences are established, persisting and predicting disease in adulthood [13,14], understanding risk-promoting dietary factors and how they interact is important to inform interventions that aim to simultaneously prevent obesity and caries in early childhood.

Beyond sugar, poor diet comprises many other risk factors for obesity (energy, saturated fat, refined grains, processed meat) and ECC (e.g., acidic foods, protective role of dairy foods) [15,16]. Therefore, it is most appropriate to examine whole diet, rather than single nutrients (e.g., sugars) or foods (e.g., sugary drinks), as a means of understanding obesity and dental caries prevention in early life. Measuring multiple dietary components together acknowledges the synergistic and correlational nature of single foods and nutrients, and reflects how people eat [17,18]. Whole-of-diet patterns can be derived using an a priori score-based approach or an a posteriori data-driven approach. Score-based (a priori) approaches are commonly based on prevailing dietary guidelines which incorporate pre-existing knowledge of several chronic diseases, whereas data-driven approaches (a posteriori) use statistical data reduction techniques such as Principal Components Analysis (PCA) to explain the total variation in diet of a population [17,18]. Each approach has advantages and disadvantages over the other. For example, as a posteriori methods generate patterns based on empirical data, without *a-priori* knowledge, they do not necessarily represent optimal patterns [19], whereas a priori approaches do not account for biological interaction among nutrients [19]. Given this, examining diet using a combination of a priori and a posteriori approaches may provide greater insight into the diet-disease relationship. Doing so using the same sample can strengthen the understanding of this relationship for both obesity and ECC.

Whole-of-diet patterns have been characterised in young children using both a priori and a posteriori approaches and their association with later health outcomes investigated [20]. Studies exploring the relationship between dietary patterns and child obesity have shown inconsistent findings [20,21], while studies exploring the relationship between dietary patterns and ECC are rare. Those few studies which have investigated the latter relationship using a posteriori-derived indices have reported inconsistent findings [22,23] with only one study, to our knowledge, (and in an Asian multi-ethnic population), doing so using a priori-derived dietary patterns (exploratory factor analysis to examine diet trajectories between 6 and 12 months of age and ECC at ages 2 and 3 years) [24]. Such inconsistencies in the evidence may be due to discrepancies in the methodological approaches used to characterize dietary patterns (a priori vs. a posteriori). Thus, using multiple methodological approaches to characterize dietary patterns in early life would be advantageous in comparing and contrasting findings, and it would provide a more detailed dietary picture for that particular population.

Given the inconsistencies in findings and scarcity of research examining the relationship between whole-of-diet in the first years of life and the outcomes obesity and ECC, (along with the benefits of utilising multiple approaches to characterize diet and the greater recognition of the CRFA), this study aimed to investigate the association between whole diets and obesity and ECC in young children. The primary aim was to describe dietary patterns in Australian toddlers at 12 months of age using a priori and a posteriori approaches and then to examine their association with obesity and ECC at 24–36 months of age. Secondary aims were to examine associations between dietary patterns and free sugars and total energy intake, and to identify the socio-demographic determinants of observed dietary patterns.

2. Materials and Methods

2.1. Data Source

This was a secondary analysis of data collected as a part of the Study of Mothers' and Infants' Life Events affecting health (SMILE), a prospective cohort study following socio-economically diverse South Australian newborns from birth to 24–36 months, described in detail elsewhere [25]. Briefly, mother–infant dyads were recruited from three major maternity hospitals between July 2013 and August 2014. Recruitment took place on postnatal wards by trained dental nurses and dental therapists within 48 h of birth. Mothers were provided with a written and verbal description of the study and only those mothers with sufficient English to comprehend the study instructions and who intended to remain living within the Adelaide region for at least 12 months were invited to participate. In total, 2147 mothers and 2181 infants, including 34 sets of twins, were recruited [25]. Children with complete dietary data (1, 2 or 3 days), socio-economic variables and outcome data were included in the secondary analysis.

2.2. Data Collection and Entry

2.2.1. Dietary Data

Children's dietary intake was collected via 1 × 24 h dietary recall (24 HDR) and 1 × 2-day estimated food record over a non-consecutive 10-day period (week and weekend days) at 12 months of age [26]. Following their child's first birthday and prior to data collection, mothers were mailed a food record and an accompanying letter advising them that a researcher would contact them to conduct the 24 HDR and to provide instructions on how to complete the food record [26,27]. A trained dietitian conducted the 24 HDR via telephone using a five-step multi-pass method [28]. Following the recall, dietitians allocated each mother two days in the subsequent week (10-day period) to record their child's dietary intake in the food record. The food record contained a one-day food record example, and pictures of food portion sizes and common household measures to assist mothers in estimating serve sizes in the food recall and record [26,27].

Dietary data were double-entered into Foodworks 8 by a team of trained nutritionists/dietitians (Xyris Software, 2012–2016, Brisbane, QSL, Australia) as paired (3-day; 1 × 24 HDR and 1 × 2-day food record) and unpaired data (single 24 HDR) using data entry protocols for standardisation. Participants were included if they had at least one complete day of dietary intake data available. Data were analysed using the AUSNUT 2011–2013 food composition database [29], and food groups and servings were classified using the Australian Dietary Guideline (ADG) numeric classification system [25,26]. Owing to the rapidly changing infant and toddler food market, some infant foods (n = 187) consumed by the SMILE cohort did not exist in the AUSNUT 2011–2013 database. Accordingly, these foods were added to the database using information sourced from manufacturer's websites and product nutrition information panels, mapped to a similar product in AUSNUT 2011–2013 for missing micronutrient values, and an appropriate 8-digit AUSNUT code allocated [26,27] (see Devenish et al. 2019 [30] for more details).

2.2.2. Child and Maternal Sociodemographic Data

Sociodemographic data (including maternal age, smoking status, pre-pregnancy weight status, education attainment, annual household income and child gender) were collected from mothers at recruitment via standardised self-completed questionnaires [25]. Data on child age (at 24 HDR), breastfeeding duration and the age at which children were introduced to solids were obtained from a series of postal, online and face-to-face surveys at 3, 6, 12 and 24 months [25].

2.2.3. Dental Data

Once children reached 24 months of age, they were invited (with their mothers), to participate in a dental examination. Dental examinations were conducted by a small team of specially trained dentists under standardised conditions [31,32]. Standard clinical indices were used; these had been developed at the Australian Research Centre for Population Oral Health (ARCPOH) and based on US National Institute of Dental and Craniofacial Research (NIDCR) protocol and the International Caries Detection and Assessment System (ICDAS) [33] were used. Non-cavitated or cavitated carious lesions, filling, missing tooth surfaces due to decay, non-carious developmental conditions and gingival conditions were recorded [25]. In the current analysis, ECC was characterised as present or absent, based on the presence of 1 or more cavitated surfaces at age 2 years.

2.2.4. Anthropometric Data

Child weight and height data were collected at the dental examination using standardised methodology and equipment including digital scales and a portable stadiometer [25]. Pre-pregnancy maternal height and weight were self-reported in the baseline questionnaire. Body mass index (BMI) (kg/m^2) was calculated for both the mother and child and weight status was categorised using World Health Organization (WHO) age-and gender-specific cut-offs [25].

2.3. *Dietary Pattern Analysis*

2.3.1. Principal Components Analysis (PCA)

A-posteriori dietary patterns were extracted using Principal Components Analysis (PCA). Prior to this, a total of 2303 food and beverage items were categorised into meaningful and interpretable groups for use as input variables. Items were grouped based on their nutrient profile, the WHO free sugars recommendations [34], the Australian Guide to Healthy Eating (AGHE) [35] and the Australian Dietary Guidelines (ADG) [36]. Food groups that were not representative of usual toddler intake (i.e., dietary supplements, cooking agents and alcoholic beverages) were excluded. Fifty-eight food groups were created and used as input variables for PCA.

PCA was conducted on all available dietary intake data. That is, participants with 1, 2 or 3-days of dietary data were included. Multiple days of dietary data were combined using mean intake across the days involved. The correlation matrix, Kaiser–Myer–Olkin measure of sampling adequacy, Bartlett's test of sphericity and communalities were all inspected to determine whether a meaningful PCA could be performed [37]. All criteria were met demonstrating that all food groups contributed to the extracted patterns and, therefore, none were removed for subsequent analysis. Orthogonal (varimax) rotation was used to improve interpretability of the component loadings. The number of dietary patterns retained was determined using eigenvalues >1.5 and examination of a break point in the scree plot [37]. Based on the scree plot a two-factor (first break) and a seven-factor (second break) solution were considered. The seven factor solution did not meet the criteria for eigenvalues >1.5 and was not interpretable and thus not considered further. Patterns were named according to foods with loadings >0.25 to aid interpretability [38,39]. A dietary pattern score was calculated for each participant for each pattern by summing the product of a standardised gram of each item consumed by its factor loading. Patterns were normally distributed (mean 0, SD 1).

2.3.2. The Dietary Guideline Index for Children and Adolescents (DGI-CA)

A priori dietary patterns were derived by applying the DGI-CA, a validated diet quality index score for children and adolescents aged 4–16 years [40], updated [41] to reflect adherence to the 2013 ADGs and extended here to include the recommended daily serves for 12–24-month-olds [42]. The tool comprises 11 indicators based on compliance with the dietary guidelines; one reflects diet variety, one reflects dietary moderation and nine reflect diet adequacy and diet quality. The total DGI-CA score is a sum of each indicator; it is converted to a score between 0 and 100, with higher scores reflecting greater adherence to the dietary guidelines.

2.4. Statistical Analysis

Statistical analysis was conducted using SPSS version 25 (IBM SPSS Statistics for Windows, New York, NY, USA). Categorical data are presented as frequency (%) and continuous data as mean ± SD (as all were normally distributed). A Chi-square test (categorical) and independent t-test (continuous data) were employed to assess the statistical difference in sample characteristics between the total sample (n = 1170) and the final regression analysis sample (n = 680, see below). Standard linear regression was employed to investigate the associations between PCA-derived dietary patterns and DGI-CA scores with various outcome variables; (1) socio-demographic factors, (2) free sugars intake (grams), (3) energy intake (kilojoules) and (4) BMI Z-scores. Binary logistic regression was employed to investigate the relationships of dietary patterns and DGI-CA scores with the presence of dental caries. Multivariable models were adjusted for the following confounders: IRSAD (Index of Relative Socio-Economic Advantage and Disadvantage) deciles, one of four Socio-Economic Indexes for Areas (SEIFA) indices that ranks areas across Australia on a continuum of disadvantage (lowest score = 1) to advantage (highest score = 10), as a proxy for socio-economic position (SEP) [43], annual household income, maternal age, smoking status during pregnancy, weight status, education attainment, number of parents in the household, child's age (at 24 HDR) and gender, and child's age at which introduced to solids and at which breastfeeding ceased [38,40,44,45]. Due to missing data, the final regression analysis sample size was $n = 680$, which met the required sample size of $n = 225$ for assessing 15 predictors based on the ratio of 15 participants to 1 predictor [37]. Regression assumptions were checked through assessing the normality, linearity and variance of residuals [37]. The level of statistical significance was set at $p < 0.05$. To determine the magnitude of the associations, unstandardized regression coefficients (B), odds ratios and 95% confidence interval (CI) were used.

3. Results

The characteristics of children and their mothers are described in Table 1. Dietary intake data were provided for 1170 children (46% female) with a mean age (at 24 HDR) of 13.1 (range 12–22) months. Most (62.1%) children were healthy weight, with 6.2% having overweight, 2.0% having obesity, and 0.4% underweight (29% missing). Few (8.8%) children had dental caries. The majority of mothers were partnered, university educated, employed prior to giving birth, not overweight or obese, and non-smokers during pregnancy. Mothers who provided complete dietary data but did not provide complete baseline or dental or weight outcome data were younger (analysis sample vs incomplete sample, mean = 30.8 vs. 30.1 years), and more educated (57.9% vs. 49.2% attended some university or above) but otherwise largely representative of the sample with complete data (Table 1).

3.1. A Posteriori and A Priori Dietary Patterns

Two a posteriori dietary patterns were extracted using PCA (Table 2). The proportion of variance explained by both patterns was 7.9%. The first was characterised by vegetables, fresh fruit, non-white bread, cheese and non-discretionary red meat and poultry, all of which are common family-based items. Hence, this pattern was termed a *family diet* pattern. The second pattern was termed *cow's milk and discretionary combination* because it was characterised by cow's milk, fluoridated water, white bread, cheese and discretionary foods including processed meat, sugary products, sugar sweetened beverages and discretionary potato products. A priori dietary patterns were determined using the DGI-CA. The mean ± SD DGI-CA score was 56 ± 13 with 0% of children achieving the maximum possible score of 100 (data not shown). There were no statistically significant or meaningful differences between the final analysis sample and incomplete sample for dietary pattern scores (*family diet*: analysis sample vs incomplete sample, mean = 0.0 ± 0.9 vs. 0.0 ± 1.1; *cow's milk and discretionary combination*: 0.0 ± 1.0 vs. 0.0 ± 1.0) and DGI-CA scores (57 ± 13 vs. 55 ± 13).

Table 1. Characteristics of mother-child dyads in the sample with complete dietary data and sample with complete outcome and explanatory variables.

Characteristics	Total Sample [a] n = 1170, n (%)		Analysis Sample [b] *n* = 680, *n* (%)	
Child Characteristics				
Age at time of 24 HDR (months) [c,d]	13.1	0.9	13.1	0.8
Gender				
Female	540	46.2	313	46.0
Breastfeeding duration (weeks) [e]				
<17	254	21.7	176	25.9
17–25	107	9.1	80	11.8
26–51	261	22.3	198	29.1
>52	316	27.0	226	33.2
Age of introduction to solids (weeks) [f]				
<17	235	20.1	147	21.6
17–25	692	59.1	454	66.8
>26	121	10.3	79	11.6
Weight status [g,h]				
Underweight	5	0.4	5	0.7
Healthy weight	727	62.1	593	87.2
Overweight	73	6.2	59	8.7
Obesitye	23	2.0	23	3.4
Maternal and household characteristics				
Age at birth [e,f]	30.5	5.1	30.8	5.0
Household income [c,d] (annual)				
<40,000	162	14.0	83	12.2
40,100–80,000	369	31.8	216	31.8
80,100–120,000	357	30.8	216	31.8
>120,000	272	23.4	165	24.3
IRSAD [d,i]				
Deciles 1–2 (most disadvantaged)	195	16.7	98	14.4
Deciles 3–4	247	21.1	150	22.1
Deciles 5–6	235	20.1	137	20.1
Deciles 7–8	220	18.8	141	20.7
Deciles 9–10 (most advantaged)	262	22.4	154	22.6
Two parent household [f]				
Yes	1090	93.2	641	94.3
Smoking status during pregnancy [d]				
Yes	78	6.7	37	5.4
Weight status [d,i]				
Underweight	47	4.0	28	4.1
Healthy	572	48.9	350	51.5
Overweight	262	22.4	168	24.7
Obesitye	211	18.0	134	19.7
Education attainment [d]				
High school/vocational	524	44.8	286	42.1
Some university or above	635	54.3	394	57.9
Work status prior to birth [d]				
Employed	875	74.8	531	78.1

[a] Sample with complete dietary data but incomplete outcome or explanatory variables. [b] Sample with complete outcome and explanatory variables. [c] Values presented as mean (SD). All other values presented as frequency (%). [d] Less than 5% missing data. [e] 20% missing data. [f] Less than 15% missing data. [g] 29% missing data. [h] Weight status categories according to body mass index (BMI) (kg/m^2); Underweight <18.5 kg/m^2, Healthy weight 18.5–24.9 kg/m^2, Overweight 25–29.9 kg/m^2, Obese >30 kg/m^2. [i] IRSAD: Index of Relative Socio-Economic Advantage and Disadvantage. HDR: hour dietary recall.

Table 2. Varimax-rotated food group loadings on each of the dietary patterns at 12 months extracted by Principal Components Analysis (PCA).

Foods	Percent Consumingd (%) [b]	Dietary Patterns [a]	
		Family Foods	Cow's Milk Discretionary
Vegetables: other non-discretionary	64.4	**0.534**	0.086
Fruit: Fresh	90.0	**0.513**	0.073
Vegetables: Orange	60.2	**0.502**	−0.154
Vegetables: Green and Brassica	56.2	**0.488**	−0.034
Meat: Red	28.9	**0.305**	0.005
Poultry and feathered game	39.3	**0.295**	0.006
Bread: non-white	42.1	**0.290**	0.247
Potato: non-discretionary	42.2	**0.260**	−0.015
Cereal: Breakfast with no added sugar	58.9	0.250	−0.045
Infant food: commercial sweet	62.0	−0.238	0.043
Flours and Grains	60.4	0.225	−0.207
Fish: non-discretionary	21.2	0.223	−0.076
Infant food: commercial savoury	13.3	−0.221	−0.152
Dairy yoghurt: whole fat	19.6	0.219	−0.040
Eggs	28.3	0.216	0.002
Sauces and condiments	28.6	0.201	0.097
Fruit juice: non-discretionary	9.7	−0.186	0.074
Fruit juice: discretionary	3.7	−0.142	0.045
Infant drinks	1.8	−0.137	−0.007
Dairy milk: reduced fat	3.8	−0.130	0.130
Beverages: other discretionary	1.8	−0.091	0.001
Vegetables MD: discretionary	3.0	0.053	0.034
Fruit: stewed and MD	3.2	0.051	0.035
Fruit: packaged with added sugar	1.8	0.049	0.015
Meat: MD non-discretionary	20.6	0.033	−0.028
Vegetables: MD non-discretionary	3.8	−0.032	−0.030
Dairy milk: flavoured	1.9	0.029	0.002
Infant formula and breastmilk	71.0	−0.207	**−0.682**
Dairy milk: Whole fat	71.0	−0.007	**0.504**
Water: domestic	96.8	0.247	**0.426**
Meat: processed	32.8	0.010	**0.397**
Sugar and sugary products	23.4	−0.135	**0.330**
Cheese	57.5	**0.279**	**0.309**
Potato: discretionary	16.0	−0.188	**0.289**
Bread: white	48.7	−0.236	**0.272**
Sugar sweetened beverages: discretionary	1.5	−0.165	**0.259**
Margarine and oils	27.0	0.117	0.250
Sweet biscuits and cakes	40.9	−0.001	0.244
Fish: discretionary	6.8	0.036	0.234
Confectionary	6.7	−0.178	0.217
Nuts and seeds	19.7	0.147	0.211
Bread: sweet	9.5	−0.064	0.210
Fruit: dried	19.6	0.031	0.206
Cereal: other discretionary	35.1	−0.107	0.205
Cereal: savoury non-discretionary	43.0	0.039	0.173
Butter	38.6	−0.021	0.168
Water: other	2.4	−0.027	0.167
Fruit: packaged with no added sugar	8.3	−0.049	0.143
Flavoured yoghurt and custard	27.9	0.051	0.138
Poultry: MD non-discretionary	15.6	0.064	0.132
Cereal fruit and nut bars	4.7	−0.065	0.129
Dairy: other discretionary	9.6	−0.099	0.105
Poultry: MD discretionary	1.1	−0.046	0.096
Dairy Alternatives: non-discretionary	3.9	0.078	0.095
Soups	9.3	0.005	−0.091
Legumes and Beans	10.9	0.025	0.073
Cereal: Breakfast with added sugar	5.6	0.003	0.039
Meat: MD discretionary	0.3	−0.021	0.030

Abbreviations: PCA: principal component analysis; MD: mixed dishes. [a] Loadings ≥ 0.25 in bold to aid labelling of dietary patterns. [b] Total number of participants consuming the food or beverage.

3.2. *Association between Dietary Patterns and Adiposity or Dental Caries*

After adjustment for covariates, no significant or clinically meaningful associations were found between dietary pattern scores or DGI-CA scores and BMI Z-scores or presence of dental caries (Table 3).

Table 3. Associations between dietary patterns at 12 months and BMI Z-scores, BMI-weight category, dental caries at 24–36 months, after adjusting for covariates [a].

	BMI Z-Score [b]			Dental Caries [c]			
	B	95% CI	*p*-Value	OR	Wald	95% CI	*p*-Value
Diet Patterns [d]							
Family Diet	0.031	−0.059, 0.120	0.500	0.830	1.346	0.605, 1.137	0.246
Cow's milk and discretionary combination	0.022	−0.068, 0.111	0.632	0.889	0.554	0.653, 1.212	0.457
DGI-CA scores *(Scale: 0–100)*	0.007	0.000, 0.013	0.053	0.987	1.287	0.966, 1.009	0.257

Abbreviations: BMI, body mass index, 95%CI, 95% confidence interval. [a] Maternal (age at birth, Index of Relative Socio-Economic Advantage and Disadvantage (IRSAD), household income, two parent household, smoking status, weight status, education attainment and work status prior to birth) and child (age at 24 HDR, gender, breastfeeding duration and age introduced to solids) confounders were adjusted for in analysis. [b] Results were obtained using standard linear regression models with child BMI Z-scores as outcome variable and diet pattern scores, DGI-CA scores and all respective covariates as independent predictors. [c] Defined as the presence of 1 or more cavitates surfaces. Results were obtained by binary logistic regression models with dental status as the outcome variable and diet pattern scores, DGI-CA scores and all respective covariates as independent predictors. [d] Dietary pattern scores are standardized scores with a mean and standard deviation of 0 ± 1.

3.3. *Association between Dietary Patterns and Free Sugars or Energy Intakes*

Dietary pattern scores and DGI-CA scores were independently associated with free sugars and energy intake at 12 months after adjusting for covariates (Table 4). A 1 SD higher *family diet* pattern score was associated with a 5.5 g lower free sugars intake, while a 10 point higher DGI-CA score would equate to a 4 g lower free sugars intake. Conversely a 1 SD higher *cow's milk and discretionary combination* pattern score was associated with a 9.7 g higher free sugars intake, and a 1310 kJ greater energy intake, almost double that predicted by higher family diet pattern scores (779kJ). A 10 point higher DGI-CA scores was associated with a 380 kJ higher energy intake.

Table 4. Associations between dietary patterns at 12 months and intake of free sugars (g) and total energy intake (kJ), after adjusting for covariates [a].

	Free Sugars (g)			Energy Intake (kJ)		
	B	95% CI	*p*-Value	b	95% CI	*p*-Value
Diet Patterns [b]						
Family Diet	−5.461	−7.088, −3.834	<0.001	779.112	461.090, 1097.134	<0.001
Cow's milk and discretionary combination	9.767	8.140, 11.394	<0.001	1310.417	992.307, 1628.526	<0.001
DGI-CA scores (Scale: 0–100)	−0.393	−0.529, −0.258	<0.001	37.784	12.301, 63.266	0.004

Abbreviations: BMI, Body Mass Index, 95%CI, 95 Percent Confidence Interval. [a] Results were obtained using standard linear regression models with child BMI Z-scores as outcome variable and diet pattern scores, DGI-CA scores and all respective covariates as independent predictors. Maternal (age at birth, Index of Relative Socio-Economic Advantage and Disadvantage (IRSAD), household income, two parent household, smoking status, weight status, education attainment and work status prior to birth) and child (age at 24 HDR, gender, breastfeeding duration and age introduced to solids) confounders were adjusted for in analysis. [b] Dietary pattern scores are standardized scores with a mean and standard deviation of 0 ± 1.

3.4. *Predictors of Dietary Patterns and Quality*

After adjusting for covariates, several maternal (age, education, employment status, IRSAD decile, household income) and child (age at 24 HDR, age of introduction to solids, breastfeeding duration) characteristics were independently associated with dietary pattern scores and/or DGI-CA scores (Table 5). For example, some maternal university education was associated with a 0.16 higher *family diet* pattern score than for those mothers whose highest education was the completion of school or vocational education. Higher scores on this *family diet* pattern were also associated with greater socioeconomic advantage and younger mothers. Conversely, higher scores on the *cow's milk and discretionary combination* pattern were observed with older children at 24 HDR, earlier introduction to solids, earlier breastfeeding cessation, younger mothers and mothers who were unemployed prior to giving birth. Similarly, higher DGI-CA scores were observed with older children at 24 HDR, greater household income and university educated mothers.

Table 5. Multivariable associations with dietary patterns at 12 months and mother-child dyad characteristics, after adjusting for covariates (n = 680) [a].

	Dietary Patterns [i]						DGI–CA [i]		
	Family Diet			Cow's Milk and Discretionary Combination					
	B	95% CI	*p*-Value [j]	B	95% CI	*p*-Value [j]	b	95% ci	*p*-Value [j]
Child Characteristic									
Gender	−0.101	−0.242, 0.040	0.160	0.023	−0.117, 0.164	0.745	−1.079	−2.938, −0.044	0.255
Age [b]	0.067	−0.017, 0.151	0.116	0.179	0.095, 0.263	0.000	1.661	0.553, 2.769	0.003
Breastfeeding duration	0.036	−0.029, 0.100	0.275	−0.098	−0.162, −0.033	0.003	0.560	−0.291, 1.410	0.197
Age of introduction to solids	0.103	−0.026, 0.233	0.118	−0.175	−0.305, −0.046	0.008	−0.107	−1.816, 1.601	0.902
Maternal Characteristics									
Age at child's birth	−0.019	−0.033, −0.004	0.012	−0.024	−0.039, −0.010	0.001	−0.130	−0.324, 0.064	0.189
IRSAD Decile [c]	0.033	0.006, 0.060	0.016	0.002	−0.025, 0.029	0.867	0.221	−0.136, 0.577	0.225
Household Income [d]	0.071	−0.011, 0.152	0.090	0.078	−0.004, 0.159	0.062	1.967	0.888, 3.046	0.000
Two parent household [e]	0.188	−0.128, 0.505	0.243	−0.155	−0.471, 0.161	0.336	0.304	−3.873, 4.480	0.887
Smoking status during pregnancy [e]	−0.259	−0.577, 0.058	0.109	−0.039	−0.356, 0.278	0.811	−3.743	−7.931, 0.445	0.080
Weight status (Healthy weight) [f]									
Underweight	0.055	−0.305, 0.416	0.764	−0.304	−0.665, 0.056	0.098	2.277	−2.482, 7.035	0.348
Overweight	−0.048	−0.223, 0.127	0.591	0.007	−0.665, 0.056	0.934	−0.480	−2.787, 7.035	0.683
Obese	−0.064	−0.255, 0.128	0.514	0.160	−0.032, 0.351	0.102	−1.168	−3.692, 1.827	0.364
Work status prior to birth [g]	−0.095	−0.273, 0.082	0.290	0.192	0.015, 0.369	0.033	−1.434	−3.772, 0.905	0.229
Education attainment [h]	0.160	0.005, 0.315	0.043	−0.146	−0.301, 0.009	0.064	2.594	0.548, 4.640	0.013

[a] Results were obtained using standard linear regression models using diet pattern and DGI-CA scores as dependent variables and all respective covariates as independent variables. [b] Age at time of 24 HDR (12 months). [c] Index of Relative Socio-Economic Advantage and Disadvantage, IRSAD decile categorized as 1 = most disadvantaged and 10 = most advantaged. [d] Household income categorized as (1) <40 K (2) 40.1–80 K (3) 80.1–120 K (4) >120 K. [e] Categorised as yes (reference category) or no. [f] Weight status categories according to Body Mass Index (BMI) (kg/m^2); Underweight <18.5 kg/m^2, Healthy weight 18.5–24.9 kg/m^2, Overweight 25–29.9 kg/m^2, Obesity >30 kg/m^2. Healthy weight is used as reference category. [g] Work status categorized as employed (reference category) or unemployed. [h] Education attainment categorized as school/vocational or some university and above (reference category). [i] Dietary pattern scores are standardized scores with a mean and standard deviation of 0 ± 1. DGI-CA scores are on a scale between 0–100. [j] Model Fit: All linear regression models statistically significant ($p < 0.001$). Bold values represent statistically significant values ($p < 0.05$).

4. Discussion

The present study aimed to characterise whole-of-diet patterns at 12-months of age using multiple dietary pattern methods, and investigate their relationship with obesity and ECC at 24–36 months of age. No association was found between dietary patterns and obesity, or between dietary patterns and dental caries, using either the a priori DGI-CA, or a posteriori PCA approaches. However, higher free sugars and energy intakes, risk factors for both obesity and ECC, were positively associated with the *cows milk and discretionary combination* pattern (reflecting poorer-quality diet), and lower free sugars intake positively associated with both the *family diet* pattern and higher DGI-CA scores (both reflecting higher-quality diet). Dietary patterns were also predicted by maternal socio-demographic factors and child early feeding experiences in expected directions. Given this face validity of extracted dietary patterns, and their association with intermediate outcomes of free sugars and energy intake, the association between dietary patterns obesity and/or ECC may not yet have manifested and thus further longitudinal follow-up is warranted.

The lack of association between diet, obesity and dental caries in the present study is unsurprising given the inconsistent findings reported previously from investigations of both a priori and a posteriori-derived dietary patterns and measures of weight status [21,38,46–48] and dental caries [49–52] in early life. A possible explanation for the lack of association seen in the present study is that it may be too early to detect the influence of poor diet. For example, a 2014 systematic review found a positive association between energy-dense, high-fat and low-fibre dietary patterns in childhood and later overweight and obesity in high quality studies with a follow up period greater than 2 years (2–21 years) [53]. Thus, longer-term follow-up, beyond 24–36 months of age (i.e., one-year follow-up) is required. This is supported by the fact that dietary patterns were predicted by free sugars and energy intakes, as well as maternal factors (age, income, employment and education status) and early feeding experiences (breastfeeding cessation, age of introduction to solids) in expected directions, demonstrating face validity of the dietary patterns extracted using both methods. Therefore, further investigation of the relationship between dietary patterns, obesity and ECC, using the CRFA model, is warranted to clarify the utility of whole-of-diet approaches in examining obesity and dental caries in early life, or whether it is too soon in the developmental trajectory to identify any association.

The diets in this sample were similar to those observed previously in Australian [38], European [45], and US [44] toddlers. For example, the *family diet* pattern resembles the *14-month and 24-month core food* patterns in 14 (n = 552) and 24 (n = 493)-month-old Australian toddlers respectively, while the *cow's milk and discretionary pattern* shares similarities with the *basic combination* (14 months) and *non-core pattern* (24 months) [38]. Furthermore, while the DGI-CA has not been previously applied to the diets of children under 4 years, the mean DGI-CA score (56/100, indicating poor adherence to the ADGs) is also consistent with previous research in older Australian children and adolescents (4–16 years, 54/100; 4–7 year olds 61/100 [40]; 4–8 years, 51/100; 4–16 years, 54/100; [41]).

Despite no significant longitudinal association between diet and weight and dental status, both a priori and a posteriori-derived dietary patterns were associated cross-sectionally with free sugars and energy intakes; those are key risk factors for both obesity and ECC. That is, higher and lower free sugars intakes were associated with 'poorer' and 'higher' diet patterns, respectively. These findings are consistent with previous research in British [54] infants (n = 6065, 6 and 8 months of age) and Australian children and adolescents (n = 3416, 4–16 years) [40]). In contrast, although higher energy intakes were associated with poorer-quality dietary patterns (characterised a posteriori), they were also associated with higher-quality dietary patterns (characterised a priori [DGI-CA] and a-posteriori). These findings suggest that nutrient adequacy may be coupled with higher energy intakes, contradicting the currently understood concept that higher energy intakes and nutrient inadequacy occur simultaneously [40]. Further, given the association between poorer-quality dietary patterns and higher free sugars and energy intakes, it is possible that an association of dietary patterns with obesity and/or ECC could be observed with further longitudinal investigation.

Dietary patterns characterised in the present study were also associated with key socio-demographic characteristics. For example, poorer diets (derived a posteriori using PCA) were associated with earlier breastfeeding cessation and age of introduction to solids. This is consistent with previous findings in Australian [38] and European [44] toddlers and is likely explained by the influence of early feeding experiences (for example, flavour exposure from breastmilk) on later food taste and food acceptance [55,56]. Furthermore, earlier introduction of solids may coincide with an earlier introduction of discretionary foods [57], or an enhanced preference for discretionary-type foods [58]. Also consistent with previous research, poorer and higher-quality diets were associated with lower maternal employment status [40] and maternal income [40,44,59] and university-education [38,44,45,60], respectively, whilst both were associated with younger mothers [38]. Together, these findings support the well-established role of mothers in determining early experiences with health behaviours, including food and eating [21,61], highlighting potential intervention targets. Lastly, although previous research suggests diet quality decreases with child age [13,40], the present study found that older children tended to have poorer diet-quality patterns (derived a posteriori using PCA) but higher diet quality scores (derived a priori using the DGI-CA). However, the DGI-CA does not account for breast- or formula-milk and thus younger children may receive a lower overall DGI-CA score than older children who consume a greater amount and variety of foods other than milk.

4.1. Strengths and Limitations

This study is strengthened by the use of longitudinal data from the SMILE study which overcomes the possibility of reverse directionality between dietary patterns and obesity and ECC outcomes. The use of two dietary pattern approaches to assess relationships is novel and strengthens the findings, given that each provides different information about diet and the advantages and disadvantages of each approach are somewhat counteracted by the other. The use of a validated dietary index, the DGI-CA, and multivariable analysis, which has not been utilised in previous studies within the dental context, are also strengths. Lastly, despite a modest sample size, the most socially disadvantaged families were only slightly under-represented (15–17% of participants in the lowest two deciles). This is much better than most studies of this kind which are typically skewed towards the upper deciles. Nonetheless, the findings must be considered within the context of the study limitations. Energy intake was able to be estimated at only one time point (12-months of age) due to the dietary assessment method used (24-HDRand food records at 12 months), and thus only cross-sectional associations between dietary patterns and underlying free sugars and energy intakes could be investigated, precluding the determination of directionality. Another consideration is that some dental-specific (e.g., fluoride exposure, although it is unlikely that this would have varied greatly in the present sample as all were living in fluoridated areas at the time of recruitment) and obesity-specific (e.g., physical activity level) confounders were not able to be adjusted for in the multivariable analysis because they were not measured. Lastly, the limitations of PCA and the DGI-CA cannot be ignored. Principal Component Analysis is a highly subjective, multi-step process where numerous decisions are made by the researcher (for example, how data are grouped, how variables should be treated and how many patterns to retain), thus affecting the nature of the extracted patterns [18]. The DGI-CA is also limited in that it represents current dietary guidelines with disease outcomes considered individually, not concurrently. However, multiple dietary pattern approaches were utilised to account for the limitations of each.

4.2. Implications for Future Practice and Research

Although this study investigated the relationship between diet and obesity and ECC longitudinally, longer-term follow-up is warranted beyond two years of age to more fully determine the nature of the associations. While it was valuable to investigate the impact of dietary patterns characterised by PCA (a-posteriori) and the DGI-CA (a-priori) using the CRFA, it appears that exploration of dietary patterns using a more specific and tailored whole-of-diet approach might be more insightful. Reduced rank regression (RRR) and disease-specific indices are two methods that have potential in determining associations between whole diet and health outcomes such as obesity and dental caries in future studies [62]. Reduced rank regression has rarely been adopted in nutrition epidemiology; however, in the existing literature RRR-derived dietary patterns have been associated with obesity in children [48] and with cardiometobolic health in infants. Additionally, the associations between dietary patterns, free sugars and energy intakes identified in the present study highlight the potential for these nutrients to be used as response variables in RRR. Disease-specific indices offer another direction moving forward in determining the association of whole-of-diet in early life on later health outcomes, particularly in the dental context. However, to our knowledge, only one dental-specific index has been developed for the paediatric population [49], and this failed to account for the synergistic effects of positive (risk-reducing) nutrients such as calcium and phosphate (i.e., from dairy). Thus, a dental-specific index incorporating both negative (risk-promoting; free sugars) and positive (risk-reducing; calcium, phosphate) nutrients would be a useful tool to better understand the association between early life diet and ECC. Together, the use of RRR and disease-specific indices in future research could improve our understanding of the relationship between early life diet and childhood obesity and dental caries, and could ultimately inform new dietary guidelines for both obesity and dental caries prevention. Such guidelines could be useful for dentists, dietitians, child health nurses, public health workers and policymakers.

5. Conclusions

In summary, this is one of the first studies to describe early life diet using multiple methodologies and to investigate its impact on two key conditions prevalent in childhood, obesity and early childhood caries (ECC). While no association was found between a priori and a posteriori described dietary patterns, and obesity or ECC, the association with intermediate outcomes of free sugars and energy intakes is important, suggesting that obesity and/or ECC may not yet have manifested due to the short follow-up period (24–36 months). Thus, further longitudinal investigation beyond 2 years of age is warranted. Future studies utilising reduced rank regression and disease-specific indices to characterise whole diet may also contribute to a greater understanding of the impact of early life diet on obesity and ECC outcomes. This could ultimately assist in the design of new dietary guidelines and recommendations, useful for dentists, dietitians, child health nurses, public health workers and policymakers, and help to combat both childhood obesity and early childhood caries.

Author Contributions: R.K.G., J.A.S., D.H., L.G.D., J.A.S. and L.G.D. contributed to the design of the SMILE study, secured funding and coordinated the research team. C.S. conducted the secondary analysis under the supervision of R.K.G. and L.K.B.; G.D. helped design and administer the dietary assessment and contributed to preparation of the dataset. C.S. wrote the first manuscript draft which was significantly revised by L.K.B. All authors contributed to subsequent revisions of the manuscript, including interpretation of the results, and approved the final version.

Acknowledgments: The authors wish to thank all participants of the Study of Mothers and Infants Life Events (SMILE) affecting oral health study. Thank you also to Elizabeth Beaton for assisting with secondary entry of dietary data.

References

1. Kassebaum, N.J.; Bernabe, E.; Dahiya, M.; Bhandari, B.; Murray, C.J.; Marcenes, W. Global burden of untreated caries: A systematic review and metaregression. *J. Dent. Res.* **2015**, *94*, 650–658. [CrossRef] [PubMed]
2. Lopez, K.N.; Knudson, J.D. Obesity: From the agricultural revolution to the contemporary pediatric epidemic. *Congenit. Heart Dis.* **2012**, *7*, 189–199. [CrossRef] [PubMed]
3. Australian Institue of Health and Welfare. *A Picture if Overweight and Obesity in Australia 2017*; Australian Institue of Health and Welfare: Canberra, Australia, 2017.
4. Ha, D.H.; Roberts-Thomson, K.; Arrow, P.; Peres, K.; Do, L.G.; Spencer, A.J. Children's oral health status in Australia, 2012–14. In *Oral Health of Australian Children: The National Child Oral Health Study*; Adelaide University Press: Adelaide, Australia, 2016; Volume 2014.
5. Vázquez-Nava, F.; Vázquez-Rodríguez, E.M.; Saldívar-González, A.H.; Lin-Ochoa, D.; Martínez-Perales, G.M.; Joffre-Velázquez, V.M. Association between obesity and dental caries in a group of preschool children in Mexico. *J. Public Health Dent.* **2010**, *70*, 124–130. [PubMed]

6. Spiegel, K.A.; Palmer, C.A. Childhood dental caries and childhood obesity. Different problems with overlapping causes. *Am. J. Dent.* **2012**, *25*, 59–64.
7. Tseng, R.; Vann, W.F.; Perrin, E.M. Addressing childhood overweight and obesity in the dental office: Rationale and practical guidelines. *Pediatr. Dent.* **2010**, *32*, 417–423.
8. Sheiham, A.; Watt, R.G. The common risk factor approach: A rational basis for promoting oral health. *Community Dent. Oral Epidemiol.* **2000**, *28*, 399–406. [CrossRef]
9. Skafida, V.; Chambers, S. Positive association between sugar consumption and dental decay prevalence independent of oral hygiene in pre-school children: A longitudinal prospective study. *J. Public Health* **2017**, *40*, e275–e283. [CrossRef]
10. Moynihan, P.; Tanner, L.; Holmes, R.; Hillier-Brown, F.; Mashayekhi, A.; Kelly, S.; Craig, D. Systematic review of evidence pertaining to factors that modify risk of early childhood caries. *JDR Clin. Transl. Res.* **2019**, *4*, 202–216. [CrossRef]
11. Bovi, A.P.D.; Di Michele, L.; Laino, G.; Vajro, P. Obesity and Obesity Related Diseases, Sugar Consumption and Bad Oral Health: A Fatal Epidemic Mixtures: The Pediatric and Odontologist Point of View. *Transl. Med. UniSa* **2017**, *16*, 11.
12. Hooley, M.; Skouteris, H.; Millar, L. The relationship between childhood weight, dental caries and eating practices in children aged 4–8 years in A ustralia, 2004–2008. *Pediatr. Obes.* **2012**, *7*, 461–470. [CrossRef]
13. Birch, L.; Savage, J.S.; Ventura, A. Influences on the development of children's eating behaviours: From infancy to adolescence. *Can. J. Diet. Pract. Res.* **2007**, *68*, s1. [PubMed]
14. Movassagh, E.Z.; Baxter-Jones, A.D.; Kontulainen, S.; Whiting, S.J.; Vatanparast, H. Tracking dietary patterns over 20 years from childhood through adolescence into young adulthood: The Saskatchewan Pediatric Bone Mineral Accrual Study. *Nutrients* **2017**, *9*, 990. [CrossRef] [PubMed]
15. Adegboye, A.R.; Tomaz, M.; Jeavons, C.A.; Heitmann, B.L. Intake of dairy foods and oral health: Review of epidemiological data. *Dan. Dent. J.* **2017**, *120*, 884–891.
16. Moynihan, P.; Petersen, P.E. Diet, nutrition and the prevention of dental diseases. *Public Health Nutr.* **2004**, *7*, 201–226. [CrossRef]
17. Kant, A.K. Dietary patterns and health outcomes. *J. Am. Diet. Assoc.* **2004**, *104*, 615–635. [CrossRef] [PubMed]
18. Moeller, S.M.; Reedy, J.; Millen, A.E.; Dixon, L.B.; Newby, P.; Tucker, K.L.; Krebs-Smith, S.M.; Guenther, P.M. Dietary patterns: Challenges and opportunities in dietary patterns research: An Experimental Biology workshop, April 1, 2006. *J. Acad. Nutr. Diet.* **2007**, *107*, 1233–1239.
19. Hu, F.B. Dietary pattern analysis: A new direction in nutritional epidemiology. *Curr. Opin. Lipido.* **2002**, *13*, 3–9. [CrossRef]
20. Smithers, L.G.; Golley, R.K.; Brazionis, L.; Lynch, J.W. Characterizing whole diets of young children from developed countries and the association between diet and health: A systematic review. *Nutr. Rev.* **2011**, *69*, 449–467. [CrossRef]
21. Marshall, S.; Burrows, T.; Collins, C.E. Systematic review of diet quality indices and their associations with health-related outcomes in children and adolescents. *J. Hum. Nutr. Diet.* **2014**, *27*, 577–598. [CrossRef]
22. Chaffee, B.W.; Feldens, C.A.; Rodrigues, P.H.; Vítolo, M.R. Feeding practices in infancy associated with caries incidence in early childhood. *Community Dent. Oral Epidemiol.* **2015**, *43*, 338–348. [CrossRef]
23. İnan-Eroğlu, E.; Özşin-Özler, C.; Erçim, R.E.; Büyüktuncer, Z.; Uzamış-Tekçiçek, M.; Güçiz-Doğan, B. Is diet quality associated with early childhood caries in preschool children? A descriptive study. *Turk. J. Pediatr.* **2017**, *59*, 537–547. [CrossRef] [PubMed]
24. Hu, S.; Sim, Y.F.; Toh, J.Y.; Saw, S.M.; Godfrey, K.M.; Chong, Y.-S.; Yap, F.; Lee, Y.S.; Shek, L.P.-C.; Tan, K.H. Infant dietary patterns and early childhood caries in a multi-ethnic Asian cohort. *Sci. Rep.* **2019**, *9*, 852. [CrossRef] [PubMed]
25. Do, L.G.; Scott, J.A.; Thomson, W.M.; Stamm, J.W.; Rugg-Gunn, A.J.; Levy, S.M.; Wong, C.; Devenish, G.; Ha, D.H.; Spencer, A.J. Common risk factor approach to address socioeconomic inequality in the oral health of preschool children–a prospective cohort study. *BMC Public Health* **2014**, *14*, 429. [CrossRef] [PubMed]
26. Scott, J.; Davey, K.; Ahwong, E.; Devenish, G.; Ha, D.; Do, L. A comparison by milk feeding method of the nutrient intake of a cohort of australian toddlers. *Nutrients* **2016**, *8*, 501. [CrossRef]
27. Beaton, E.; Wright, J.; Devenish, G.; Do, L.; Scott, J. Relative Validity of a 24-h Recall in Assessing Intake of Key Nutrients in a Cohort of Australian Toddlers. *Nutrients* **2018**, *10*, 80. [CrossRef]

28. Australian Bureau of Statistics. 4363.0.55.001—Australian Health Survey: Users' Guide, 2011–2013. 24-h Dietary Recall 2014. Available online: http://www.abs.gov.au/ausstats/abs@.nsf/Lookup/0D6B1FE95EAB8FF3CA257CD2001CA113?opendocument (accessed on 18 March 2016).
29. Food Standards Australia and New Zealand. *AUSNUT 2011-13—Australian Food Composition Database*; Food Standards Australia and New Zealand: Canberra, Australia, 2014. Available online: http://www.foodstandards.gov.au/science/monitoringnutrients/ausnut/Pages/default.aspx (accessed on 18 November 2019).
30. Ismail, A.I.; Sohn, W.; Tellez, M.; Amaya, A.; Sen, A.; Hasson, H.; Pitts, N.B. The International Caries Detection and Assessment System (ICDAS): An integrated system for measuring dental caries. *Community Dent. Oral Epidemiol.* **2007**, *35*, 170–178. [CrossRef]
31. NIDCR. *National Health and Nutrition Examination Survey Dental Examiners Procedures Manual*; National Center for Health Statistics: Hyattsville, MD, USA, 2002.
32. World Health Organisation. *Oral Health Surveys: Basic Methods*; World Health Organisation: Geneva, Switzerland, 2013.
33. World Health Organisation. *Guideline: Sugars Intake For Adults And Children*; WHO: Geneva, Switzerland, 2015.
34. National Health and Medical Research Council. *Australian Guide to Healthy Eating*; NHMRC: Canberra, Australia, 2013.
35. National Health and Medical Research Council. *Australian Dietary Guidelines*; NHMRC: Canberra, Australia, 2013.
36. Pallant, J. *SPSS Survival Manual: A Step by Step Guide to Data Analysis Using SPSS*, 4th ed.; Allen & Unwin: Crows Nest, NSW, Australia, 2011.
37. Bell, L.K.; Golley, R.K.; Daniels, L.; Magarey, A.M. Dietary patterns of Australian children aged 14 and 24 months, and associations with socio-demographic factors and adiposity. *Eur. J. Clin. Nutr.* **2013**, *67*, 638. [CrossRef]
38. Northstone, K.; Emmett, P. The associations between feeding difficulties and behaviours and dietary patterns at 2 years of age: The ALSPAC cohort. *Matern. Child Nutr.* **2013**, *9*, 533–542. [CrossRef]
39. Golley, R.K.; Hendrie, G.A.; McNaughton, S.A. Scores on the Dietary Guideline Index for Children and Adolescents Are Associated with Nutrient Intake and Socio-Economic Position but Not Adiposity–3. *J. Nutr.* **2011**, *141*, 1340–1347. [CrossRef]
40. Golley, R.K.; Hendrie, G.A. Dietary Guideline Index for Children and Adolescents: What is the impact of the new dietary guidelines? *Nutr. Diet.* **2014**, *71*, 210–212. [CrossRef]
41. National Health and Medical Research Council. *Eat for Health Educator Guide*; NHMRC: Canberra, Australia, 2013.
42. Australian Bureau of Statistics. 2033.0.55.001-Census of Population and Housing: Socio-Econimic Indexes for Areas (SEIFA), Australia. 2011. Available online: http://www.abs.gov.au/AUSSTATS/abs@.nsf/allprimarymainfeatures/8C5F5BB699A0921CCA258259000BA619?opendocument (accessed on 27 May 2018).
43. Kiefte-de Jong, J.C.; de Vries, J.H.; Bleeker, S.E.; Jaddoe, V.W.; Hofman, A.; Raat, H.; Moll, H.A. Socio-demographic and lifestyle determinants of 'Western-like'and 'Health conscious' dietary patterns in toddlers. *Br. J. Nutr.* **2013**, *109*, 137–147. [CrossRef] [PubMed]
44. Robinson, S.; Marriott, L.; Poole, J.; Crozier, S.; Borland, S.; Lawrence, W.; Law, C.; Godfrey, K.; Cooper, C.; Inskip, H. Dietary patterns in infancy: The importance of maternal and family influences on feeding practice. *Br. J. Nutr.* **2007**, *98*, 1029–1037. [CrossRef] [PubMed]
45. Shin, K.O.; Oh, S.Y.; Park, H.S. Empirically derived major dietary patterns and their associations with overweight in Korean preschool children. *Br. J. Nutr.* **2007**, *98*, 416–421. [CrossRef] [PubMed]
46. Friedman, L.S.; Lukyanova, E.M.; Serdiuk, A.; Shkiryak-Nizhnyk, Z.A.; Chislovska, N.V.; Zvinchuk, A.V.; Oliynyk, I.; Hryhorczuk, D. Social-environmental factors associated with elevated body mass index in a Ukrainian cohort of children. *Int. J. Pediatr. Obes.* **2009**, *4*, 81–90. [CrossRef]
47. Voortman, T.; Leermakers, E.T.; Franco, O.H.; Jaddoe, V.W.; Moll, H.A.; Hofman, A.; van den Hooven, E.H.; Kiefte-de Jong, J.C. A priori and a posteriori dietary patterns at the age of 1 year and body composition at the age of 6 years: The Generation R Study. *Eur. J. Epidemiol.* **2016**, *31*, 775–783. [CrossRef]
48. Evans, E.W.; Hayes, C.; Palmer, C.A.; Bermudez, O.I.; Naumova, E.N.; Cohen, S.A.; Must, A. Development of a pediatric cariogenicity index. *J. Public Health Dent.* **2013**, *73*, 179–186. [CrossRef]

49. Nunn, M.E.; Braunstein, N.S.; Krall Kaye, E.A.; Dietrich, T.; Garcia, R.I.; Henshaw, M.M. Healthy eating index is a predictor of early childhood caries. *J. Dent. Res.* **2009**, *88*, 361–366. [CrossRef]
50. Zaki, N.A.; Dowidar, K.M.; Abdelaziz, W.E. Assessment of the Healthy Eating Index-2005 as a predictor of early childhood caries. *Int. J. Paediatr. Dent.* **2015**, *25*, 436–443. [CrossRef]
51. Marshall, T.A.; Broffitt, B.; Eichenberger-Gilmore, J.; Warren, J.J.; Cunningham, M.A.; Levy, S.M. The roles of meal, snack, and daily total food and beverage exposures on caries experience in young children. *J. Public Health Dent.* **2005**, *65*, 166–173. [CrossRef]
52. Ambrosini, G.L. Childhood dietary patterns and later obesity: A review of the evidence. *Proc. Nutr. Soc.* **2014**, *73*, 137–146. [CrossRef]
53. Golley, R.K.; Smithers, L.G.; Mittinty, M.N.; Brazionis, L.; Emmett, P.; Northstone, K.; Campbell, K.; McNaughton, S.A.; Lynch, J.W. An Index Measuring Adherence to Complementary Feeding Guidelines Has Convergent Validity as a Measure of Infant Diet Quality–3. *J. Nutr.* **2012**, *142*, 901–908. [CrossRef] [PubMed]
54. Mennella, J.A.; Forestell, C.A.; Morgan, L.K.; Beauchamp, G.K. Early milk feeding influences taste acceptance and liking during infancy. *Am. J. Clin. Nutr.* **2009**, *90*, 780S–788S. [CrossRef] [PubMed]
55. Scott, J.; Chih, T.; Oddy, W. Food variety at 2 years of age is related to duration of breastfeeding. *Nutrients* **2012**, *4*, 1464–1474. [CrossRef] [PubMed]
56. Koh, G.A.; Scott, J.A.; Oddy, W.H.; Graham, K.I.; Binns, C.W. Exposure to non-core foods and beverages in the first year of life: Results from a cohort study. *Nutr. Diet.* **2010**, *67*, 137–142. [CrossRef]
57. Howard, A.J.; Mallan, K.M.; Byrne, R.; Magarey, A.; Daniels, L.A. Toddlers' food preferences. The impact of novel food exposure, maternal preferences and food neophobia. *Appetite* **2012**, *59*, 818–825. [CrossRef] [PubMed]
58. Kranz, S.; Hartman, T.; Siega-Riz, A.M.; Herring, A.H. A diet quality index for American preschoolers based on current dietary intake recommendations and an indicator of energy balance. *J. Am. Diet. Assoc.* **2006**, *106*, 1594–1604. [CrossRef]
59. Ystrom, E.; Niegel, S.; Vollrath, M.E. The impact of maternal negative affectivity on dietary patterns of 18-month-old children in the Norwegian Mother and Child Cohort Study. *Matern. Child Nutr.* **2009**, *5*, 234–242. [CrossRef]
60. Darmon, N.; Drewnowski, A. Does social class predict diet quality? *Am. J. Clin. Nutr.* **2008**, *87*, 1107–1117. [CrossRef]
61. Hoffmann, K.; Schulze, M.B.; Schienkiewitz, A.; Nöthlings, U.; Boeing, H. Application of a new statistical method to derive dietary patterns in nutritional epidemiology. *Am. J. Epidemiol.* **2004**, *159*, 935–944. [CrossRef]
62. Leermakers, E.T.; van den Hooven, E.H.; Franco, O.H.; Jaddoe, V.W.; Moll, H.A.; Kiefte-de Jong, J.C.; Voortman, T. A priori and a posteriori derived dietary patterns in infancy and cardiometabolic health in childhood: The role of body composition. *Clin. Nutr.* **2018**, *37*, 1589–1595. [CrossRef]

2

Effects of Lifestyle Modification Interventions to Prevent and Manage Child and Adolescent Obesity

Rehana A. Salam [1], Zahra A. Padhani [1], Jai K. Das [1], Amina Y. Shaikh [1], Zahra Hoodbhoy [1], Sarah Masroor Jeelani [2], Zohra S. Lassi [3] and Zulfiqar A. Bhutta [4,*]

1 Division of Women and Child Health, Aga Khan University Hospital, Karachi 74800, Pakistan; rehana.salam@aku.edu (R.A.S.); zahra.feroz@aku.edu (Z.A.P.); jai.das@aku.edu (J.K.D.); amina.shaikh@hotmail.com (A.Y.S.); zahra.hoodbhoy@aku.edu (Z.H.)

2 Department of Trauma & Orthopaedics, Macclesfield District General Hospital, East Cheshire NHS Trust Victoria Rd, Macclesfield SK10 3BL, UK; saarc93@yahoo.com

3 Robinson Research Institute, University of Adelaide, Adelaide, SA 5005, Australia; zohra.lassi@adelaide.edu.au

4 Centre for Global Child Health, the Hospital for Sick Children, Toronto, ON M5G 1X8, Canada

* Correspondence: zulfiqar.bhutta@sickkids.ca.

Abstract: The objective of this review was to assess the impact of lifestyle interventions (including dietary interventions, physical activity, behavioral therapy, or any combination of these interventions) to prevent and manage childhood and adolescent obesity. We conducted a comprehensive literature search across various databases and grey literature without any restrictions on publication, language, or publication status until February 2020. We included randomized controlled trials and quasi-experimental studies from both high income countries (HIC) and low-middle-income countries (LMICs). Participants were children and adolescents from 0 to 19 years of age. Studies conducted among hospitalized children and children with any pre-existing health conditions were excluded from this review. A total of 654 studies (1160 papers) that met the inclusion criteria were included in this review. A total of 359 studies targeted obesity prevention, 280 studies targeted obesity management, while 15 studies targeted both prevention and management. The majority of the studies (81%) were conducted in HICs, 10% of studies were conducted in upper middle income countries, while only 2% of the studies were conducted in LMICs. The most common setting for these interventions were communities and school settings. Evidence for the prevention of obesity among children and adolescents suggests that a combination of diet and exercise might reduce the BMI *z*-score (MD: −0.12; 95% CI: −0.18 to −0.06; 32 studies; 33,039 participants; I^2 93%; low quality evidence), body mass index (BMI) by 0.41 kg/m^2 (MD: −0.41 kg/m^2; 95% CI: −0.60 to −0.21; 35 studies; 47,499 participants; I^2 98%; low quality evidence), and body weight (MD: −1.59; 95% CI: −2.95 to −0.23; 17 studies; 35,023 participants; I^2 100%; low quality evidence). Behavioral therapy alone (MD: −0.07; 95% CI: −0.14 to −0.00; 19 studies; 8569 participants; I^2 76%; low quality evidence) and a combination of exercise and behavioral therapy (MD: −0.08; 95% CI: −0.16 to −0.00; 9 studies; 7334 participants; I^2 74%; low quality evidence) and diet in combination with exercise and behavioral therapy (MD: −0.13; 95% CI: −0.25 to −0.01; 5 studies; 1806 participants; I^2 62%; low quality evidence) might reduce BMI *z*-score when compared to the control group. Evidence for obesity management suggests that exercise only interventions probably reduce BMI *z*-score (MD: −0.13; 95% CI: −0.20 to −0.06; 12 studies; 1084 participants; I^2 0%; moderate quality evidence), and might reduce BMI (MD: −0.88; 95% CI: −1.265 to −0.50; 34 studies; 3846 participants; I^2 72%) and body weight (MD: −3.01; 95% CI: −5.56 to −0.47; 16 studies; 1701 participants; I^2 78%; low quality evidence) when compared to the control group. and the exercise along with behavioral therapy interventions (MD: −0.08; 95% CI: −0.16 to −0.00; 8 studies; 466 participants; I^2 49%; moderate quality evidence), diet along with behavioral therapy interventions (MD: −0.16; 95% CI: −0.26 to −0.07; 4 studies; 329 participants; I^2 0%; moderate quality evidence), and combination of diet, exercise and behavioral therapy (MD: −0.09; 95% CI: −0.14 to −0.05; 13 studies; 2995 participants; I^2 12%; moderate quality evidence) also probably decreases BMI *z*-score when compared to the control group. The existing evidence is most favorable for a combination of interventions, such as diet along with exercise and exercise along with behavioral therapy for obesity prevention and exercise alone, diet along with exercise, diet along with behavioral therapy, and a combination of diet, exercise, and behavioral therapy for obesity management. Despite the growing obesity epidemic in LMICs, there is a significant dearth of obesity prevention and management studies from these regions.

Keywords: obesity; interventions; children; adolescents

---

1. Introduction

Obesity is a major public health crisis for children and adults across the world [1]. The Global Nutrition Report 2019 highlights that about 40.1 million children globally are overweight and at the same time, overweight, and obesity are increasing rapidly in nearly every country in the world, with no signs of slowing [2]. It is estimated that in 2015, approximately 10% of children and adults globally were obese [3]. The non-communicable disease risk factor collaboration reported that the global prevalence of obesity in boys increased from 0.7% in 1975 to 5.6% in 2016, while in girls the increase was from 0.9% to 7.8% in boys during the same time duration [4]. Data from the National Health and Nutrition Examination Survey (NHANES) reported that in United States, obesity in boys aged 2–5 years had a steep incline from 1999–2016, while there was an increase in overweight girls aged 16–19 years [5]. Similar trends were noted in the data obtained from the United Kingdom, where the obesity epidemic continued to rise in the adolescent population [6]. Low middle income countries (LMICs) are plagued with the "double burden of disease" epidemic [7]. Popkin et al. have demonstrated a significant increase in body mass index (BMI) and waist circumference in individuals from LMICs including Asia and Africa [8]. The prevalence of overweight and obesity in adolescents in LMICs was 15% and 6% respectively [9]. This was particularly noted in Asian regions, Latin America, and Africa [4]. Childhood obesity is known to be associated with a myriad of morbidities, such as atherosclerosis, hypertension, diabetes, metabolic syndrome etc. [10]. The rising obesity epidemic and its associated complications led to the World Health Organization Commission on Ending Childhood Obesity recommending three strategic areas for action [11]. These include prevention through heath education, treatment for childhood obesity, and advocacy regarding healthier environments [11].

Childhood obesity interventions include lifestyle modifications, pharmacological, and surgical interventions [12]. For the purpose of this review, we restricted the interventions to lifestyle modifications only, including dietary interventions, physical activity interventions, and behavioral therapy. Lifestyle modification with increased intake of fruits and vegetables along with recommended moderate physical activity form the mainstay for primary prevention of childhood obesity [13]. Pineda et al. have demonstrated that changes in the school food environment, such as a ban on sugar sweetened beverages and increased availability of fruits and vegetables has led to a significant decrease in obesity prevalence [14]. Nutrition education, as well as school meal policy changes, have been the driving forces behind the reduction in obesity reported in these studies [14]. Physical activity interventions for childhood obesity include promotion of exercise and reduction in sedentary behavior. School-based exercise interventions have been shown to be associated with a lower body mass index (BMI) in children as compared to their inactive counterparts [15]. Reducing sedentary behavior by restricting television and computer time is known to prevent excessive weight gain in children [16]. These interventions ensure that there is no excessive caloric gain thus preventing obesity. Behavioral interventions, such as cognitive behavioral therapy (CBT) are known to be effective in addressing several health conditions including adult and childhood obesity [17]. This technique encourages participants to self-regulate their diet and activity routines to improve their weight management. These interventions are largely implemented in school or community settings, where children and adolescents are available and follow up is convenient over a long period [18–22]. Schools tend to be an ideal location for intervention due to the facilities available and easy access to this particular age group; they also offer time slots and equipment facility to encourage adequate physical activity [23,24]. Other delivery platforms include after-school settings, sports clubs, or within family settings [24].

Multiple reviews and meta-analyses exist evaluating the efficacy of interventions to prevent and manage obesity in children and adolescent [12,25–28]. With the variety of interventions and the ever increasing number of reviews, it is difficult to generate conclusions regarding which interventions are relatively more effective, compared to others for preventing and managing obesity in this age group [24]. Moreover, the results of the existing meta-analyses do not always point in the same direction. A recent meta-synthesis has attempted moderator analyses to explain why some interventions are more effective than others; however, it is limited to a few factors [24]. Furthermore, the majority of the existing systematic reviews have restricted their inclusions to randomized controlled trials (RCTs) alone and focused too much on effectiveness aspect without focusing on the various contextual factors that might potentially impact the effectiveness of these interventions. Although RCTs are considered to be the gold standard when evaluating effectiveness, complementing RCT data with observational studies is sometimes imperative when evaluating complex lifestyle and behavioral interventions [29–33]. Behavioral interventions are complex and influenced by various individual and environmental factors that could potentially impact the uptake and effectiveness of these interventions.

This review aims to summarize up-to-date evidence for both children and adolescents. In addition, we also assessed the studies included in our review with the lens of the PROGRESS framework (place, race, occupation, gender, religion, education, socioeconomic status, and social status). The findings from this review will provide a basis to guide public health program planners to adapt these interventions (alone or in combination) based on identifying factors that may affect how some groups engage with the intervention or the method of implementation along with an insight to the public health researchers on whether outcomes differed by relevant socio-demographic characteristics and whether the intervention was effective for disadvantaged groups.

2. Materials and Methods

2.1. *Objectives*

The objective of this review was to assess the impact of lifestyle interventions (including dietary interventions, physical activity, behavioral therapy, or any combination of these interventions) along with the contextual factors to prevent and manage childhood and adolescent obesity.

2.2. *Types of Studies and Participants*

Keeping in mind the objective of this work, we included primary studies using randomized control trials (individual and cluster) and quasi-experimental studies from both high income countries (HIC) and LMICs. Participants were children and adolescents aged 0 to 19 years. Studies conducted among hospitalized children were excluded from this review. We also excluded children with any pre-existing health conditions (e.g., diabetes and kidney disease).

2.3. Types of Interventions

The interventions included in this review included the following interventions conducted in any settings including schools or communities:

1. Dietary interventions including nutrition education and provision of balanced meals;
2. Physical activity including promotion of physical exercise and reduction in sedentary behaviors;
3. Behavioral therapy;
4. Combination of any of these interventions.

Single interventions were analyzed separately from those studies, where a combination of interventions was being used. The control group comprised of no intervention or standard of care (whatever is applicable in the study setting). We did not include studies comparing any two of the above mentioned intervention. We only included studies with a minimum duration of 12 weeks for intervention and follow-up.

2.4. Types of Outcome Measures

The primary outcomes of this study included BMI *z*-scores, BMI, change in body weight, and adverse events (including symptoms associated with low calorie diet). The secondary outcomes included prevalence of overweight and obesity, percentage body fat change, skin fold thickness, waist circumference, health-related quality of life, self-esteem, and cost effectiveness of the intervention. Explanatory secondary outcomes included intensity of physical activity and total caloric consumption. We included studies that reported either subjectively measured or self/-parent-reported outcomes.

2.5. Search Methods

We used a comprehensive search strategy to identify eligible studies in Cochrane Controlled Trials Register (CENTRAL), MEDLINE, EMBASE, CINAHL, PsycINFO, the World Health Organization (WHO) nutrition databases (http://www.who.int/nutrition/databases/en/), Social Science Index, and Dissertation Abstracts International. The trials registry (Clinicaltrials.gov) was also searched for ongoing trials. We searched Google along with key nutrition agencies databases, such as Nutrition International, the Global Alliance for Improved Nutrition, the World Food Program, and HarvestPlus, to search for non-indexed, grey literature to locate relevant program evaluations. We also screened the reference lists of all included studies and relevant reviews to identify any additional trials that were not found by the electronic searches. We did not apply any restrictions based on publication, language, or publication status. We included studies published in or after 1990. The search was conducted up to February 2020.

2.6. Data Collection and Analysis

Two pairs of review authors (ZAP and AYS; ZH and RAS) independently assessed potential study eligibility using predefined screening criteria. We retrieved the full text of all studies which passed this first level of screening. Disagreements were resolved through discussion with third review author (JKD and RAS) until a consensus was reached. Reasons for exclusion of studies was documented. We extracted data on the study background (time and country where the study was conducted), description of study participants, study design, description of study arms, sample size in each arm, baseline characteristics of the groups, description of intervention, and control groups along with the primary and secondary outcomes listed above.

We performed statistical analysis using RevMan 5 [34]. The included studies were classified as either prevention or management studies and then further classified according to the type of intervention and then analyzed accordingly. We analyzed dichotomous data using risk ratio (RR) with 95% confidence intervals (CI) while for continuous data, we used the mean difference (MD) with 95% CI. We used the standardized mean difference (SMD) with 95% CI to combine trials that measured the same outcome, but used different methods of measurement. We assessed heterogeneity among studies in population interventions or outcomes visually using forest plots. Secondly, heterogeneity between trial results were tested using a standard Chi^2 test, to assess whether observed differences in results are compatible with chance alone [35]. We reported statistical heterogeneity as I^2, Q, and tau^2 for all random-effects meta-analyses. We conducted separate meta-analysis based on the studies assessing obesity prevention and obesity management and type of interventions (dietary intervention, physical activity, behavioral therapy, or any combination of these) within these comparisons. We anticipated heterogeneity within included studies and also performed sensitivity analysis based on study quality. Sensitivity analysis was conducted for all the primary outcomes by removing the studies judged to be at high or unclear risk of bias for sequence generation and incomplete outcome data and the estimates were reported with and without sensitivity analysis.

2.7. *Quality Assessment*

Two pairs of review authors (ZH and ZAP; and AYS and RAS) independently assessed quality of studies, and risk of bias for each study. For randomized studies, we used the Cochrane Risk of Bias tool recommended by the Cochrane Handbook for Systematic Reviews of Interventions [35], which assesses selection, performance, detection, attrition, and reporting bias. Each component was rated as 'high', 'low', or 'unclear' risk of bias. For non-randomized studies, we used the Cochrane Effective Practice and Organization of Care (EPOC) risk of bias criteria (based on additional criteria including baseline characteristics, outcome measurements, protection against contamination, intervention independent of other changes, shape of intervention effect pre-specified, and intervention unlikely to affect data collection) and rated the studies as low risk, high risk, or unclear risk [36]. The quality of evidence was summarized according to the outcomes as per Grading of Recommendations, Assessment, Development and Evaluation (GRADE) criteria [37]. Grades of 'high', 'moderate', 'low', and 'very low' were used for grading the overall evidence [38]. For non-randomized studies, the quality of evidence was updated based on large magnitude of effect, dose response, and effect of all plausible confounding factors reducing, which suggests a spurious effect. Two reviewers discussed ratings, reached consensus, and disagreements were resolved by consulting a third reviewer. We developed a summary of findings table to show the effects for the primary outcomes.

3. Results

3.1. *Results of the Search*

The search identified 40,775 records from outlined search engines. After the removal of 5446 duplicates, the remaining 35,329 records underwent title and abstract screening. We included 654 studies (1160 papers) for data extraction, and meta-analysis (see Figure 1 for study flow diagram). The major reasons for excluding studies from full text screening stage included wrong study design, wrong comparison group and duration of intervention being <12 weeks.

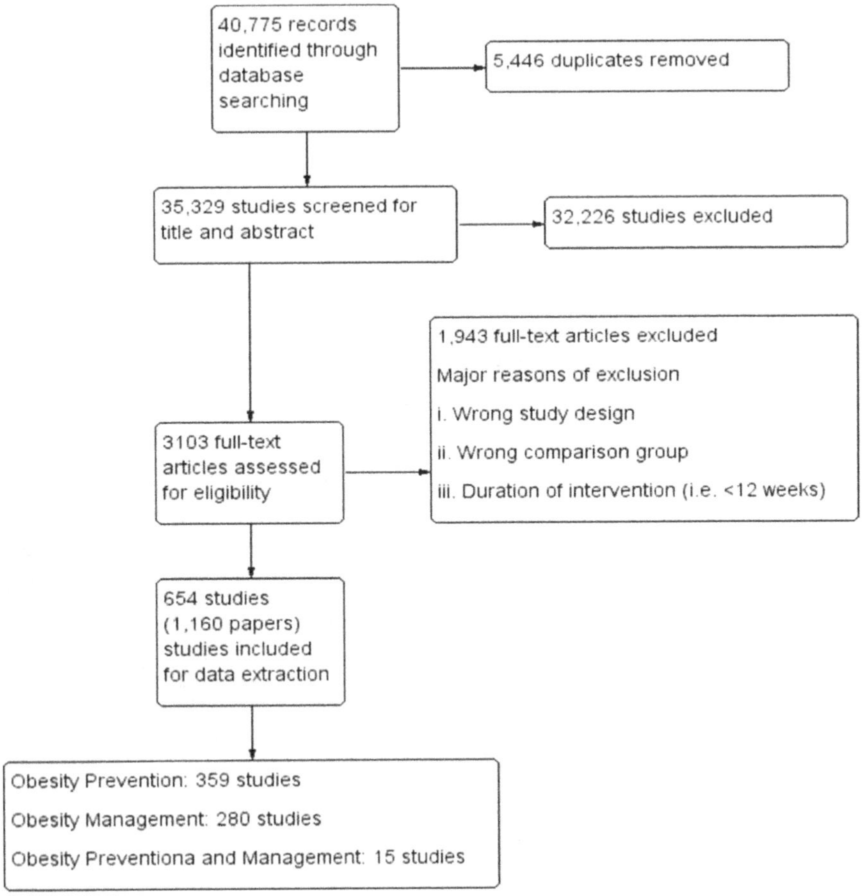

Figure 1. Study flow diagram.

3.2. Description of Included Studies

Out of the 654 included studies, a total of 359 studies focused on obesity prevention; a total of 280 studies targeted obesity management, while 15 studies targeted both prevention and management. The following interventions were assessed for obesity prevention:

1. Diet only interventions—34 studies;
2. Exercise only interventions—57 studies;
3. Behavioral therapy only intervention—89 studies;
4. Diet and Exercise interventions—99 studies;
5. Diet and Behavioral therapy interventions—7 studies;
6. Exercise and behavioral therapy interventions—47 studies;
7. Diet, exercise and behavioral therapy interventions—26 studies.

The following interventions were assessed for obesity management:

1. Diet only interventions—17 studies;
2. Exercise only interventions—59 studies;
3. Behavioral therapy only intervention—63 studies;
4. Diet and Exercise interventions—57 studies;
5. Diet and Behavioral therapy interventions—5 studies;
6. Exercise and behavioral therapy interventions—30 studies;
7. Diet, exercise and behavioral therapy interventions—49 studies.

Among the included studies, a total of 515 studies were RCTs and 139 studies were quasi-experimental studies. Majority of the included studies (n = 531, 81.1%) were conducted in HICs, while 70 studies (10.6%) studies were conducted in Upper Middle Income Countries (UMICs) and 13 studies (2%) were conducted in LMICs. Characteristics of all the included studies are summarized in Supplementary Table S1.

3.3. *Risk of Bias*

3.3.1. For Randomized Control Trials

The Cochrane Risk of Bias tool was used to assess the quality of the included RCTs. Six studies were judged to be at high risk of bias for random sequence generation, while 221 studies were judged to be at unclear risk of bias since these studies did not specify the methods used to generate random sequence. A total of 288 studies were judged to be at low risk of bias for sequence generation, since appropriate methods were used to generate a random sequence. Thirteen studies were judged to be at high risk of bias for allocation concealment since they did not adequately conceal the allocation, while 423 studies did not specify the methods used to conceal allocation and hence were judged to be at unclear risk of bias. A total of 79 were judged to be at low risk of bias for allocation concealment since adequate methods were used to conceal the allocation. Blinding of participants and personnel was adequately done in 81 studies. A total of 162 studies were judged to be at high risk of blinding of participants and personnel, since no blinding was done, while 272 studies failed to report on blinding of participants and personnel. Blinding of outcome assessors was successfully done in 103 studies; however, 89 studies failed to blind outcome assessors and 323 studies did not report on blinding of the outcome assessors and hence were judged to be at unclear risk. A total of 314 studies were judged to be at low risk of bias for incomplete outcome data, while 142 studies had high attrition rates and were judged to be at high risk of bias for attrition. Attrition could not be calculated due to insufficient information in 59 studies and hence were judged to be at unclear risk of bias. A total of 211 studies were at low risk for selective reporting since they had referred to the pre-published protocol or trial registration details, while 304 studies were judged to be at unclear risk for selective reporting since it could not be assessed due to lack of availability of pre-published protocol or trial registration number. The majority of the studies (n = 496) were judged to be at low risk for any other bias while 19 studies were judged to be at high risk for other biases. Figure 2 depicts the summary risk of bias graph for the included RCTs.

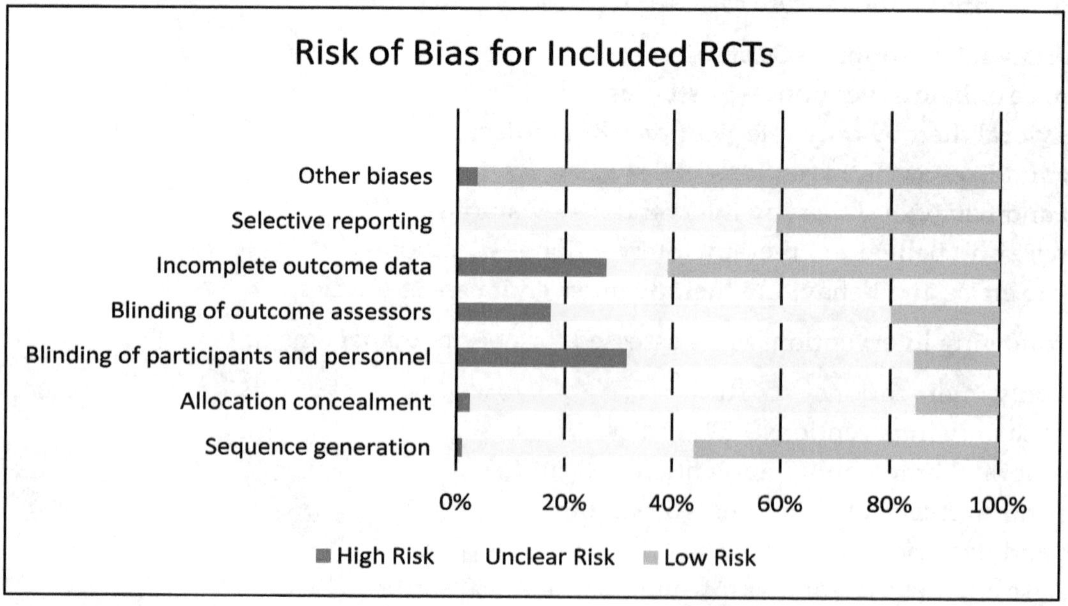

Figure 2. Summary risk of bias for included randomized controlled trials (RCTs).

3.3.2. For Quasi-Experimental Studies

The EPOC criteria was used to assess the quality of the quasi-experimental studies. All the included quasi-experimental studies were judged to be at high risk for sequence generation. A total of 38 studies were judged to be at high risk of bias for allocation concealment while insufficient information did not permit judgement in 101 studies. Baseline outcome measurements were similar across groups in 73 studies. A total of 32 studies were judged to be at high risk for similarity in baseline measurements while there was insufficient data in 34 studies and hence were judged to be at unclear risk of bias. Baseline characteristic were similar across groups in 77 studies, while in 27 studies the baseline characteristics were not similar across the groups and hence were labelled as high risk. There was insufficient information in 35 studies regarding baseline characteristics and hence were judged to be at unclear risk. A total of 68 studies were judged to be at low risk of bias for attrition while 34 studies did not report on attrition and were judged to be at unclear risk. The attrition rate was high in 37 studies and were judged to be at high risk of bias. Knowledge of allocation was adequately prevented in 11 studies; it was not prevented in 39 studies, while in 89 studies there was insufficient information and hence these were judged to be at unclear risk. A total of 31 studies were adequately protected from contamination; 11 studies did not prevent contamination between groups while 97 studies did not provide sufficient information on protection against contamination. Majority of the quasi-experimental studies (n = 121) were judged to be at unclear risk for selective reporting due to lack of published protocols or study registration numbers while 18 studies were judged to be at low risk for selective reporting. A total of 135 studies were free from other risk of bias while only four studies were judged to be at high risk for any other biases. Figure 3 depicts the summary risk of bias graph for the included quasi-experimental studies.

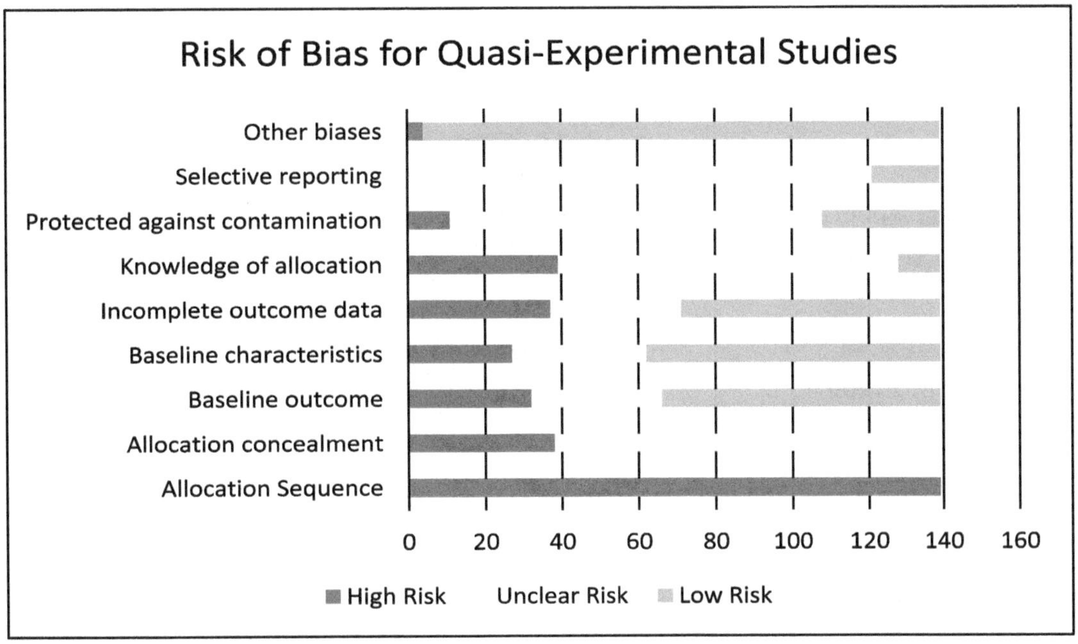

Figure 3. Summary risk of bias for included quasi-experimental studies.

3.4. *PROGRESS Findings*

The findings from the PROGRESS are summarized in Table 1:

Table 1. The summary of findings from the PROGRESS.

PROGRESS-Plus Factors	Summary of Reported Factors
Place of residence/setting	No. studies conducted in high-income countries (HICs): 533 No. studies conducted in upper-middle-income countries (UMICs): 70 No. studies conducted in lower-middle-income countries (LMICs): 13 40 studies had no country stated.
Race/ethnicity/culture/language	Almost half of the included studies specified details under this domain while reporting the baseline characteristics of the study population.
Occupation	This is one of the most under-reported categories in the studies probably since the study population were children and adolescents. Very few studies reported the occupation of the parents of the enrolled chidlren and adolescents.
Gender/sex	This category was reported in almost every study, although few did not provide the specific distribution of the sample by sex when participants from both sexes were included. Most studies were conducted with children and adolescents, but some also included only adolescents or only children.
Religion	This is also one of the under-reported categories in the studies. Very few studies reported on this domain.
Education	Since many studies were carried out in school settings, majority of such studies reported the level of education as preschool/elementary, primary or secondary.
Socioeconomic status	This factor was also poorly reported in the published data of the included studies. Moreover, various studies used different definitions of the socio-economic status. Majorly, the studies reported income, class, or the areas of residence (rural/urban/mixed) under this domain.
Social capital	Few studies directly reported any measurement of social capital. Indirectly, some studies reported that participants were recruited through schools, clinics, hospitals and sports/recreation centres, thus indicating that participants had at least one social connection or network.
Plus (other characteristics)	All studies reported on age, as this factor is essential for their analysis. Many reported the participants' Body Mass Index (BMI) and other body measures e.g., height, weight, skinfold thickness. Studies including parents also reported parent education, occupation, income and marital status although very infrequently.
Recruitment methods	Most studies recruited their participants through similar strategies: schools, mailings, printed ads and flyers distributed in school campuses, community centres, clinics or hospitals, through advertisement on local radio and television. Most of the studies took place in HICs and in children and/or adolescents, hence the use of schools and community centres.

3.5. *Effects of Interventions*

3.5.1. Comparison 1: Obesity Prevention

A total of 359 studies focused on obesity prevention. Studies reported primary outcomes including studies reported BMI, BMI *z*-score, and body weight. None of the included studies reported any adverse events. Among secondary outcomes, included studies reported prevalence of overweight/obesity, percentage body fat change, skin fold thickness, waist and hip circumference, health related quality of life, and cost effectiveness.

Primary Outcomes

The analysis shows that combined diet and exercise interventions might reduce BMI *z*-score (MD: −0.12; 95% CI: −0.18 to −0.06; 32 studies; 33,039 participants; I^2 93%; low quality evidence; Figure 4), BMI by 0.41 kg/m^2 (MD: −0.41 kg/m^2; 95% CI: −0.60 to −0.21; 35 studies; 47, 499 participants; I^2 98%; low quality evidence) and bodyweight by 1.59 kg (MD: −1.59; 95% CI: −2.95 to −0.23; 17 studies; 35,023 participants; I^2 100%; low quality evidence; Figure 5) when compared to control group. The BMI *z*-score might also reduce by behavioral therapy only (MD: −0.07; 95% CI: −0.14 to −0.00; 19 studies; 8569 participants; I^2 76%; low quality evidence; Figure 6); combined exercise and behavioral therapy (MD: −0.08; 95% CI: −0.16 to −0.00; 9 studies; 7334 participants; I^2 74%; low quality evidence), and diet in combination with exercise and behavioral therapy (MD: −0.13; 95% CI: −0.25 to −0.01; 5 studies; 1806 participants; I^2 62%; low quality evidence; Figure 7) when compared to the control group.

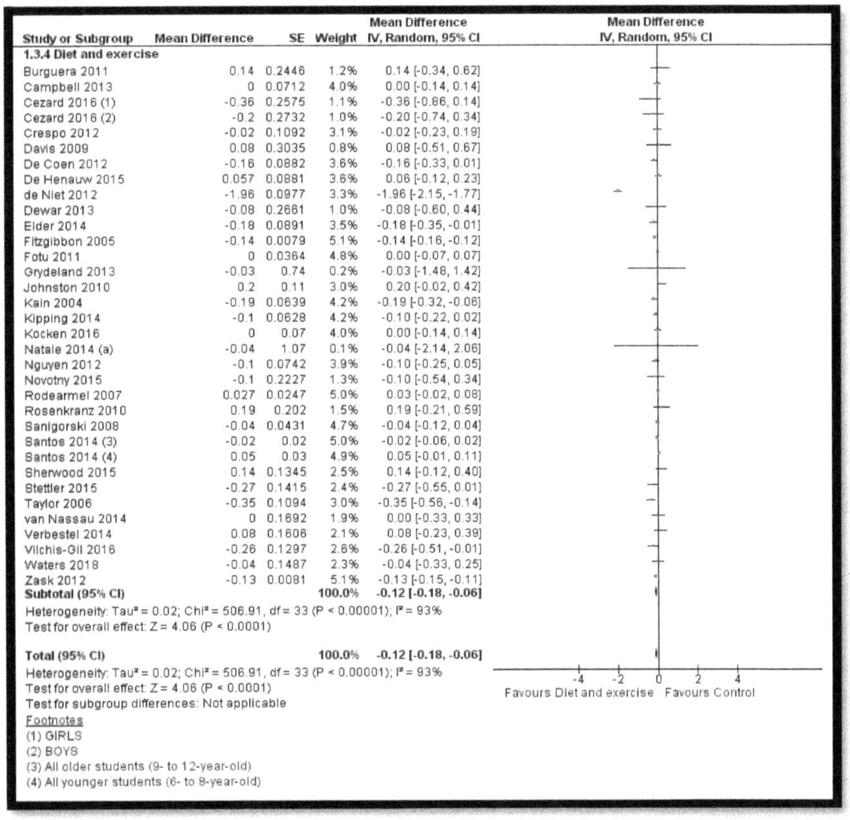

Figure 4. Forest plot for the effect of combined diet and exercise interventions for obesity prevention on body mass index (BMI) *z*-score.

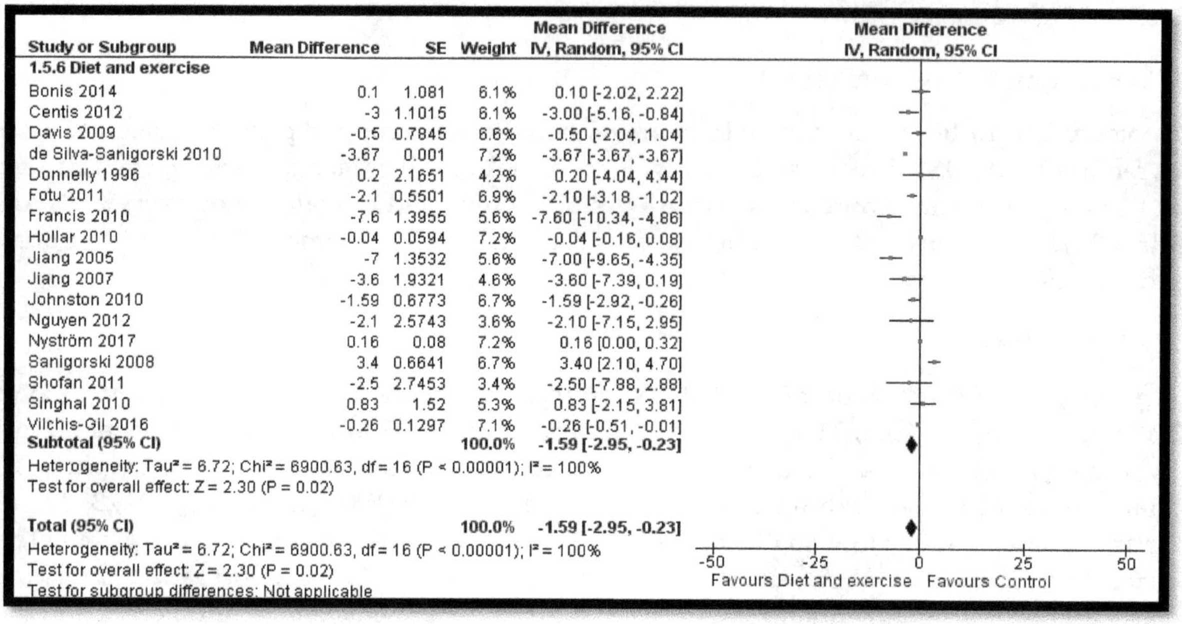

Figure 5. Forest plot for the effect combined diet and exercise interventions for obesity prevention on body weight.

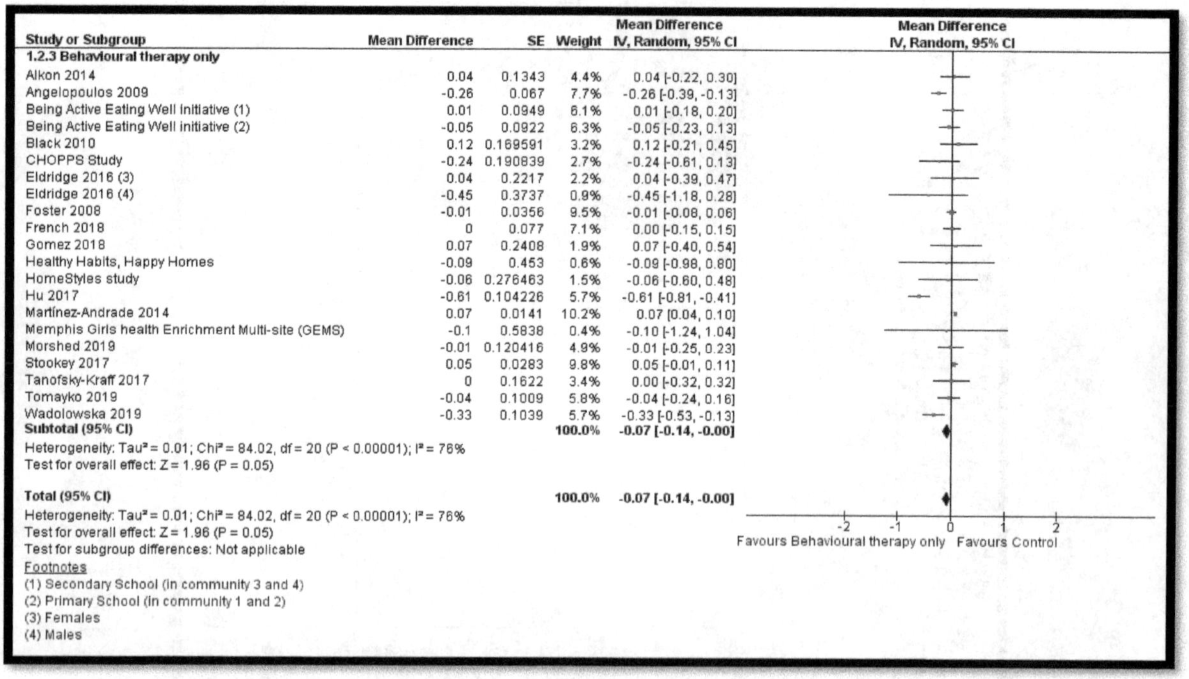

Figure 6. Forest plot for the effect of behavioural therapy interventions for obesity prevention on body mass index (BMI) *z*-score.

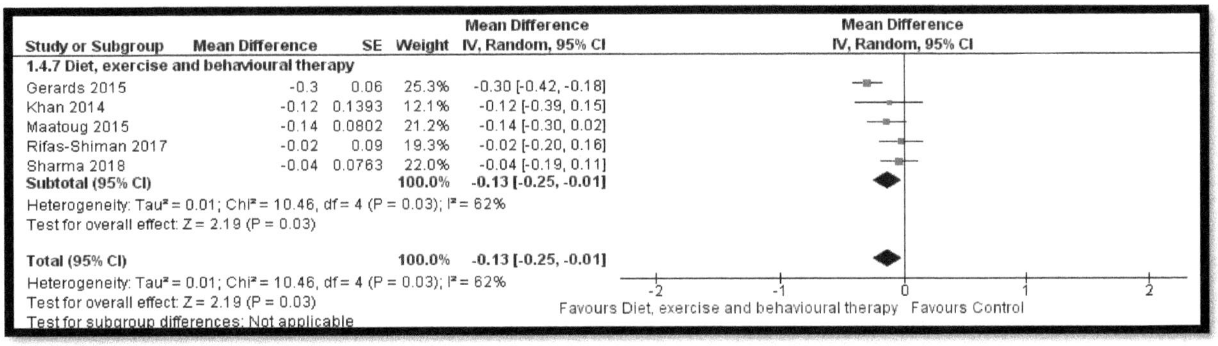

Figure 7. Forest plot for the effect of combined diet, exercise and behavioral therapy interventions for obesity prevention on body mass index (BMI) *z*-score.

There was no difference of effect of diet only and exercise only interventions on BMI *z*-score, BMI, or bodyweight when compared to the control group. Diet in combination with behavioral therapy intervention had no difference on BMI *z*-score when compared to the control group, while there was no difference in effect of behavioral therapy alone, exercise in combination with behavioral therapy intervention, and diet in combination with exercise and behavioral therapy intervention on BMI when compared to the control group.

Sensitivity Analysis for the Primary Outcomes

In order to explore the heterogeneity, we conducted sensitivity analysis by removing the studies that were quasi-experimental or at high risk or unclear risk of bias for sequence generation and incomplete outcome data. There was no changes in the estimates for the outcome of BMI in the sensitivity analysis. However, the previous effect of diet in combination with exercise and behavioral therapy on BMI *z*-score disappeared after removing studies at high risk of bias or quasi experimental studies (MD: −0.16; 95% CI: −0.36, 0.04; 3 studies; 644 participants; I^2 72%). There was asignificant reduction for behavioral therapy alone on body weight by 0.8 kg after removing studies at high risk of bias or quasi experimental studies (MD: −0.80; 95% CI: −1.57, −0.04; 4 studies; 931 participants; I^2 76%).

Secondary Outcomes

Combined diet and exercise interventions might reduce percentage of body fat by 0.95 kg compared to controls (MD: −0.95; 95% CI: −1.28 to −0.61; 10 studies; 19,643 participants; I^2 80%; low quality evidence). Combined exercise and behavioral therapy might reduce the skinfold thickness (triceps) (MD: −1.33; 95% CI −1.89 to −0.76; five studies; 2944 participants) and increase physical activity intensity (MD: 0.84; 95% CI: 0.09 to 1.59; 14 studies; 5924 participants). We are uncertain of the effect of any of the obesity prevention interventions on any of the other secondary outcomes including prevalence of overweight, prevalence of obesity, waist circumference and health-related quality of life (Figures S1–S8).

A few of the included studies assessed cost effectiveness of the interventions for obesity prevention, mainly in the school settings. The cost-effectiveness study of the "Join the Healthy Boat" program evaluating state-wide implementation of the health promotion in primary schools in Germany [39] suggested that the positive impacts of the study were achieved at affordable costs and with proven cost-effectiveness. The findings from the economic evaluation of the Physical Activity 4 Everyone (PA4E1) intervention [40], which was a multi-component intervention implemented in secondary schools located in low-income communities also suggested that PA4E1 was a cost effective intervention for increasing the physical activity levels and reducing unhealthy weight gain in adolescence. The cost effectiveness analysis of the CHIRPY DRAGON study suggested that this school and family based obesity prevention programme was not only effective but highly cost effective in reducing BMI z scores in primary-school–aged children in China [41]. The economic evaluation of the Healthy Caregivers-Healthy Children (HC2) program, which is an early childcare center-based obesity prevention program, suggested that the HC2 intervention shows potential for generating cost savings [42]. One study (the WAVES study) [43] assessing the cost-effectiveness of a multi-faceted school-based obesity prevention intervention targeting children aged 6–7 years suggested that more research to explore obesity prevention within schools as part of a wider systems approach to obesity prevention are needed. One study also assessed the cost-effectiveness of a large, multifaceted, community-based capacity-building demonstration program (Be Active Eat Well (BAEW)) and suggested that BAEW was affordable and cost-effective [44].

3.5.2. Comparison 2: Obesity Management

A total of 280 studies assessed obesity management interventions. Studies reported primary outcomes including BMI, BMI *z*-score, and body weight. None of the included studies reported any adverse events. Among secondary outcomes, included studies reported prevalence of overweight/obesity, percentage body fat change, skin fold thickness, waist and hip circumference, health related quality of life, and cost effectiveness.

Primary Outcomes

The analysis shows that exercise only interventions probably reduces BMI *z*-score (MD: −0.13; 95% CI: −0.20 to −0.06; 12 studies; 1084 participants; I^2 0%; moderate quality evidence; Figure 8), and might reduce BMI (MD: −0.88; 95% CI: −1.26 to −0.50; 34 studies; 3846 participants; I^2 72%; Figure 9) and body weight (MD: −3.01; 95% CI: −5.56 to −0.47; 16 studies; 1701 participants; I^2 78%; low quality evidence; Figure 10) when compared to the control group. The exercise along with behavioral therapy interventions (MD: −0.08; 95% CI: −0.16 to −0.00; 8 studies; 466 participants; I^2 49%; moderate quality evidence; Figure 11), diet along with behavioral therapy interventions (MD: −0.16; 95% CI: −0.26 to −0.07; 4 studies; 329 participants; I^2 0%; moderate quality evidence; Figure 12) and combination of diet, exercise and behavioral therapy (MD: −0.09; 95% CI: −0.14 to −0.05; 13 studies; 2995 participants; I^2 12%; moderate quality evidence; Figure 13) also probably decreases BMI *z*-score when compared to the control group. There was no difference of effect of diet only or diet in combination with exercise on BMI *z*-score when compared to the control group 9 (Figures S9–S16). Behavioral therapy alone might reduce BMI (MD: −0.44; 95% CI: −0.78 to −0.11; 26 studies; 3642 participants; I^2 82%; Figure 14), and a combination of diet and exercise interventions might reduce the bodyweight (MD: −2.07; 95% CI: −2.90 to −1.24; 24 studies; 4415 participants; I^2 86%; low quality evidence; Figure 15).

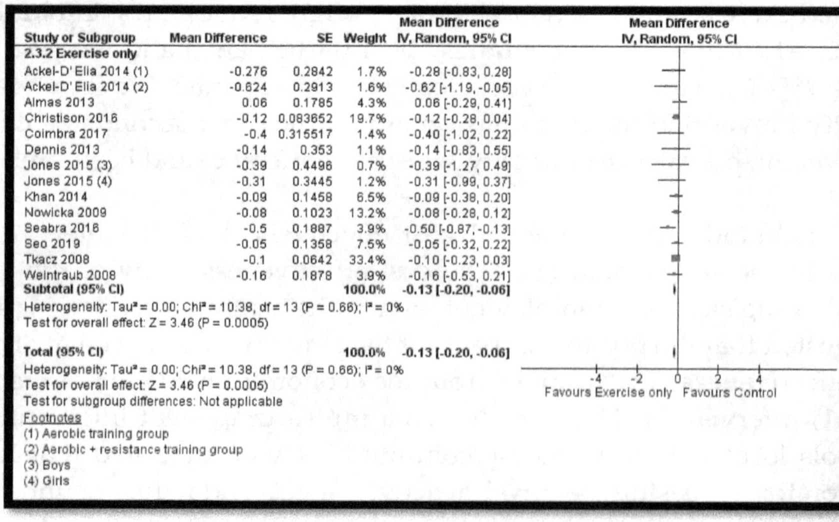

Figure 8. Forest plot for the effect of exercise only interventions for obesity management on body mass index (BMI) *z*-score.

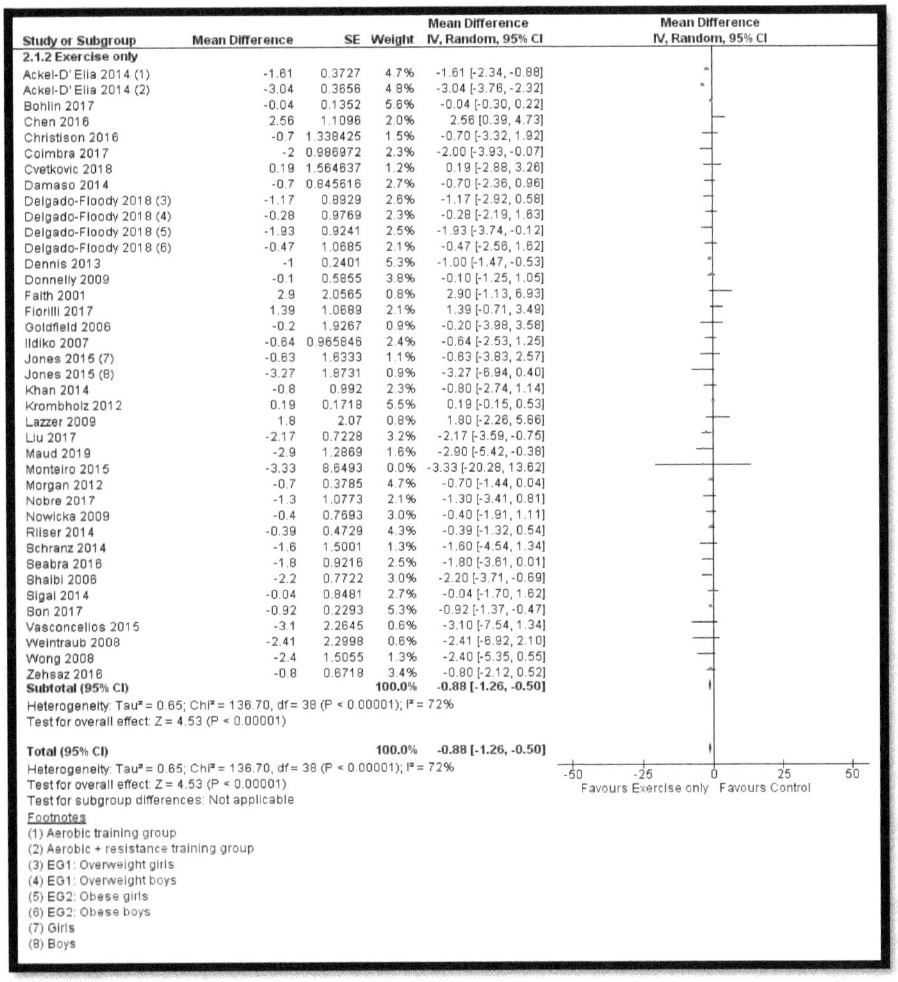

Figure 9. Forest plot for the effect of exercise only interventions for obesity management on body mass index (BMI).

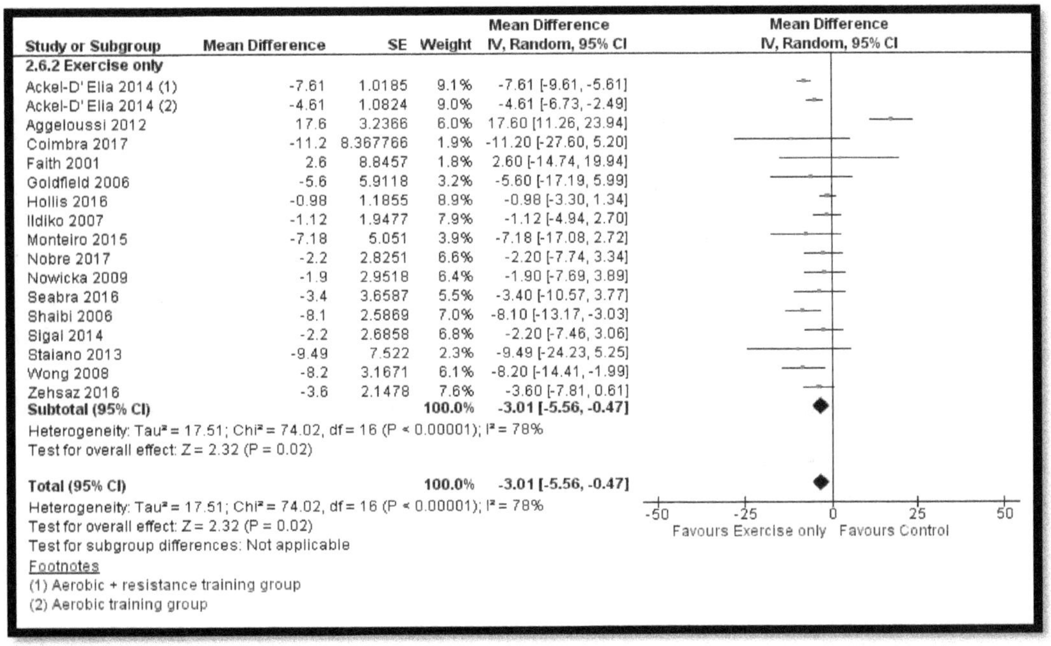

Figure 10. Forest plot for the effect of exercise only interventions for obesity management on body weight.

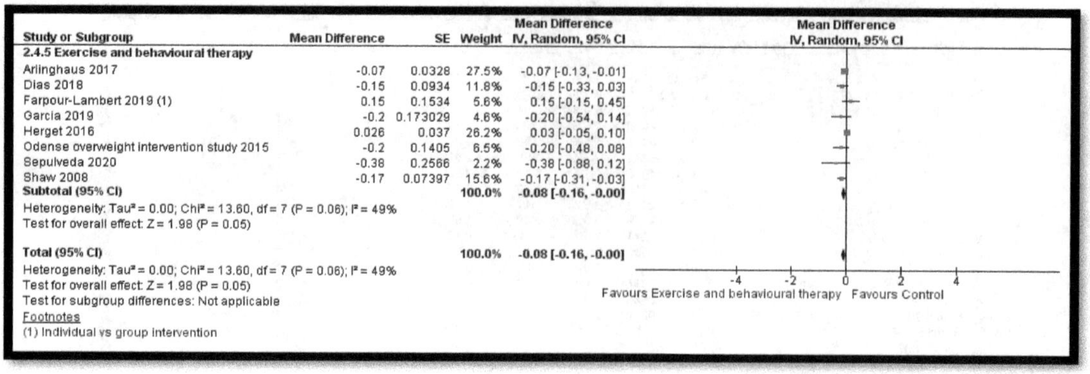

Figure 11. Forest plot for the effect of exercise and behavioural therapy interventions for obesity management on body mass index (BMI) *z*-score.

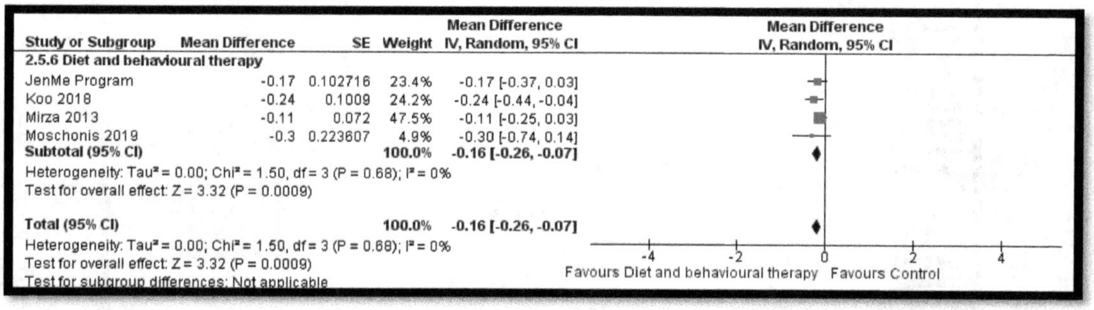

Figure 12. Forest plot for the effect of diet and behavioural therapy interventions for obesity management on body mass index (BMI) *z*-score.

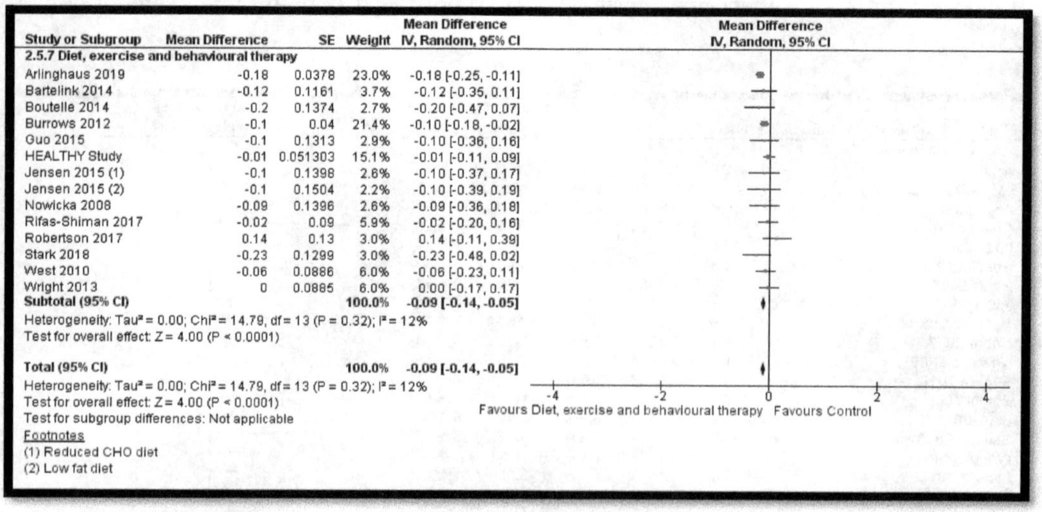

Figure 13. Forest plot for the effect of diet, exercise and behavioural therapy interventions for obesity management on body mass index (BMI) *z*-score.

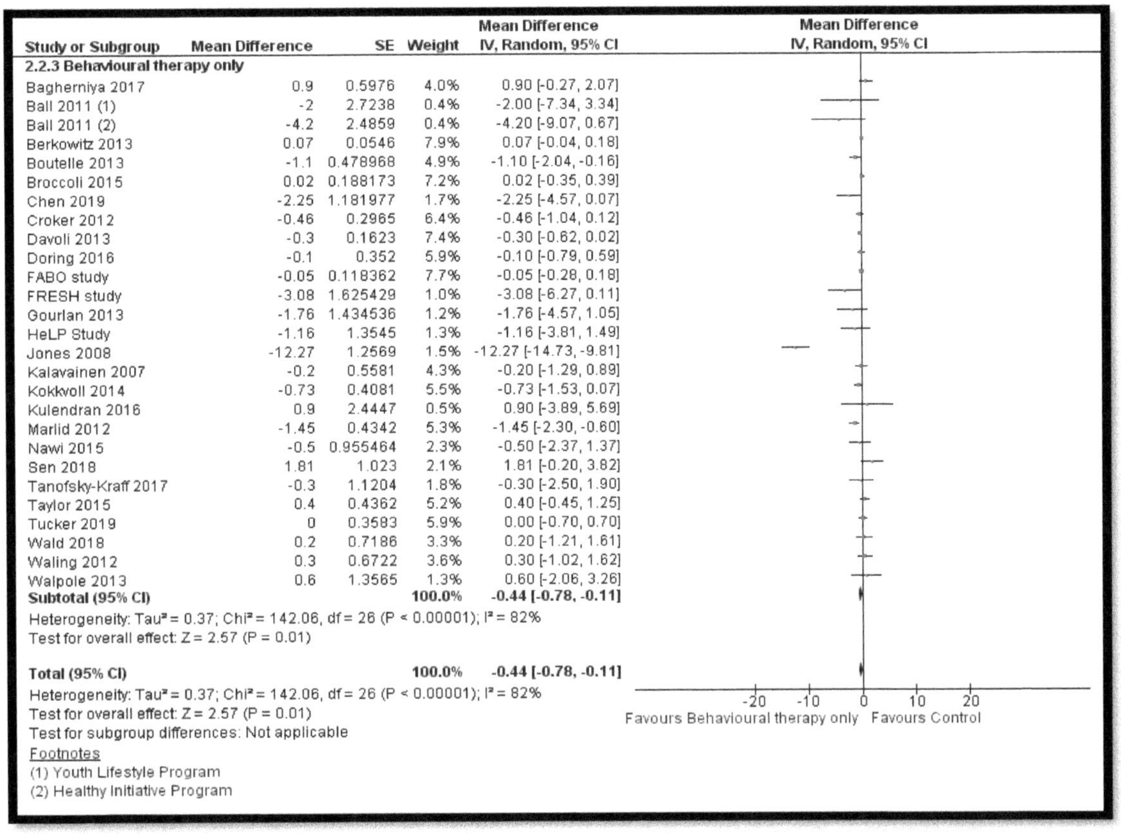

Figure 14. Forest plot for the effect of behavioural therpy only interventions for obesity management on body mass index (BMI).

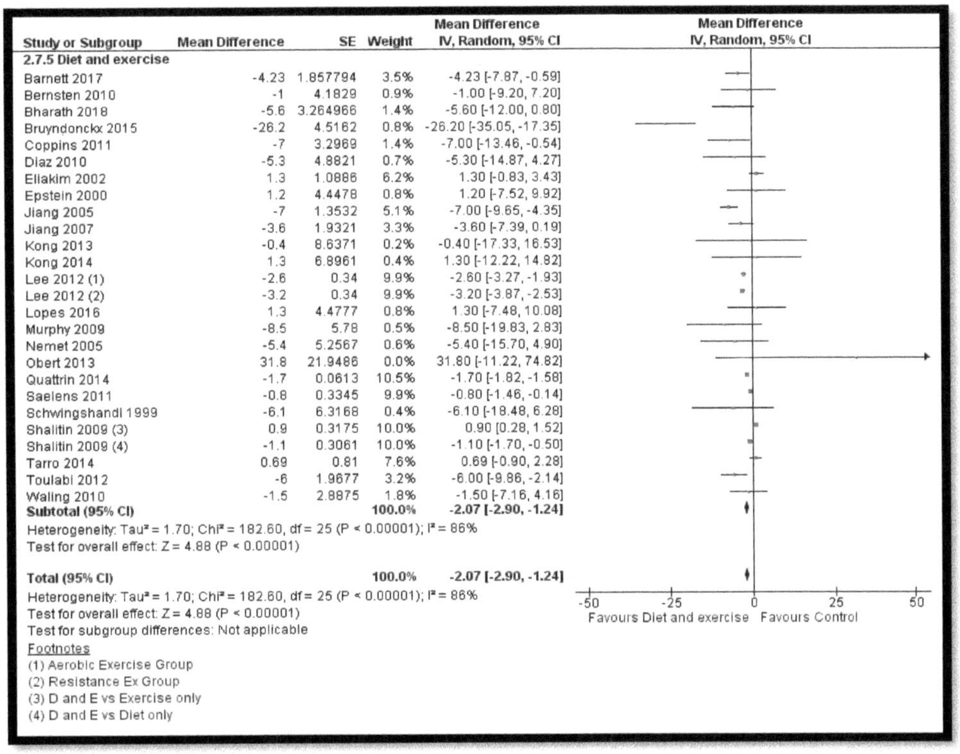

Figure 15. Forest plot for the effect of diet and exercise interventions for obesity management on body weight.

There is no difference of effect of diet only, exercise in combination with behavioral therapy, diet in combination with behavioral therapy, or diet in combination with exercise and behavioral therapy on BMI and bodyweight when compared to the control group. There was also no difference of effect of diet in combination with exercise on BMI and behavioral therapy alone on bodyweight when compared to the control group.

Sensitivity Analysis for the Primary Outcomes

In order to explore the heterogeneity, we conducted sensitivity analysis for the primary outcomes by removing the quasi experimental studies and the studies at high or unclear risk of bias for sequence generation and incomplete outcome data. After sensitivity analysis, there was significant reduction in BMI with diet along with exercise interventions which was previously statistically non-significant (MD: −0.5; 95% CI: −0.85 to −0.16; I^2 87%). There was a significant reduction in BMI with the combination of diet, exercise, and behavioral therapy interventions (MD: −0.51; 95% CI: −0.89 to −0.13; I^2 82%). For BMI *z*-score, diet along with exercise interventions also showed significant effect on BMI *z*-score (previously non-significant) (MD: −0.09; 95% CI: −0.18 to −0.01; I^2 91%). There was no change in body weight after sensitivity analysis.

Secondary Outcomes

Exercise only interventions might reduce percentage body fat (MD: −1.36; 95% CI: −2.32 to −0.39; 25 studies; 1635 participants; I^2 78%). Diet in combination with exercise (MD: −2.03; 95% CI: −3.50 to −0.56; 8 studies; 2234 participants; I^2 87%; low quality evidence) and a combination of diet, exercise and behavioral therapy (MD: −1.54; 95% CI: −2.56 to −0.52; 11 studies; 3018 participants; I^2 63%; low quality evidence) might reduce waist circumference. Behavioral therapy only might reduce the total caloric consumption (MD: −131.58; 95% CI: −188.16 to −75.01; 6 studies; I^2 13%; 919 participants). There was no effect of any intervention on any other secondary outcomes including prevalence of overweight, prevalence of obesity and skin fold thickness (Figure S11).

Few studies reported the cost-effectiveness of obesity prevention interventions. Three studies [45–47] compared the cost-effectiveness of Family-Based Group Treatment for Child and Parental Obesity, suggesting that for families with overweight/obese children and parents, family based therapy might be a low cost strategy compared to treating the parent and child separately. Study assessing the economic evaluation of the Families for Health program focusing on a parenting approach, designed to help parents develop their parenting skills to support lifestyle change within the family suggested that the program was neither effective nor cost-effective for the management of obesity in children aged 6–11 years, in comparison with usual care [48]. The economic evaluation of a childhood obesity intervention with electronic decision support for clinicians and self-guided behavior-change support for parents suggested that these interventions might be more cost-effective than previous clinical interventions [49]. An economic evaluation was conducted for the Whānau Pakari [50], which was a home-based, 12-month multi-disciplinary child obesity intervention programme, suggesting that such programs had lower programme costs per child, greater reach, with similar impacts. However, one study assessing the cost-effectiveness of group treatment compared with routine counseling in obese children suggested that family-based group treatment was more costly compared with individual routine counseling and the salaries were the major component of the total costs [51]. One study assessing the cost-utility of a motivational multicomponent lifestyle-modification intervention in a community setting (the Healthy Eating Lifestyle Programme (HELP)) [52] suggested that there was no evidence that the program was more effective than a single educational session in improving quality of life in a sample of adolescents with obesity. A study assessing the cost-effectiveness of an intensive weight-loss intervention for children compared with a low-intensity intervention suggested that, compared with the standard care, the camp group was more costly [53]. The cost effectiveness of the Live, Eat and Play (LEAP) study suggested that the intervention led to higher costs to families and the health care sector, which could have been devoted to other uses that do create benefits to health and/or family well-being [54].

4. Discussion

This review was a comprehensive review on obesity prevention and management interventions in children and adolescents from HICs as well as LMICs. The review summarizes findings from a total of 654 studies from 1160 papers. A total of 359 of the included studies focused on obesity prevention while 280 studies focused on obesity management. About 15 studies focused on both treatment and prevention. Majority of the studies (about 81%) were conducted in HIC; about 10% of the included studies were conducted in UMICs while only 2% of the included studies were conducted in LMIC settings. The interventions evaluated for obesity prevention and management included diet only interventions; exercise only interventions; behavioral therapy only interventions; diet along with exercise, diet along with behavioral therapy, exercise along with behavioral therapy and a combination of diet, exercise and behavioral therapy. About 515 studies were RCTs, while 139 studies were quasi-experimental studies. Among RCTs, the majority of the studies were judged to be at low risk of bias for sequence generation and incomplete outcome data while majority of the studies were labelled as unclear risk for blinding and selective reporting due to insufficient information provided. Among quasi-experimental studies, almost all the studies were judged to be at high risk for sequence generation, while the majority of the studies were judged to be at unclear risk for allocation concealment, prevention of knowledge of the intervention, contamination, and selective reporting. Due to the nature of the intervention, majority of the studies could not achieve blinding of the participants and personnel. Overall, the outcomes were judged to be of moderate to low quality due to study limitations, high heterogeneity. and imprecision. Among the PROGRESS factors, studies reported on a few factors, including place of residence/setting; gender/sex; education and recruitment methods. The least reported factors were found to be race/ethnicity/culture/language; occupation; religion; socioeconomic status; and social capital.

For primary outcomes, evidence for the prevention of obesity among children and adolescents suggests that a combination of diet and exercise might reduce the BMI, BMI *z*-score and body weight. Behavioral therapy alone and a combination of exercise and behavioral therapy might reduce BMI *z*-score. Sensitivity analysis suggested that behavioral therapy might also reduce body weight. For the secondary outcomes, combined diet and exercise interventions might reduce percentage of body fat while combined exercise and behavioral therapy might reduce the skinfold thickness (triceps) and increase physical activity intensity. There was no effect of any other intervention on any of the other outcomes.

For obesity management, evidence suggests that Exercise only interventions, diet along with behavioral therapy interventions and a combination of diet, exercise and behavioral therapy probably decreases BMI *z*-score. Sensitivity analysis suggests that diet along with exercise might also reduce BMI *z*-score. Exercise only and behavioral therapy only might reduce BMI while the sensitivity analysis suggests that diet along with exercise and a combination of diet, exercise and behavioral therapy might also reduce BMI in overweight/obese children and adolescents. Exercise only interventions and diet along with exercise might reduce body weight. There was no effect of any other intervention on any of the other outcomes.

Despite there being several isolated and combination of interventions available for addressing childhood and adolescent obesity, this review demonstrated that in dealing with obesity might require a combination of interventions rather than each intervention on its own. Primary prevention of obesity in children and adolescents has been a major public health challenge for several decades [55]. Lifestyle modifications form the mainstay of primary prevention for this condition [55]. The current review highlighted that combination of dietary and exercise interventions might led to significant reductions in BMI, BMI z score and body weight. This change is likely mediated by increase in energy expenditure as indicated by the increase in physical activity intensity while there was no change in the total caloric consumption. Vissers et al. also reported that diet and exercise interventions had a greater impact on adipose tissue as compared to diet alone [56], thus indicating the role of energy expenditure in weight loss.

For obesity management, lifestyle modification along with pharmacological and surgical interventions have been proposed; however the focus of this review was limited to lifestyle modifications only. A recent review of 8 trials on approximately 4000 obese children indicated that diet and exercise interventions for 6 months helped reduced BMI z scores and other markers of metabolic dysfunction such as fasting plasma glucose in these children [57]. Our findings indicate that adding behavioral modifications such as family based therapy or cognitive behavioral therapy (CBT) to dietary and exercise interventions might have an impact on BMI and skinfold thickness along with BMI z scores. Family based therapy where parents and children are actively involved in making healthier nutrition and physical activity choices is one of the most robust interventions for childhood obesity [58]. Complementing family based therapy with CBT where individuals are encouraged to change attitudes and behaviors that sustain a current behavior have also proven to be beneficial in this age group [59]. Thus, a comprehensive "body and mind" intervention may result in a greater impact on improving body composition [60].

This review serves as an umbrella review of the existing evidence for childhood and adolescent obesity prevention and management. It synthesizes global evidence from the RCTs and quasi-experimental studies along with the PROGRESS factors. This review included anthropometric as well as other outcomes such as health related quality of life and cost effectiveness of the interventions. However, this review only provides a basis for what works and what does not work for childhood and adolescent obesity. Future reviews in the domain should further microscopically evaluate these findings in terms of effectiveness in specific subgroups of population and types of intervention. Childhood obesity is a known risk factor for adult obesity and other non-communicable diseases leading to morbidity and mortality. This may potentially lead to loss of human capital and economic challenges at the family and community level [61]. Future work in this domain should assess the impact of these interventions on outcomes other than anthropometry like quality of life and health economic evaluations to better inform policy makers [61]. There was a significant dearth of literature on obesity management and prevention from LMICs. This lack of evidence continues to exist despite the well documented rise of obesity in LMICs, hence, the findings from this review may have limited applicability in such regions.

5. Conclusions

The existing evidence is most favorable for a combination of interventions, such as diet and exercise in obesity prevention and diet, exercise, and behavioral therapy for obesity management. Despite the growing obesity epidemic in LMICs, there is significant dearth of obesity prevention and management studies from these regions. Future studies in this domain should focus on combinations of interventions with an appropriate follow up period to generate robust evidence on weight and related parameters, with evidence from LMICs.

Supplementary Materials: Impact of obesity prevention interventions on prevalence of overweight, Figure S2: Impact of obesity prevention interventions on prevalence of obesity, Figure S3: Impact of obesity prevention interventions on percentage body fat change, Figure S4: Impact of obesity prevention interventions on skinfold thickness (Tricep), Figure S5: Impact of obesity prevention interventions on waist circumference, Figure S6: Impact of obesity prevention interventions on health-related quality of life, Figure S7: Impact of obesity prevention interventions on physical activity intensity, Figure S8: Impact of obesity prevention interventions on total caloric consumption, Figure S9: Impact of obesity management interventions on prevalence of overweight, Figure S10: Impact of obesity management interventions on prevalence of obesity, Figure S11: Impact of obesity management interventions on percentage body fat change, Figure S12: Impact of obesity management interventions on skinfold thickness (Tricep), Figure S13: Impact of obesity management interventions on waist circumference, Figure S14: Impact of obesity management interventions on health-related quality of life, Figure S15: Impact of obesity management interventions on physical activity intensity,

Figure S16: Impact of obesity management interventions on total caloric consumption, Table S1: Characteristics of included studies.

Author Contributions: All review authors contributed to the development of the review. R.A.S., Z.H., Z.S.L., S.M.J., A.Y.S., and Z.A.P. selected which studies to include, obtained copies of the studies, and extracted data from the studies. A.Y.S., Z.A.P., R.A.S. and J.K.D. entered data into RevMan, carried out the analysis, and interpreted the results. J.K.D., Z.H., R.A.S., and Z.A.B. drafted the final review. All authors have read and agreed to the published version of the manuscript.

Acknowledgments: We would like to acknowledge Karim Rizwan Nathani, Kashif Mukhtar, Yamna Jadoon, and Wajeeha Tariq for their contributions towards screening and extractions for the review.

References

1. Karnik, S.; Kanekar, A. Childhood obesity: A global public health crisis. *Int. J. Prev. Med.* **2012**, *3*, 1.
2. The Global Nutrition Report. 2019 [cited 2020 05/06/2020]. Available online: https://globalnutritionreport.org/ (accessed on 10 May 2019).
3. Friedrich, M. Global obesity epidemic worsening. *JAMA* **2017**, *318*, 603. [CrossRef] [PubMed]
4. Abarca-Gómez, L.; A Abdeen, Z.; Hamid, Z.A.; Abu-Rmeileh, N.M.; Acosta-Cazares, B.; Acuin, C.; Adams, R.J.; Aekplakorn, W.; Afsana, K.; A Aguilar-Salinas, C.; et al. Worldwide trends in body-mass index, underweight, overweight, and obesity from 1975 to 2016: A pooled analysis of 2416 population-based measurement studies in 128·9 million children, adolescents, and adults. *Lancet* **2017**, *390*, 2627–2642. [CrossRef]
5. Skinner, A.C.; Ravanbakht, S.N.; Skelton, J.A.; Perrin, E.M.; Armstrong, S.C. Prevalence of Obesity and Severe Obesity in US Children, 1999–2016. *Pediatrics* **2018**, *141*, e20173459. [CrossRef] [PubMed]
6. van Jaarsveld, C.H.; Gulliford, M.C. Childhood obesity trends from primary care electronic health records in England between 1994 and 2013: Population-based cohort study. *Arch. Dis. Child.* **2015**, archdischild-2014-307151. [CrossRef] [PubMed]
7. World Health Organization. Obesity and Overweight Factsheet. [cited 2020 03/06/2020]. 2017. Available online: https://www.who.int/news-room/fact-sheets/detail/obesity-and-overweight (accessed on 11 May 2019).
8. Popkin, B.M.; Slining, M. New dynamics in global obesity facing low-and middle-income countries. *Obes. Rev.* **2013**, *14*, 11–20. [CrossRef] [PubMed]
9. Yang, L.; Bovet, P.; Ma, C.; Zhao, M.; Liang, Y.; Xi, B. Prevalence of underweight and overweight among young adolescents aged 12–15 years in 58 low-income and middle-income countries. *Pediatric Obes.* **2019**, *14*. [CrossRef]
10. Roth, C.L.; Jain, V. *Rising Obesity in Children: A Serious Public Health Concern*; Springer: Berlin/Heidelberg, Germany, 2018.
11. World Health Organization. *Consideration of the Evidence on Childhood Obesity for the Commission on Ending Childhood Obesity: Report of the Ad Hoc Working Group on Science and Evidence for Ending Childhood Obesity*; World Health Organization: Geneva, Switzerland, 2016.
12. Luttikhuis, H.O.; Baur, L.; Jansen, H.; A Shrewsbury, V.; O'Malley, C.; Stolk, R.P.; Summerbell, C.D. WITHDRAWN: Interventions for treating obesity in children. *Cochrane Database Syst. Rev.* **2019**, *3*, CD001872. [CrossRef]
13. Pandita, A.; Sharma, D.; Pandita, D.; Pawar, S.; Tariq, M.; Kaul, A. Childhood obesity: Prevention is better than cure. *Diabetes, Metab. Syndr. Obesity: Targets Ther.* **2016**, *9*, 83–89. [CrossRef]
14. Pineda, E.; Swinburn, B.; Sassi, F. Effective school food environment interventions for the prevention of childhood obesity: Systematic review and meta-analysis. *Lancet* **2019**, *394*, S77. [CrossRef]
15. Mei, H.; Xiong, Y.; Xie, S.; Guo, S.; Li, Y.; Guo, B.; Zhang, J. The impact of long-term school-based physical activity interventions on body mass index of primary school children—A meta-analysis of randomized controlled trials. *BMC Public Heal.* **2016**, *16*, 205. [CrossRef] [PubMed]
16. Viitasalo, A.; Eloranta, A.-M.; Lintu, N.; Väistö, J.; Venäläinen, T.; Kiiskinen, S.; Karjalainen, P.; Peltola, J.; Lampinen, E.-K.; Haapala, E.A.; et al. The effects of a 2-year individualized and family-based lifestyle intervention on physical activity, sedentary behavior and diet in children. *Prev. Med.* **2016**, *87*, 81–88. [CrossRef] [PubMed]

17. Hofmann, S.G.; Asnaani, A.; Vonk, I.J.J.; Sawyer, A.T.; Fang, A. The Efficacy of Cognitive Behavioral Therapy: A Review of Meta-analyses. *Cogn. Ther. Res.* **2012**, *36*, 427–440. [CrossRef] [PubMed]
18. Graf, C.; Rost, S.V.; Koch, B.; Heinen, S.; Falkowski, G.; Dordel, S.; Bjarnason-Wehrens, B.; Sreeram, N.; Brockmeier, K.; Christ, H.; et al. Data from the StEP TWO programme showing the effect on blood pressure and different parameters for obesity in overweight and obese primary school children. *Cardiol. Young* **2005**, *15*, 291–298. [CrossRef] [PubMed]
19. Hofsteenge, G.H.; Weijs, P.J.; Waal, H.A.D.-V.D.; De Wit, M.; Chinapaw, M.J. Effect of the Go4it multidisciplinary group treatment for obese adolescents on health related quality of life: A randomised controlled trial. *BMC Public Heal.* **2013**, *13*, 939. [CrossRef]
20. Schranz, N.; Tomkinson, G.; Parletta, N.; Petkov, J.; Olds, T. Can resistance training change the strength, body composition and self-concept of overweight and obese adolescent males? A randomised controlled trial. *Br. J. Sports Med.* **2014**, *48*, 1482–1488. [CrossRef]
21. Toulabi, T.; Nikoo, M.K.N.; Amini, F.; Nazari, H.; Mardani, M. The influence of a behavior modification interventional program on body mass index in obese adolescents. *J. Formos. Med Assoc.* **2012**, *111*, 153–159. [CrossRef]
22. Vos, R.C.; Wit, J.M.; Pijl, H.; Kruyff, C.C.; Houdijk, M.C. The effect of family-based multidisciplinary cognitive behavioral treatment in children with obesity: Study protocol for a randomized controlled trial. *Trials* **2011**, *12*, 110. [CrossRef]
23. De Bourdeaudhuij, I.; Van Cauwenberghe, E.; Spittaels, H.; Oppert, J.-M.; Rostami, C.; Brug, J.; Van Lenthe, F.; Lobstein, T.; Maes, L. School-based interventions promoting both physical activity and healthy eating in Europe: A systematic review within the HOPE project. *Obes. Rev.* **2011**, *12*, 205–216. [CrossRef]
24. Kobes, A.; Kretschmer, T.; Timmerman, G.; Schreuder, P. Interventions aimed at preventing and reducing overweight/obesity among children and adolescents: A meta-synthesis. *Obes. Rev.* **2018**, *19*, 1065–1079. [CrossRef]
25. Luttikhuis, H.O.; Baur, L.; Jansen, H.; A Shrewsbury, V.; O'Malley, C.; Stolk, R.P.; Summerbell, C. Cochrane review: Interventions for treating obesity in children. *Evid.-Based Child Heal. A Cochrane Rev. J.* **2009**, *4*, 1571–1729. [CrossRef]
26. Mead, E.; Brown, T.; Rees, K.; Azevedo, L.B.; Whittaker, V.; Jones, D.; Olajide, J.; Mainardi, G.M.; Corpeleijn, E.; O'Malley, C.; et al. Diet, physical activity and behavioural interventions for the treatment of overweight or obese children from the age of 6 to 11 years. *Cochrane Database Syst. Rev.* **2017**, *2017*. [CrossRef] [PubMed]
27. Waters, E.; De Silva-Sanigorski, A.; Burford, B.J.; Brown, T.; Campbell, K.J.; Gao, Y.; Armstrong, R.; Prosser, L.; Summerbell, C.D. Interventions for preventing obesity in children. *Cochrane Database Syst. Rev.* **2011**, CD001871. [CrossRef]
28. Colquitt, J.L.; Loveman, E.; O'Malley, C.; Azevedo, L.B.; Mead, E.; Al-Khudairy, L.; Ells, L.J.; Metzendorf, M.-I.; Rees, K. Diet, physical activity, and behavioural interventions for the treatment of overweight or obesity in preschool children up to the age of 6 years. *Cochrane Database Syst. Rev.* **2016**, *2016*. [CrossRef] [PubMed]
29. Faraoni, D.; Schaefer, S.T. Randomized controlled trials vs. observational studies: Why not just live together? *BMC Anesthesiol.* **2016**, *16*, 102. [CrossRef] [PubMed]
30. Black, N. Why we need observational studies to evaluate the effectiveness of health care. *BMJ* **1996**, *312*, 1215–1218. [CrossRef] [PubMed]
31. Hannan, E.L. Randomized clinical trials and observational studies: Guidelines for assessing respective strengths and limitations. *JACC Cardiovasc. Interv.* **2008**, *1*, 211–217. [CrossRef]
32. Oakley, A.; Strange, V.; Bonell, C.; Allen, E.; Stephenson, J. Process evaluation in randomised controlled trials of complex interventions. *BMJ* **2006**, *332*, 413–416. [CrossRef]
33. Mulder, R.; Singh, A.B.; Hamilton, A.; Das, P.; Outhred, T.; Morris, G.; Bassett, D.; Baune, B.T.; Berk, M.; Boyce, P.; et al. The limitations of using randomised controlled trials as a basis for developing treatment guidelines. *Évid. Based Ment. Heal.* **2017**, *21*, 4–6. [CrossRef]
34. Cochrane, T. *Review Manager (RevMan) 5.3.*; The Nordic Cochrane Centre: Copenhagen, Denmark, 2008.
35. Higgins, J.P.; Green, S. *Cochrane Handbook for Systematic Reviews of Interventions*; John Wiley & Sons: Hoboken, NJ, USA, 2011; Volume 4.
36. Practice, E.; Care, O.O. *EPOC Resources for Review Authors*; Norwegian Knowledge Centre for the Health Services: Oslo, Norway, 2015.

37. Guyatt, G.; Oxman, A.D.; E Vist, G.; Kunz, R.; Falck-Ytter, Y.; Alonso-Coello, P.; Schünemann, H.J. GRADE: An emerging consensus on rating quality of evidence and strength of recommendations. *BMJ* **2008**, *336*, 924–926. [CrossRef]
38. Balshem, H.; Helfand, M.; Schünemann, H.J.; Oxman, A.D.; Kunz, R.; Brozek, J.; Vist, G.E.; Falck-Ytter, Y.; Meerpohl, J.J.; Norris, S. GRADE guidelines: 3. Rating the quality of evidence. *J. Clin. Epidemiol.* **2011**, *64*, 401–406. [CrossRef] [PubMed]
39. Kesztyüs, D.; Lauer, R.; Kesztyüs, T.; Kilian, R.; Steinacker, J.M.; on behalf of the "Join the Healthy Boat" Study Group. Costs and effects of a state-wide health promotion program in primary schools in Germany – the Baden-Württemberg Study: A cluster-randomized, controlled trial. *PLOS ONE* **2017**, *12*, e0172332. [CrossRef]
40. Sutherland, R.; Reeves, P.; Campbell, E.; Lubans, D.R.; Morgan, P.J.; Nathan, N.; Wolfenden, L.; Okely, A.D.; Gillham, K.; Davies, L.; et al. Cost effectiveness of a multi-component school-based physical activity intervention targeting adolescents: The 'Physical Activity 4 Everyone' cluster randomized trial. *Int. J. Behav. Nutr. Phys. Act.* **2016**, *13*, 94. [CrossRef] [PubMed]
41. Li, B.; Pallan, M.; Liu, W.J.; Hemming, K.; Frew, E.; Lin, R.; Martin, J.; Zanganeh, M.; Hurley, K.; Cheng, K.K.; et al. The CHIRPY DRAGON intervention in preventing obesity in Chinese primary-school–aged children: A cluster-randomised controlled trial. *PLoS Med.* **2019**, *16*, e1002971. [CrossRef] [PubMed]
42. McCollister, K.E.; Tolbert, D.V.; Mishra, S.; Natale, R.; Uhlhorn, S.; Messiah, S.E. Cost Analysis of a Childcare Center-Based Intervention to Prevent Obesity in the Preschool Years. *J. Compr. Pediatr.* **2015**, *6*, 6. [CrossRef]
43. Canaway, A.; Frew, E.; Lancashire, E.; Pallan, M.; Hemming, K.; Adab, P.; On behalf of the WAVES trial investigators. Economic evaluation of a childhood obesity prevention programme for children: Results from the WAVES cluster randomised controlled trial conducted in schools. *PLoS ONE* **2019**, *14*, e0219500. [CrossRef] [PubMed]
44. Moodie, M.; Herbert, J.K.; De Silva-Sanigorski, A.M.; Mavoa, H.M.; Keating, C.L.; Carter, R.C.; Waters, E.; Gibbs, L.; Swinburn, B.A. The cost-effectiveness of a successful community-based obesity prevention program: The be active eat well program. *Obesity* **2013**, *21*, 2072–2080. [CrossRef] [PubMed]
45. Epstein, L.H.; Paluch, R.A.; Wrotniak, B.H.; Daniel, T.O.; Kilanowski, C.; Wilfley, D.; Finkelstein, E. Cost-Effectiveness of Family-Based Group Treatment for Child and Parental Obesity. *Child. Obes.* **2014**, *10*, 114–121. [CrossRef] [PubMed]
46. Goldfield, G.; Epstein, L.; Kilanowski, C.; Paluch, R.; Kogut-Bossler, B. Cost-effectiveness of group and mixed family-based treatment for childhood obesity. *Int. J. Obes.* **2001**, *25*, 1843–1849. [CrossRef]
47. Quattrin, T.; Cao, Y.; Paluch, R.A.; Roemmich, J.N.; Ecker, M.A.; Epstein, L.H. Cost-effectiveness of Family-Based Obesity Treatment. *Pediatrics* **2017**, *140*, e20162755. [CrossRef]
48. Robertson, W.; Fleming, J.; Kamal, A.; Hamborg, T.; A Khan, K.; Griffiths, F.; Stewart-Brown, S.; Stallard, N.; Petrou, S.; Simkiss, D.; et al. Randomised controlled trial evaluating the effectiveness and cost-effectiveness of 'Families for Health', a family-based childhood obesity treatment intervention delivered in a community setting for ages 6 to 11 years. *Heal. Technol. Assess.* **2017**, *21*, 1–180. [CrossRef] [PubMed]
49. Sharifi, M.; Franz, C.; Horan, C.M.; Giles, C.M.; Long, M.W.; Ward, Z.; Resch, S.C.; Marshall, R.; Gortmaker, S.L.; Taveras, E.M. Cost-Effectiveness of a Clinical Childhood Obesity Intervention. *Pediatrics* **2017**, *140*, e20162998. [CrossRef] [PubMed]
50. Anderson, Y.C.; Leung, W.; Grant, C.C.; Cave, T.L.; Derraik, J.G.; Cutfield, W.S.; Pereira, N.M.; Hofman, P.L.; Sullivan, T.A. Economic evaluation of a multi-disciplinary community-based intervention programme for New Zealand children and adolescents with obesity. *Obes. Res. Clin. Pr.* **2018**, *12*, 293–298. [CrossRef] [PubMed]
51. Kalavainen, M.; Karjalainen, S.; Martikainen, J.; Korppi, M.; Linnosmaa, I.; Nuutinen, O. Cost-effectiveness of routine and group programs for treatment of obese children. *Pediatr. Int.* **2009**, *51*, 606–611. [CrossRef] [PubMed]
52. Panca, M.; Christie, D.; Cole, T.J.; Costa, S.; Gregson, J.; Holt, R.; Hudson, L.D.; Kessel, A.S.; Kinra, S.; Mathiot, A.; et al. Cost-effectiveness of a community-delivered multicomponent intervention compared with enhanced standard care of obese adolescents: Cost-utility analysis alongside a randomised controlled trial (the HELP trial). *BMJ Open* **2018**, *8*, e018640. [CrossRef]

53. Larsen, K.T.; Huang, T.; Møller, N.C.; Andersen, L.B.; Sørensen, J. Cost-effectiveness of a day-camp weight-loss intervention programme for children: Results based on a randomised controlled trial with one-year follow-up. *Scand. J. Public Heal.* **2017**, *45*, 666–674. [CrossRef]
54. Wake, M.; Gold, L.; McCallum, Z.; Gerner, B.; Waters, E. Economic Evaluation of a Primary Care Trial to Reduce Weight Gain in Overweight/Obese Children: The LEAP Trial. *Ambul. Pediatr.* **2008**, *8*, 336–341. [CrossRef]
55. Zylke, J.W.; Bauchner, H. Preventing Obesity in Children: A Glimmer of Hope. *JAMA* **2018**, *320*, 443–444. [CrossRef]
56. Vissers, D.; Hens, W.; Hansen, D.; Taeymans, J. The Effect of Diet or Exercise on Visceral Adipose Tissue in Overweight Youth. *Med. Sci. Sports Exerc.* **2016**, *48*, 1415–1424. [CrossRef]
57. Lien, A.S.-Y.; Tsai, J.-L.; Lee, J.-T.; Wu, M.-Y.; Jiang, Y.-D.; Yen, H.-R. A Systematic Review and Meta-Analysis of the Effect of Lifestyle Modification on Metabolic Control in Overweight Children. *Evid.-Based Complement. Altern. Med.* **2017**, *2017*, 1–12. [CrossRef]
58. Coppock, J.H.; Ridolfi, D.R.; Hayes, J.F.; Stpaul, M.; Wilfley, D.E. Current Approaches to the Management of Pediatric Overweight and Obesity. *Curr. Treat. Options Cardiovasc. Med.* **2014**, *16*, 343. [CrossRef] [PubMed]
59. Miri, S.F.; Javadi, M.; Lin, C.-Y.; Griffiths, M.D.; Björk, M.; Pakpour, A.H. Effectiveness of cognitive-behavioral therapy on nutrition improvement and weight of overweight and obese adolescents: A randomized controlled trial. *Diabetes Metab. Syndr. Clin. Res. Rev.* **2019**, *13*, 2190–2197. [CrossRef] [PubMed]
60. Wilfley, D.E.; Hayes, J.F.; Balantekin, K.N.; Van Buren, R.J.; Epstein, L.H. Behavioral interventions for obesity in children and adults: Evidence base, novel approaches, and translation into practice. *Am. Psychol.* **2018**, *73*, 981–993. [CrossRef] [PubMed]
61. Sonntag, D. Why Early Prevention of Childhood Obesity Is More Than a Medical Concern: A Health Economic Approach. *Ann. Nutr. Metab.* **2017**, *70*, 175–178. [CrossRef]

3

Prevalence and Predictors of Overweight and Obesity among Young Children in the Children's Healthy Living Study on Guam

Rachael T. Leon Guerrero [1,*], L. Robert Barber [1], Tanisha F. Aflague [1], Yvette C. Paulino [1], Margaret P. Hattori-Uchima [1], Mark Acosta [1], Lynne R. Wilkens [2] and Rachel Novotny [3]

[1] Office of Research & Sponsored Programs, University of Guam, Mangilao, Guam 96923, USA; bbarber@triton.uog.edu (L.R.B.); taflague@triton.uog.edu (T.F.A.); paulinoy@triton.uog.edu (Y.C.P.); muchima@triton.uog.edu (M.P.H.-U.); macosta@triton.uog.edu (M.A.)

[2] University of Hawaii Cancer Center, Honolulu, HI 96813, USA; lynne@cc.hawaii.edu

[3] College of Tropical Agriculture and Human Resources, University of Hawaii At Manoa, Honolulu, HI 96822, USA; novotny@hawaii.edu

* Correspondence: rachaeltlg@triton.uog.edu.

Abstract: This study is part of the Children's Healthy Living program in U.S. Affiliated Pacific region. The objectives were to estimate overweight and obesity (OWOB) prevalence and identify possible related risk factors among ethnic groups in Guam. In 2013, 865 children (2–8 years) were recruited via community-based sampling from select communities in Guam. Children's demographic and health behavior information; dietary intake; and anthropometric measurements were collected. Logistic regression, odds ratio, t-tests, and chi-square tests were used to determine differences and assess covariates of OWOB. The results indicate that 58% of children were living below the poverty level, 80% were receiving food assistance, and 51% experienced food insecurity. The majority of children surveyed did not meet recommendations for: sleep duration (59.6%), sedentary screen-time (83.11%), or fruit (58.7%) and vegetable (99.1%) intake, and consumed sugar sweetened beverages (SSB) (73.7%). OWOB affected 27.4% of children. Children affected by OWOB in this study were statistically more likely ($p = 0.042$) to suffer from sleep disturbances ($p = 0.042$) and consume marginally higher amounts (p value = 0.07) of SSB compared to children with healthy weight. Among Other Micronesians, children from families who considered themselves 'integrated' into the culture were 2.05 (CI 0.81–5.20) times more likely to be affected by OWOB. In conclusion, the OWOB prevalence among 2–8-year-olds in Guam was 27.4%; and compared with healthy weight children, children with OWOB were more likely to have educated caregivers and consume more SSBs. Results provide a basis for health promotion and obesity prevention guidance for children in Guam.

Keywords: child obesity; Guam; Children's Healthy Living (CHL); islander; Pacific; Micronesia

---

1. Introduction

Childhood overweight and obesity (OWOB) is a global epidemic affecting many countries [1–5], including the United States (US) and the US Affiliated Pacific region (USAP). In the US a high prevalence of OWOB among racial/ethnic minority groups for children 2–19 years is reported, specifically Non-Hispanic black (19.5%) and Hispanic (21.9%), yet Native Hawaiian or Other Pacific Islanders are not included [1,2]. Novotny and colleagues conducted a systematic review of childhood OWOB in the USAP region and estimated that the prevalence of OWOB for children 2–8 years was 21%, and that the prevalence increased to 39% by age 8 [6]. Similarly, the proportion of obese children increased from 10% at age 2 years to 23% at age 8 years, with the highest prevalence of obesity in both Guam and American Samoa [6]. The systematic review found that in Guam, OWOB prevalence (39%) among children ages 3 to 5 years [6] exceeded the US national average (23%) for children aged 2 to 5 years [1,2].

Guam is a U.S. Territory located in the northwestern Pacific Ocean, approximately 3700 miles west of Hawaii, 6000 miles west of California, and 1300 miles southeast of Japan. CHamorus are the original inhabitants of Guam [7,8], and are typically grouped with other Pacific Islanders. However, the current population of Guam is characterized by substantial ethnic variation [9]: 37% CHamoru, 26% Filipino, 12% other Pacific Islander, 11% other ethnicity, 7% White, and 7% other Asian. This ethnic diversity evolved through centuries of colonization and migration that continues today [10] and may modify the burden and predictors of OWOB among CHamorus. Factors related to OWOB are sleep, physical activity, psychosocial, life course exposure, SES, and diet [11,12] that for many racial/ethnic groups in Guam is influenced by this history [12,13]. OWOB prevalence among adults is higher among CHamorus compared to other ethnic groups on Guam [11]. In a study among adults in the two largest ethnic populations in Guam then (2008) and now, CHamorus and Filipinos, there was a significant difference in energy density of diets between the two groups, where CHamorus had a higher energy and added sugar intake [11]. In 2009 and 2010, prevalence of OWOB was highest among CHamorus followed by Other Micronesians reported in one of the first reports to disaggregate BRFSS data by ethnicity [14].

Children who are overweight or obese have a higher risk of being overweight or obese adults [15] with an increased risk of chronic diseases later in life [16]. However, there is limited information about young children in Guam, and data are needed to understand the burden of and determine the appropriate intervention for childhood OWOB. Therefore, the purpose of this study is to estimate the prevalence of OWOB among children in Guam and identify demographic or other risk factors targeted by the Children's Healthy Living (CHL) program for overweight and obesity in CHamoru children.

2. Methods

The Children's Healthy Living Program for Remote Underserved Minority Populations in the Pacific Region (CHL) program is a partnership of universities and local organizations across the remote USAP (Alaska, American Samoa, Commonwealth of the Northern Marianas, Federated States of Micronesia, Republic of Marshall Islands, Republic of Palau, Hawaii, and Guam) working to prevent childhood obesity in the Pacific. Detailed information on the study design of the CHL program can be found elsewhere [17,18]. Briefly, approximately 900 children (2–8 years) and their parents/caregivers from each participating USAP jurisdiction were recruited to participate in the study at both baseline and 24-month follow-up. On Guam, a total of 865 children were recruited at baseline (2013) and 696 children were recruited from the same communities at 24-month follow-up. This paper will focus on baseline data of the 865 children on Guam recruited from communities (Agana Heights, Sinajana, Agat, Santa Rita, Yigo, Yona, Talafofo, and Dededo) selected due to their size, representation of indigenous (CHamoru) residents, and isolation and cohesiveness (for purpose of intervention) [17]. Behavioral targets of the CHL program were increasing sleep, water intake, fruit and vegetable intake, physical activity and decreasing sugar sweetened beverage intake and sedentary behavior [17].

Child participants were recruited primarily at early childhood education centers (e.g., Guam Head Start program, daycares, and public elementary schools) and community-based settings (e.g., municipal centers and public housing areas) on Guam. Data collection occurred over a minimum of two visits at these recruitment sites. Further details on recruitment is described elsewhere [17,18]. Child participants with parents' consent and who provided assent were assessed.

At the first visit, parents/caregivers completed surveys on demographic information (i.e., child age, place of birth, race/ethnicity, and sex; household composition and food security; parent/caregiver educational level and income); cultural identity of the parent/caregiver; and general health status, early life feeding behaviors, and sedentary screen-time and sleep behavior germane to the child. They also received instructions for completing a two-day food and activity log at home during the week. Sleep quality was measured with the Tayside Children's Sleep Questionnaire (TCSQ) [19] and sleep duration [20] was reported by the parent/caregiver as hours asleep at night and during naps. Other surveys were adapted from previous studies [17] with some local terminology added for participant clarity.

Detailed information was collected in CHL on race/ethnic groups, allowing for multiple groups to be selected; classification prioritized ethnic groups indigenous to the jurisdiction. On Guam, the indigenous ethnic group is CHamoru [7,8]. If more than one race/ethnicity was indicated for the child and CHamoru was selected, the child was categorized as CHamoru. If a child identified as not CHamoru and as one of the other Micronesian Pacific Island ethnic groups, such as Chuukese, Palauan, Yapese, Carolinian, Marshallese, or Kosraean, that child was categorized as 'Other Micronesian', because the only other Pacific Island ethnic groups identified in the Guam sample were from Micronesia and not Polynesia (e.g., Native Hawaiians or Samoans). These other Micronesian Pacific Islander groups were grouped together as their numbers were small and they were all from neighboring Micronesian islands.

Food insecurity was determined by asking one question from the US Department of Agriculture's Core Food Security Module: "In the past 12 months how often does money for food run out by the end of the month?" (never, seldom, sometimes, most times, always, don't know, or no response [21]. In this study, options of don't know or no response were treated as missing values. Household food insecurity was considered present if the respondent chose sometimes, most times, or always. Parent's cultural identity, or "acculturation," was determined using their responses reported on a cultural affiliation questionnaire, which assesses one of four modes of acculturation, from two cultural identity subscales (i.e., respondent's ethnic group and the US): traditional (high ethnic and low US subscale scores), integrated (high ethnic and high US subscale scores), assimilated (low ethnic and high US subscale scores), or marginalized (low ethnic and low US scores) [22]. The same scoring system was used as described by Kaholokula and others [22].

After providing assent, each child was measured for weight, height, and waist circumference (WC) by trained and standardized research staff [23] and described in detail elsewhere [17]. These measures were used to compute Body Mass Index (BMI) [weight (kg)/height(m)^2], WC (cm) to height (cm) ratios, and subsequent BMI z-score, BMI-for-age-percentiles, and waist circumference- for-age percentiles [24,25]. BMI percentiles and z-scores were calculated according to CDC reference data [26] and BMI categories were assigned accordingly: underweight (<5th percentile), healthy weight (5th–84th percentile), overweight (85th–94th percentile), and obese (≥95th percentile). Children were considered to have OWOB if their BMI percentile was greater than the 85th percentile for age and sex. Cutoff values for biologically implausible values defined as <−5 or >4 standard deviations (SD) for height-for-age z-score and <−4 or >8 SD for BMI z-score (according to CDC reference data) were removed from the analysis. Child participants were considered to have abdominal obesity if their WC was greater than the International Diabetes Federation [27] cut-point.

Fruit, vegetable, and beverage intake were estimated using data recorded in the child's two-day food logs reported by the child's parent/caregiver and data collection methods are described in detail elsewhere [17]. Parents/caregivers were asked to complete the food log of everything their children ate or drank for two randomly assigned non-consecutive days, which included weekdays and weekend days, between visit one and two, approximately 6 days apart. Assignment of recording days was based on the day of the child's first visit (Monday–Saturday). Parents/caregivers were instructed in record keeping techniques with the aid of food models, service ware, and measuring utensils. During visit two, research staff reviewed the food log with the parents/caregivers (e.g., for completeness of food entries, portion size estimation, food preparation methods, and/or accuracy of recording data). Trained staff entered the food log data into the Pacific Tracker3 (PacTrac3), which includes a food composition database developed in collaboration with the University of Hawaii Cancer Center for use in the Pacific region [28–30]. For this study, PacTrac3 data were used to classify beverage type (i.e., sugar-sweetened beverages (SSB), milk, or water), fruit, and vegetable, as well as, calculate intake (e.g., cups/day, grams/day). All soft drinks, fruit drinks (fruit flavored or containing less than 100% juice), sports drinks, energy drinks, sweetened tea, and sweetened coffee reported were classified as SSB. Milk intake in cups was calculated for food log entries and included all fluid milk (cow and/or goat), chocolate milk, lactose-reduced milk, lactose-free milk, filled milk, dry milk, and evaporated milk. Fruit, vegetable, milk, water, and SSB intake per day was adjusted for within person variance and then averaged over the two days of records, weighted for weekday and weekend days.

Compensation for study participation was provided at visits one and two [17]. The CHL program was funded by the United States Department of Agriculture (USDA), Agriculture and Food Research Initiative. Ethical approval for this project was granted by both the University of Guam Committee on Human Research Subjects (IRB) (CHRS#12-74) and the University of Hawaii Institutional Review Board (CHS#18915); written consent was given by all parents and oral assent was given by all child participants prior to their inclusion, in accordance with the Declaration of Helsinki.

Statistical analyses were performed using IBM SPSS Statistics version 26 (IBM Corporation, Armonk, NY, USA). Data analysis included the calculation of percentages for ordinal and nominal data, and means and standard errors for the interval and continuous data. *t*-tests and chi-square tests were used to test for differences in continuous and categorical variables, respectively, between BMI groups and ethnic groups. Binary logistic regression models of OWOB assessed its relationship with several potential covariates, adjusted for sex, age, and ethnicity and with the variance corrected for clustering of children within communities. Odds ratios and 95% CI were the primary statistics reported from the models. ORs were calculated for each of the following child factors from all ethnic groups combined and in CHamoru and Other Micronesian children separately: child age, sex, ever breastfed, sleep, sedentary screen-time, vegetable intake, fruit intake, water intake, and SSB intake; and parent/caregiver education, acculturation and marital status; and household income, food insecurity, food assistance, and household size. Does-response was assessed using a trend variable assigned consecutive integers (1, 2, ...) to each ordered category. These factors were selected among demographic and lifestyle-related variables because they have been reported to be risk factors for OWOB among children [17,25,31,32] and/or were behaviors of interest for the CHL Program. p values < 0.05 were considered statistically significant, whereas p values of 0.05 to 0.10 were described as borderline significant.

3. Results

3.1. Demographics

The descriptive characteristics of child participants at baseline are summarized by ethnicity in Table 1. The average age of child participants was 5.79 years (sem 0.062). The majority of child participants were male (51.7%), 2–5 years old (53.8%), CHamoru ethnicity (64.8%), born on Guam (84.5%), from households where parents were not married (60.7%) or there were 3 or more children (76.2%), and considered as being 'integrated' (79.9%) as reported by parent/caregiver.

Overall, more than half of participating children (57.9%) came from families whose annual income was less than $20,000, which was slightly below the poverty level for a 3-person household in 2015 [33]. A significantly higher ($p < 0.001$) proportion of Other Micronesian children (82.9%) came from families whose annual income was less than $20,000 compared to CHamoru (54.2%), Filipino (43.24%) and Other (40%) children. Parents of Filipino children reported significantly higher ($p < 0.001$) education attainment levels compared to both CHamoru and Other Micronesians.

3.2. OWOB Prevalence

OWOB prevalence among child participants in this study is 27.4%. A significantly ($p = 0.03$) higher proportion of Other Micronesian children were affected by obesity (BMI $\geq$ 95th percentile) compared to CHamoru children (18.3% versus 11.0%) (Table 1).

Table 1. Characteristics * of child participants from Guam in the Children's Healthy Living (CHL) Program by ethnicity.

	Total	CHamoru (*n* = 561)	Other Micronesians (*n* = 223)	Filipino (*n* = 81)	Other (*n* = 10)	*p* Value
Child Participant						
Age, years	5.79 ± 0.062	5.80 ± 0.078	5.66 ± 0.123	5.99 ± 0.062	6.24 ± 0.670	
2–5 years old	465 (53.76%)	296 (52.76%)	123 (57.76%)	42 (51.85%)	4 (40%)	0.418
6–8 years old	400 (46.24%)	265 (47.23%)	90 (42.25%)	39 (48.14%)	6 (60%)	
Birthplace						0.0001
Guam	723 (84.46%)	488 (88.09%)	170 (80.19%)	62 (76.54%)	3 (33.33%)	
U.S. Mainland	52 (6.08%)	36 (6.50%)	9 (4.25%)	3 (3.70%)	4 (44.44%)	
Saipan, CNMI	34 (3.97%)	28 (5.05%)	5 (2.36%)	1 (1.24%)	0 (0%)	
Other Islands in Micronesia	28 (3.27%)	0 (0%)	28 (13.21%)	0 (0%)	0 (0%)	
Philippines	15 (1.75%)	0 (0%)	0 (0%)	15 (18.52%)	0 (0%)	
Other	4 (0.47%)	2 (0.36%)	0 (0%)	0 (0%)	2 (22.22%)	
Ever Breastfed?						0.0006
Yes	557 (67.19%)	341 (62.80%)	155 (78.68%)	53 (67.09%)	8 (80%)	
No	272 (32.81%)	202 (37.20%)	42 (21.32%)	26 (32.91%)	2 (20%)	
Child fed both breastmilk & infant formula						0.8223
Yes	443 (54.23%)	291 (54.09%)	102 (53.40%)	46 (58.23%)	4 (44.45%)	
No	374 (45.77%)	247 (45.91%)	89 (46.60%)	33 (41.77%)	5 (55.55%)	
Child age (months) when weaned from breastmilk	9.76 ± 0.438	8.63 ± 0.519	12.48 ± 0.958	8.511 ± 1.165	18.0 ± 3.928	
Average Sleep Duration (h/d)	8.61 ± 0.078	8.86 ± 0.086 †	7.75 ± 0.200	8.99 ± 0.206 †	9.05 ± 0.273	0.0001
TCSQ Sleep Score	6.34 ± 0.205	6.583 ± 0.246	6.011 ± 0.4621	5.231 ± 0.554	8.00 ± 3.386	
Met Sleep Recommendations F						0.0136
Yes	343 (40.35%)	240 (43.09%)	63 (30.58%)	35 (43.75%)	5 (50%)	
No	507 (59.65%)	317 (56.91%)	143 (69.42%)	45 (65.25%)	5 (50%)	
Average Screen-time (hr/d)	5.29 ± 0.132	5.13 ± 0.154 §	5.45 ± 0.308	6.24 ± 0.425	3.59 ± 0.550	
Met Screen-time Recommendations Ω						0.0069
Yes	124 (16.89%)	82 (16.73%)	39 (22.54%)	3 (4.61%)	0 (0%)	
No	610 (83.11%)	408 (83.27%)	134 (77.46%)	62 (95.39%)	6 (100%)	
Height (cm)	110.56 ± 0.46	109.07 ± 0.59	111.31 ± 1.71	112.98 ± 1.22	114.75 ± 5.03	
Weight (kg)	21.05 ± 0.25	20.78 ± 0.31	21.50 ± 0.54	21.55 ± 0.72	22.4 ± 2.44	
Body Mass Index (kg/m^2)	16.84 ± 0.11	16.77 ± 0.14	17.09 ± 0.43	16.65 ± 0.27	16.42 ± 0.61	
BMI z-score	0.402 ± 0.039	0.352 ± 0.048 †	0.544 ± 0.08	0.395 ± 0.132	0.189 ± 0.284	0.0397
BMI Categories ß						
Underweight	25 (2.96%)	18 (32.91%)	4 (1.93%)	3 (3.75%)	0 (0%)	0.6945
Healthy weight	595 (70.49%)	392 (71.66%)	144 (69.56%)	51 (63.75%)	8 (80%)	0.4523
Overweight, % (≥85th%ile)	113 (13.39%)	77 (14.08%)	21 (10.14%)	14 (17.50%)	1 (10%)	0.3385
Obesity, % (≥95th%ile)	111 (13.15%)	60 (10.97%)	38 (18.36%)	12 (15.0%)	1 (10%)	0.0314
OWOB by Age						
2–5 years old	107 (23.94%)	59 (20.85%)	32 (26.89%)	16 (39.02%)	0 (0%)	0.0378
6–8 years old	117 (29.47%)	78 (29.54%)	27 (30.68%)	10 (25.64%)	2 (33.33%)	0.9441
Waist Circumference (cm)	55.07 ± 0.30	54.76 ± 0.38	55.44 ± 0.58	56.104 ± 0.95	55.64 ± 2.50	

Table 1. *Cont.*

	Total	CHamoru (*n* = 561)	Other Micronesians (*n* = 223)	Filipino (*n* = 81)	Other (*n* = 10)	*p* Value
Child Participant						
Abdominal Obesity €						0.6782
Yes	76 (8.94%)	48 (8.77%)	17 (7.98%)	10 (12.50%)	1 (10%)	
No	774 (91.06%)	499 (91.23%)	196 (92.02%)	70 (87.5%)	9 (90%)	
Consumed SSB?						0.0001
Yes	497 (74.74%)	361 (81.49%)	95 (61.29%)	36 (59.01%)	5 (50%)	
No	168 (25.26%)	82 (18.51%)	60 (38.71%)	25 (40.99%)	5 (50%)	
Beverage Consumption ‡,¶						
Water (c/d)	1.47 ± 0.048	1.306 ± 0.45	1.298 ± 0.66	1.401 ± 0.105	1.522 ± 0.429	
Milk (c/d)	1.241 ± 0.024	1.280 ± 0.029 †,§	1.028 ± 0.045	1.454 ± 0.081 †	1.660 ± 0.139	
Sugar-sweet drinks (c/d)	0.845 ± 0.029	0.958 ± 0.036 †,§,‡	0.560 ± 0.050 Ø	0.727 ± 0.101	1.095 ± 0.269	
Fruit Consumption ‡ (c/d)	0.882 ± 0.021	0.88 ± 0.025	0.846 ± 0.045	0.956 ± 0.080	1.153 ± 0.240	
Vegetable Consumption ‡,¶ (c/d)	0.609 ± 0.013	0.648 ± 0.015	0.472 ± 0.026	0.651 ± 0.041	0.850 ± 0.139	
Met Recommendation for:						
Fruit Intake	257 (41.35%)	182 (41.08%)	63 (40.65%)	27 (44.26%)	3 (50%)	0.9312
Vegetable Intake	6 (0.90%)	5 (1.13%)	1 (0.65%)	0 (0%)	0 (0%)	0.8064
Parent/Caregiver/Household						
Annual Family Income Level						0.0001
<$20,000	348 (57.91%)	220 (54.18%)	92 (82.88%)	32 (43.24%)	4 (40%)	
$20,000–$34,999	182 (14.81%)	59 (14.53%)	9 (8.11%)	17 (22.97%)	4 (40%)	
$35,000–$59,999	93 (15.47%)	71 (17.49%)	5 (4.51%)	17 (22.97%)	0 (0%)	
>$60,000	71 (11.81%)	56 (13.80%)	5 (7.20%)	8 (10.82%)	2 (20%)	
Receiving any Food Assistance						0.0001
Yes	676 (80.38%)	447 (81.57%)	176 (86.70%)	47 (58.75%)	6 (60%)	
No	165 (19.62%)	101 (18.43%)	27 (13.30%)	33 (41.25%)	4 (40%)	
Type of Food Assistance						
SNAP ∂	585 (67.85%)	401 (71.61%)	146 (69.19%)	33 (40.74%)	5 (50%)	0.0001
Local Food Bank	101 (11.72%)	69 (12.32%)	28 (13.27%)	4 (4.94%)	0 (0%)	0.1319
WIC ∞	274 (31.79%)	162 (28.93%)	86 (40.76%)	22 (27.16%)	4 (40%)	0.0114
Free School Lunch/Breakfast	248 (28.77%)	202 (36.07%)	33 (15.64%)	10 (12.35%)	3 (30%)	0.0001
Food Insecurity δ						0.0001
Always/most times	127 (16.82%)	86 (17.20%)	32 (18.71%)	7 (9.46%)	2 (20%)	
Sometimes	262 (34.70%)	128 (25.6%)	96 (56.16%)	35 (47.29%)	3 (30%)	
Seldom/never	366 (48.48%)	286 (57.20%)	43 (25.15%)	32 (43.24%)	5 (50%)	
Parent/Caregiver Education						0.0001
<12th Grade	281 (32.48%)	184 (32.80%)	79 (37.08%)	17 (20.98%)	1 (10%)	
12th Grade/GED	351 (40.58%)	237 (42.24%)	97 (45.54%)	13 (16.05%)	4 (40%)	
Some college or higher	233 (26.94%)	140 (24.96%)	37 (17.38%)	32 (62.97%)	5 (50%)	
Parent Marital Status						0.0001
Married	340 (39.31%)	190 (33.89%)	90 (42.25%)	55 (67.90%)	5 (50%)	
Not Married	525 (60.69%)	371 (66.13%)	123 (57.75%)	26 (32.10%)	5 (50%)	
Number Children in Household	4.19 ± 0.077	4.29 ± 0.096 §	4.35 ± 0.164 §	3.14 ± 0.151	3.4 ± 0.306	0.0001

Table 1. *Cont.*

	Total	CHamoru ($n = 561$)	Other Micronesians ($n = 223$)	Filipino ($n = 81$)	Other ($n = 10$)	p Value
Child Participant						
Household Size						0.008
1–2 children	205 (23.78%)	127 (22.72%)	48 (22.64%)	29 (35.80%)	1 (1%)	
3–4 children	341 (39.56%)	220 (39.36%)	75 (35.38%)	39 (48.15%)	7 (70%)	
5 or more children	316 (36.66%)	212 (37.92%)	89 (41.98%)	13 (16.05%)	2 (20%)	
Acculturation ϒ						0.0565
Integrated	572 (79.89%)	388 (80.15%)	123 (75.00%)	55 (88.71%)	6 (100%)	
Traditional	101 (14.11%)	74 (15.29%)	24 (14.63%)	3 (4.84%)	0	
Assimilated	17 (2.37%)	7 (1.45%)	7 (4.27%)	3 (4.83%)	0	
Marginalized	26 (3.63%)	15 (3.10%)	10 (6.10%)	1 (1.61%)	0	

* Frequency number (%), ¶ Mean ± standard error, ‡ Consumption in cups/day, weighted for weekday/weekend days and adjusted for within person variance, † Significantly ($p < 0.05$) different from Other Micronesians § Significantly ($p < 0.05$) different from Filipino, Ø Significantly ($p < 0.05$) different from Other, F Sleep Recommendations: at least 11 h/d for 2-year-olds, at least 10 h/d for 3 to 5 year-olds, and at least 9 h/d for 6 to 10 year-olds, Ω Screen-time Recommendation of 2 h/d or less, ß BMI percentiles calculated according to CDC reference data and categories assigned as: underweight (<5th percentile), healthy weight (5th–84th percentile), overweight (85th–94th percentile), and obese (95th percentile), € Abdominal obesity defined as waist circumference greater than the International Diabetes Federation cut-point (>90.2 percentile for age and sex), ∂ USDA Supplemental Nutrition Assistance Program (SNAP), ∞ USDA Supplemental Nutrition Assistance Program for Women, Infants, and Children (WIC), δ Question from USDA Core Food Security Module "In the past 12 months how often does money for food run out by the end of the month? ϒ What category of acculturation does family consider themselves?

Table 2 shows child participant characteristics by weight status for all ethnic groups combined, and for CHamorus and Other Micronesians separately. Children affected by OWOB reported statistically higher body size parameters as measured by height, weight, WC, BMI, and BMI z-scores, compared to healthy weight children. All children with abdominal obesity, as defined by the International Diabetes Federation [27], were OWOB. Among children in the OWOB weight status, 33.8% had abdominal obesity by this cut-point. It is worth noting that the International Diabetes Federation cut-point is for older children (6–10 years old) and is limited in identifying younger children (2–5 years) with abdominal obesity.

Table 2. Characteristics of child participants from Guam in the Children's Healthy Living (CHL) Program stratified by BMI status.

Participant & Family Characteristics	Total Mean ± SE or *n*(%)	Healthy Weight * Mean ± SE or *n* (%)	OWOB * Mean ± SE or *n* (%)	*p* Value
Age				0.069
2–5 years old	437 (53.2%)	329 (55.1%)	108 (48%)	
6–8 years old	385 (46.8%)	268 (44.9%)	117 (52%)	
Sex				0.917
Boys	425 (51.7%)	308 (51.6%)	117 (52.0%)	
Girls	397 (48.3%)	289 (48.4%)	108 (48.0%)	
Child Ethnicity				0.455
CHamoru	528 (64.55%)	392 (65.88%)	137 (61.16%)	
Other Micronesians	203 (24.82%)	144 (24.20%)	59 (26.34%)	
Filipino	77 (9.41%)	51 (8.57%)	26 (11.61%)	
Other	10 (1.22%)	8 (1.34%)	2 (0.89%)	
Annual Family Income Level				0.473
<$20,000	331 (57.6%)	234 (56.9%)	97 (59.1%)	
$20,000–$34,999	86 (15%)	63 (15.3%)	23 (14%)	
$35,000–$59,999	89 (15.5%)	60 (14.6%)	29 (17.7%)	
>$60,000	69 (12%)	54 (13.1%)	15 (9.1%)	
Receiving any Food Assistance				0.768
Yes	645 (78.5%)	470 (78.7%)	175 (77.8)	
No	177 (21.5%)	127 (21.3%)	50 (22.2%)	
Type of Food Assistance				
SNAP	556 (67.9%)	408 (68.7%)	148 (65.8%)	0.426
Local Food Bank	99 (12.15%)	72 (72.7%)	27 (27.3%)	0.977
WIC	258 (31.5%)	196 (33.0%)	62 (27.6%)	0.135
Free School Lunch/Breakfast	238 (29.1%)	169 (28.5%)	69 (30.7%)	0.533
Food Insecurity				0.566
Always/most times	120 (16.7%)	88 (16.8%)	32 (16.3%)	
Sometimes	253 (35.2%)	178 (34%)	75 (38.3%)	
Seldom/never	346 (48.1%)	257 (49.1%)	89 (45.4%)	
Parent/Caregiver Education				0.052
<12th Grade	269 (32.7%)	207 (34.7%)	62 (27.6%)	
12th Grade/GED	331 (40.3%)	241 (40.4%)	90 (40%)	
Some college or higher	222 (27%%)	149 (25%)	73 (32.4%)	
Parent Marital Status				0.06
Married	326 (39.7%)	225 (37.7%)	101 (44.9%)	
Not Married	496 (60.3%)	372 (62.3%)	124 (55.1%)	
Number Children in Household	4.19 ± 0.077	4.19 ± 0.094	4.22 ± 0.152	0.838
Household Size				0.491
1–2 children	197 (24.1%)	145 (24.4%)	52 (23.1%)	
3–4 children	319 (38.9%)	224 (37.7%)	95 (42.2%)	
5 or more children	303 (37%)	225 (37.9%)	78 (34.7%)	
Birthplace				0.0070
Guam	685 (84.46%)	505 (85.45%)	180 (81.45%)	
U.S. Mainland	52 (6.41%)	37 (6.26%)	15 (6.79%)	
Saipan, CNMI	31 (3.82%)	20 (3.38%)	13 (5.88%)	
Other Islands in Micronesia	25 (3.08%)	21 (3.55%)	4 (1.81%)	
Philippines	13 (1.60%)	8 (1.35%)	5 (2.26%)	
Other	4 (0.49%)	1 (0.17%)	4 (1.82%)	

Table 2. *Cont.*

Participant & Family Characteristics	Total Mean ± SE or *n*(%)	Healthy Weight * Mean ± SE or *n* (%)	OWOB * Mean ± SE or *n* (%)	*p* Value
Acculturation				0.2913
Integrated	542 (80.30%)	394 (79.60%)	148 (82.22%)	
Traditional	94 (13.78%)	72 (14.54%)	21 (12.14%)	
Assimilated	17 (2.52%)	10 (2.02%)	7 (3.89%)	
Marginalized	23 (3.41%)	19 (3.84%)	4 (2.22%)	
Ever Breastfed?				0.2140
Yes	529 (64.59%)	373 (66.13%)	156 (70.59%)	
No	256 (35.41%)	191 (33.87%)	65 (29.41%)	
Exclusively Breastfed?				0.5655
Yes	97 (13.13%)	68 (12.69%)	29 (14.29%)	
No	642 (86.87%)	468 (87.13%)	174 (85.71%)	
Child age (mos) when weaned from breastmilk	9.76 ± 0.438 (*n* = 495)	10.22 ± 0.542	9.23 ± 0.844	0.3248
Child fed both breastmilk & infant formula				0.5135
Yes	421 (54.39%)	300 (53.67%)	121(56.28%)	
No	353 (45.61%)	259 (44.33%)	94 (43.72%)	
Average Sleep Duration (h/d)	8.62 ± 0.08	8.64 ± 0.096	8.59 ± 0.142	0.7122
TCSQ Sleep Score	6.34 ± 0.205	6.55 ± 0.257	5.59 ± 0.341	0.0421
Met Sleep Recommendations				0.725
Yes	327 (40.4%)	236 (40%)	91 (41.4%)	
No	483 (59.6%)	354 (60%)	129 (58.6%)	
Average Screen-time (h/d)	5.26 ± 0.132	5.15 ± 0.150	5.55 ± 0.270	0.1743
Met Screen-time Recommendations				0.444
Yes	117 (16.8%)	82 (16.2%)	35 (18.6%)	
No	578 (83.2%)	425 (83.8%)	153 (81.4%)	
Height (cm)	110.52 ± 0.47	108.71 ± 0.528	115.34 ± 0.912	0.0001
Weight (kg)	21.26 ± 0.26	18.77 ± 0.185	27.91 ± 0.635	0.0001
BMI, kg/m^2	16.95 ± 0.11	15.64 ± 0.038	20.45 ± 0.280	0.0001
BMI z-score	0.485 ± 0.036	0.007 ± 0.026	1.79 ± 0.045	0.0001
Waist Circumference (cm)	55.07 ± 0.457	51.93 ±0.188	64.40 ± 0.707	0.0001
Abdominal Obesity				0.0001
Yes	75 (9.2%)	0 (0%)	75 (33.60%)	
No	741 (90.8%)	591 (100%)	148 (66.40%)	
Beverage Consumption ‡				
Water (c/d)	1.31 ± 0.035	1.32 ± 0.043	1.28 ± 0.070	0.5793
Milk (c/d)	1.24 ± 0.24	1.25 ± 0.028	1.21 ± 0.048	0.5994
Sugar-sweetened drinks (c/d)	0.84 ± 0.03	0.81 ± 0.34	0.93 ± 0.061	0.0676
Vegetable Intake ‡ (c/d)	0.61 ± 0.013	0.60 ± 0.015	0.63 ± 0.027	0.2535
Fruit Intake ‡ (c/d)	0.88 ± 0.021	0.87 ± 0.025	0.89 ± 0.040	0.7324
Met Recommendation for:				
Fruit Intake	257 (41.35%)	185 (39.96%)	79 (46.20%)	0.1571
Vegetable Intake	6 (0.90%)	4 (0.86%)	2 (1.17%)	0.7242

* Healthy weight defined as BMI between 5th–84th percentile for age and sex; 'OWOB' defined as BMI greater than 85th percentile for age and sex, ‡ Consumption in cups/day, weighted for weekday/weekend days and adjusted for within person variance.

There were no significant differences in the presence of OWOB among children by sex, ethnicity, family income, food insecurity, food assistance, acculturation, screen-time, sleep duration, or intake of fruits, vegetables, water, or milk. OWOB children consumed marginally higher amounts (p value = 0.07) of SSB compared to healthy weight children. There were significant differences in the presence of OWOB among children by certain demographic characteristics, such as parent/caregiver education level, parent/caregiver marital status, and child birthplace (Table 2).

To explore further the relationship between the behavioral factors of interest and OWOB, we calculated ORs separately for CHamorus and Other Micronesians, the two largest ethnic groups in the study (Table 3). Among CHamoru children, those who were older (6–8 years) were 1.63 times more likely to be affected by OWOB than younger children (2–5 years). The highest prevalence of OWOB was seen among Filipino children (33.8%), followed by Other Micronesian children (28.9%), and CHamoru children (26.0%). OWOB was also more likely to occur among children ages 6–8 years

(30.4%) versus children between the ages of 2–5 years (24.7%). No significant associations were found except that association between OWOB and SSB intake, and OWOB and parent education level.

Table 3. Prevalence and Odds of OWOB among child participants from Guam in the Children's Healthy Living (CHL) Program.

Variable	*n*	% OWOB † (95% CI)	Adjusted OR †† (95% CI)
Overall	822	27.4 (24.3–30.4)	
Child Characteristics			
Sex			
Males	425	27.5 (23.3–31.8)	Referent
Females	397	27.2 (22.8–31.6)	1.001 (0.734–1.366)
Age			
2–5 years	437	24.7 (20.7–28.8)	Referent
6–8 years	385	30.4 (25.8–35.0)	1.337 (0.982–1.821)
Ethnicity			
CHamoru	531	26.0 (22.3–29.7)	Referent
Other Micronesians	204	28.9 (22.7–35.2)	1.186 (0.824–1.706)
Filipino	77	33.8 (23.0–44.6)	1.454 (0.870–2.430)
Other	10	20.0 (−10.2–50.2)	0.693 (0.144–3.329)
Child was breastfed?			
Yes	530	29.4 (25.5–33.3)	1.212 (0.861–1.708)
No	258	25.6 (20.2–30.9)	Referent
Child met sleep standard for his/her age group?			
Yes	327	27.8 (23.0–32.7)	0.994 (0.717–1.378)
No	483	26.7 (22.8–30.7)	Referent
Child met recommendation for screen-time of ≤ 2 h/day?			
Yes	117	29.9 (21.5–38.3)	1.184 (0.757–1.851)
No	578	26.5 (22.9–30.1)	Referent
Child met recommendation for vegetable intake for his/her age group?			
Yes	6	33.3 (−20.9–87.5)	1.342 (0.236–7.649)
No	628	26.9 (23.4–30.4)	Referent
Child met recommendation for fruit intake for his/her age group?			
Yes	264	29.9 (24.4–35.5)	1.274 (0.89–1.823)
No	370	24.9 (20.4–29.3)	Referent
SSB beverage intake ‡ (cups/day)			
(zero intake—referent)	160	21.3 (14.8–27.7)	Referent
Tertile 1 (≤0.42)	54	33.3 (20.4–46.3)	2.064 (1.024–4.160)
Tertile 2 (0.42–1.09)	208	26.4 (20.4–32.5)	1.495 (0.90–2.485)
Tertile 3 (≥1.09)	212	30.2 (24.0–36.4)	1.824 (1.106–3.007)
p-value for trend			0.022
Water beverage intake ‡ (cups/day)			
(zero intake—referent)	26	30.8 (11.8–49.8)	Referent
Tertile 1 (≤0.92)	195	26.2 (19.9–32.4)	0.827 (0.333–2.057)
Tertile 2 (0.92–1.62)	201	28.4 (22.1–34.6)	0.965 (0.388–2.401)
Tertile 3 (≥1.62)	212	25.9 (20.0–31.9)	0.819 (0.330–2.033)
p-value for trend			0.597
Parent/Caregiver/Household Characteristics			
Education Level			
Less than 12th grade (use this as reference)	269	23.1 (18.0–28.1)	Referent
12th grade/GED or higher	553	29.5 (25.7–33.3)	1.415 (1.004–1.994)
Marital Status			
Married	326	31.0 (25.9–36.0)	Referent
Not married	496	25.0 (21.2–28.8)	0.776 (0.564–1.067)
Annual household income			
<$20,000	331	29.3 (24.4–34.2)	Referent
$20,000–$34,999	86	26.7 (17.2–36.3)	0.867 (0.501–1.502)
$35,000–$59,999	89	32.6 (22.7–42.5)	1.121 (0.664–1.892)
$60,000+	69	21.7 (11.8–31.7)	0.600 (0.315–1.143)
Food Insecurity			
Yes	120	26.7 (18.6–34.7)	0.982 (0.627–1.539)
No	599	27.4 (23.8–31.0)	Referent

Table 3. *Cont.*

Variable	n	% OWOB † (95% CI)	Adjusted OR †† (95% CI)
		Receiving any food assistance	
Yes	645	27.1 (23.4–30.6)	1.027 (0.699–1.509)
No	177	28.3 (21.6–35.0)	Referent
		Number of children in household	
1–2 children	197	26.4 (20.2–32.6)	Referent
3–4 children	319	29.8 (24.7–34.8)	1.18 (0.789–1.766)
5 or more children	303	25.7 (20.8–30.7)	0.948 (0.622–1.446)
		Acculturation—Family considers themselves 'integrated' into culture	
Yes	545	27.3 (23.6–31.1)	1.162 (0.747–1.81)
No	134	24.6 (17.2–32.0)	Referent

† 'Underweight' children excluded from analysis, †† Adjusted for clustering by community, age, sex, and ethnicity, ‡ Consumption in cups/day, weighted for weekday/weekend days and adjusted for within person variance.

3.3. Nutrition Factors

The majority of child participants (80.4%) were receiving some sort of food assistance, including USDA Supplemental Nutrition Assistance Program (SNAP) (67.8%), USDA Supplemental Nutrition Assistance Program for Women, Infants, and Children (WIC) (31.8%), free or reduced school lunch/breakfast (28.8%), and/or assistance from a local food bank (11.7%). Food insecurity was also prevalent as 51.5% of participants reported that food money ran out at the end of the month either always/most times (16.8%) or sometimes (34.7%). Significantly more ($p < 0.001$) Other Micronesian child participants (74.9%) reported that food money ran out at least sometimes compared to CHamoru (42.8%), Filipino (53.7%) and Other (50%) children.

As for OWOB risk factors and CHL related nutrition behaviors, majority of children did not meet recommendations for fruit (58.7%) and vegetable (99.1%) intake and consumed SSB (73.7%). Fruit and vegetable intake did not differ significantly by ethnicity (Table 1) or by the presence of OWOB (Table 2). Mean intake of vegetables was low (0.61 c/d) and only 6 children surveyed (0.09%) consumed the recommended amount of vegetables daily, which equates to ≥1 cup equivalent for children 2 years old and ≥1.5 cup equivalent for children 3–8 years old [34–36]. Mean intake of fruits was somewhat better (0.88 c/d) and more children (41.3%) reported consuming the recommended amount of fruits daily, which equates to ≥1.5 cup equivalent for children 2–8 years old [34].

When asked if the child participant was ever breastfed as a baby, about two-thirds (67%) of all parents/caregivers responded yes. Only 13.1% of children were exclusively breastfed (not shown in table), while 54.2% of children surveyed were fed both breastmilk and infant formula as an infant. CHamoru children (21.32) reported being significantly less likely to be ever breastfed compared to Other Micronesian children (37.2%). Of those children who were ever breastfed, Other Micronesian children were weaned at a significantly older age (12.48 m) compared to children from other ethnic groups. Breastfeeding during infancy, whether exclusive or mixed with infant formula feeding did not differ by the presence of OWOB. Age at weaning also did not differ by presence of OWOB. Among those who were exclusively breastfed, mean age at weaning was significantly higher compared to mixed fed infants (19.27 ± 1.19 m versus 7.56 ± 0.04 m). Risk of OWOB increased significantly with SSB intake. The relationship between presence of OWOB and increasing SSB intake was not monotonic, the ORs (95% CI) for SSB intake for the tertile groups for consumers compared to those with zero intake of SSB were 2.06 (1.02–4.16), 1.50 (0.90–2.48), and 1.82 (1.11–3.01). Only 25% of children surveyed consumed the recommended amount of "zero intake" of SSB [37], and one-third of child participants consumed at least 1.1 cups of SSB per day. Correlation analysis showed that SSB intake was positively and significantly associated with BMI and waist circumference. Among CHamoru children, the relationship between SSB intake and body size was stronger, as SSB intake among CHamoru children was positively and significantly associated with BMI ($r = 0.18$, $p = 0.0002$), waist circumference ($r = 0.16$, $p = 0.0007$), and BMI z-score ($r = 0.11$, $p = 0.023$). In Table 3, although SSB intake was not significantly associated with OWOB for Other Micronesian children, it was significant for CHamoru children. The relationship again was not monotonic, the ORs (95% CI) for SSB intake for the tertile groups of consumers compared to those with zero intake of SSB were 3.15 (1.1–9.08), 2.84 (1.28–6.30) and 3.19 (1.46–6.95).

3.4. Sleep and Screen-Time

Less than half of all children surveyed (40.4%) met the sleep duration recommendations [20]; those recommendations being at least 8–11 h/day for children under the age of 5 years, and 8–10 h per day for children 5 years and older. Sleep duration did not differ by the presence of OWOB, yet we observed TCSQ sleep quality scores (Table 2) were significantly lower ($p = 0.0421$) among children affected by OWOB compared to children with healthy weight (5.59 ± 0.34 versus 6.55 ± 0.26, respectively), meaning that children with OWOB were statistically more likely to suffer from sleep disturbances. Only 30.58% of Other Micronesian children met sleep recommendations (Table 1), which was significantly ($p = 0.014$) less than children from other ethnic groups. Other Micronesian children reported TCSQ sleep quality scores that were lower ($p = 0.056$) compared to children from the other ethnic groups.

The recommended daily screen-time for children is less than 2 h per day [38]. Only one sixth of the children surveyed (16.9%) met this recommendation and meeting screen-time recommendations did not differ between healthy weight children and children affected by OWOB. Average screen-time was slightly more than 5 h per day. When comparisons were made across four ethnic groups, there was a significant difference ($p = 0.007$) in the proportion of children that met the screen-time recommendation: CHamorus (16.7%), Other Micronesian (22.5%), Filipinos (4.6%), and Other (0%). There was also a significant difference in the average daily screen-time among the ethnic groups: CHamorus (5.13 h), Other Micronesians (5.45 h), Filipinos (6.24 h), and Other (3.59 h) (Table 1).

3.5. Acculturation

The majority of study participants (80%) considered their cultural affiliation as integrated, meaning a bicultural orientation where the respondent retains their ethnic cultural identity at the same time moving to join the dominant society (i.e., the US) [22,39]. About 15% of both CHamorus and Other Micronesians considered their cultural affiliation traditional, where the respondent retains their ethnic identity and does not recognize or identify with cultural characteristics of the US [22,39]. The Other Micronesians (6.1%) were most likely of all ethnic groups represented in this study to report having marginalized cultural affiliation, meaning the respondent does not maintain his/her ethnic cultural characteristics and excludes or withdraws him/herself from the dominant society (i.e., the U.S.) [22,39]. Acculturation did not differ by the presence of OWOB (Table 2). However, we observed that among Other Micronesians, children from families who considered their cultural affiliation as integrated into the culture were 2.05 times more likely to be affected by OWOB (CI 0.81–5.20) (Table 3).

4. Discussion

Pacific Islanders were one of the fastest growing racial/ethnic groups in the US in 2000 to 2010 [40], but little is known about OWOB for young children (under 11 year) in the Pacific region [41]. The current prevalence of OWOB in the US is 25% among children between 2–5 years and 32.8% among children between 6–8 years [42]. Findings in this current study on Guam were consistent with previous reports [43] and similar to the US. Unlike previous reports, this study revealed ethnic differences in OWOB presence among children in Guam. Filipino and Other Micronesian had the highest OWOB (33%) and obesity (18%) prevalence compared to other children in Guam.

Some recent studies have shown that obesity among various Pacific Islander groups, such as Samoans, may be linked to specific genes influencing adiposity [40,41,44]; and Pacific Islanders of Polynesian, Micronesian, and Melanesian origin may all carry certain alleles associated with higher body weight, BMI, and risk of obesity [41,45]. Waist circumference-to-height ratio (WHR) and WC have been used as markers of body adiposity in adults and, in children and adolescents (8–18 years), WHR was determined to be better at predicting adiposity [46–48]. One third of this study's participants

(33.8%) were observed to have both, abdominal obesity and OWOB. On the other hand, healthy weight children did not have abdominal obesity (0%). This aligns with other studies that found adiposity indicators, like WC, were associated with being overweight [47]. This is alarming as the location and distribution of body fat are associated with cardiovascular and other disease risks that is likely to continue into adulthood [49–51].

Given the steady rise in obesity over the past few decades on a global scale, environmental (macro and micro) factors promoting obesity are a more likely predominant explanation for racial/ethnic disparities in childhood obesity [52], such as the increase in obesity seen on Guam and other islands in the Pacific. A majority of children in this study exhibited several behaviors that are obesity risk factors such as low intake of fruits and vegetables, high intake of SSB, low sleep duration, and high amounts of sedentary screen-time [52].

From the micro-environment of children, which includes their families and households, in this study, the majority of child participants came from households where their parent/caregivers were unmarried (60.7%) and with at least three or more children (76.2%). Those two factors, compounded by the fact that most of the parents in this study also reported low annual incomes, can lead to an unfavorable home environment. Research shows that family and home environments, whether directly or indirectly, may contribute to the development of child OWOB [53–55], possibly through maternal depression and stress. Further study and more specific questions regarding parent/caregiver psychological health is needed to determine impact of family environment on the presence of OWOB among children in Guam.

Surprisingly, 59.65% of the children surveyed did not meet the recommended sleep duration for their age. Research indicates that short sleep duration puts children at risk for obesity and other metabolic, cardiovascular, and behavior disorders [56–58]. This study did not find sleep duration to differ significantly between children with OWOB and those with healthy weight, possibly due to misinterpretation of the question on sleep duration. Given some of the very low reported levels of sleep hours per day for some of the children and limited English comprehension of the islander parents/caregivers, it is possible that nap times during the day may have been the reported time, rather than sleep over the 24-h period. Future studies should separate questions for nap time sleep from night sleep in determining USAP children's sleep duration and include more qualitative non-subjective measurements for sleep duration. In terms of sleep quality, children affected by OWOB in this study were statistically more likely to suffer from sleep disturbances. This aligns with the research linking poor sleep quality with OWOB and an increased risk for cognitive and behavioral problems [56–58]. Research also links reduced sleep quality with high SSB intake, and in bed screen-time [59].

The proportion of children exceeding screen-time recommendation in this study (83%) was comparable to the 87% reported among a prospective birth cohort of children born in New York led by researchers from the NIH Eunice Kennedy Shriver National Institute of Child Health and Human Development [60]; however, the birth cohort included children below two years of age, which is an age group not represented in the Guam study. Additionally, while screen-time increased with preschool age in the birth cohort, the total hours decreased to below the recommended two hours by 7–8 years old possibly due to school activities [60].

Screen-time has been shown to be associated with other behaviors, especially sleep. Twenge and colleagues [61] found an inverse association, increased screen-time and reduced sleep duration among a population-based sample of 0–17 year-olds in the United States [61]. In the current study, the order of screen-time, from highest to lowest duration, by ethnic group was Filipino (6.24 h), Other Micronesians (5.45 h), CHamorus (5.13 h), and Other (3.59 h). Interestingly, this order was reversed with the TCSQ sleep quality score, where Filipinos reported the highest quality sleep (5.23), and Others reported the lowest quality (8.0), but the pattern was not the same with sleep duration. Researchers are beginning to better understand the impact of screen-time on sleep behaviors. For example, Guerrero and colleagues [62] found a relationship between increased screen-time and increased social problems (e.g., rule-breaking, social problems, aggressive behavior, and thought problems), and the relationship was mediated by sleep duration (every hour increase in sleep = 8.8% to 16.6% decrease in problem behaviors) among 9–10 year-old in the Adolescent Brain Cognitive Development study [63]. Behavioral problems, although complex, are real issues plaguing children and should be considered when building wellness models for healthy families and healthy communities. Further studies on screen-time among children in Guam are warranted.

Childhood behavioral problems have been linked to racial socialization and cultural resilience [64]. Similarly, cultural affiliation, or low acculturation (i.e., traditional), is associated with lower rates of obesity and sedentary behaviors in children from migrant populations [39]. Although CHamorus in this study are not likely migrants, the long history of colonization in Guam lends to multidimensional acculturation for CHamorus and Guamanians alike in the presence of the colonial society (i.e., the US). This considered, CHamoru children had the highest proportion of parents identifying as traditional and the lowest rates of obesity compared to other ethnic groups in this study. Additionally, Filipino children identified most as integrated had the highest average screen-time (hr/d) compared to other ethnic groups. These findings align with previous studies that have found traditional or low acculturation to be protective against obesity and related risk factors [39,65,66]. A greater acculturation (i.e., assimilation) has also shown to be a predictor of lower fruit and vegetable intake among adult populations [67,68]. Therefore, obesity interventions or health programs in Guam should include cultural values and practices to maintain or reinforce healthy cultural behaviors unique to each and shared across ethnic group(s).

Both fruit and vegetable consumption among child participants in this study were low and failed to meet the recommendations set forth by the USDA Dietary Guidelines [34]. Little is known about the food intake, particularly fruits and vegetables, of children on Guam. Pobocik and colleagues [69,70] studied the food intake of over 1000 elementary school-aged children on Guam and reported fruit and vegetable consumption was well below the recommended intake levels [69]. Leon Guerrero and Workman [71] studied health behaviors of adolescents on Guam and reported that only 24.7% of those surveyed reported consumption at least one serving of fruit and/or vegetable, and none reported consuming the recommendations for fruit and vegetable intake set forth by the Dietary Guidelines. Children on Guam are not unlike children from the US mainland. A recent study looking at diet quality by BMI category of US children found that in general, all children's diets in the United States were poor and in need of improvement, regardless of BMI status, age, sex, race/ethnicity, and poverty-to-income ratio classification [72].

CHamorus and Filipinos were less likely to exclusively breastfeed and tended to breastfeed for shorter durations, compared to other Micronesians and Other ethnic groups; mixed feeding was common in all ethnic groups and associated with earlier weaning as would be expected. No relationship of feeding method with overweight and obesity was detected. Breastfeeding is the biologic norm, important for infant nutrition and healthy growth, and protective for child obesity [73–75], although not demonstrated here. Likely other socio-economic (e.g., income) and behavioral factors (e.g., SSB intake) not controlled in this comparison confound the association in this study.

Several studies have shown an association between SSB intake and adverse health outcomes in children, particularly overweight, obesity, unhealthy weight gain, and central adiposity [76–78]. Other longitudinal data indicated that children consuming as little as one SSB serving per day were 55% more likely to be OWOB compared to children with limited SSB consumption [79]. Wojcicki and colleagues looked at the effect of SSB consumption on leukocyte telomere length in preschool children [80]. After adjusting for age sex, and BMI, SSB intake among the preschool children was significantly related to shorter leukocyte length. Shorter telomere length has been associated with a number of adverse health outcomes such as type 2 diabetes, stroke, and myocardial infarction because shortened telomeres start the inflammatory cascade through increased production of cytokines, thus adversely impacting cellular health [80]. SSB consumption during early childhood may not lead immediately to OWOB, as there may be an age effect. It may take a number of years of SSB consumption before the development of OWOB or metabolic changes associated with obesity [77,80–82]. SSB intake may also be a marker of a food and beverage intake pattern and other lifestyle factors that are associated with obesity.

High intake of SSB is common on Guam, and SSBs are readily available in food stores. In a previous study looking at dietary intake of CHamoru and Filipino adults living on Guam, Leon Guerrero and colleagues [11] found that CHamoru adults reported consuming between 7–9% of food energy from SSBs (7% for women and 9% for men). In this same study [11], SSBs were the second largest contributor to energy intake for CHamoru adults; and third largest contributor to energy intake for Filipino adults.

Like most other islands in the Pacific, Guam relies heavily on imported processed foods. A 2013 survey of processed foods available in the Pacific Islands [83] showed that Guam recorded the highest number of available processed food products compared to the other Pacific islands surveyed, with over 2100 products available to Guam consumers. High intake of SSBs is not only a problem for children affected by OWOB. The child participants surveyed on Guam, whether or not they were affected by OWOB, consumed a high amount of SSBs, putting them at risk for developing adverse cardiometabolic outcomes as they grow older.

There were some limitations to this study. The small sample size of Other Micronesian and especially Filipino children made ethnic group comparisons difficult. Some parents/caregivers, Other Micronesians in particular, spoke English as a second language and had limited English comprehension; making it difficult to comprehend and respond to survey tools. This may have affected accuracy of results. Generalizations are limited due to non-randomized cluster sampling. However, recruitment of children at the community-based settings in Guam communities was designed to ensure appropriate representation by age, sex, ethnicity, and geographic location. Since this study reports cross-sectional data, causal association of OWOB with behavioral or demographic factors cannot be conclusively inferred; longitudinal examination is needed to confirm causality. Despite the limitations, we were able to recruit and assess a large sample of children (n = 865) from several communities across the island that were representative of the major ethnic groups on Guam. Anthropometric measurements of children surveyed provided a reliable assessment of OWOB status among children on Guam.

In conclusion, the child participants surveyed on Guam, whether or not they are currently affected by OWOB, are at a high risk for developing OWOB in adulthood, as well as other chronic diseases. Specifically, for OWOB risk factors and CHL behaviors, the majority of children surveyed did not meet recommendations for: sleep duration (59.6%), sedentary screen-time (83.11%), or fruit (58.7%) and vegetable (99.1%) intake and consumed SSB (73.7%). The study found children affected by OWOB in this study, were statistically more likely ($p = 0.042$) to suffer from sleep disturbances, and consumed marginally higher amounts (p value = 0.07) of SSB compared to children with healthy weight. The study identified indicators of potentially stressful home situations among participant families that include: high prevalence of the child participants being cared for by a single parent (60.7%), families with three or more children (76.2%), and high prevalence of some level of food insecurity (59.6%) among participant families. These family stressors may also contribute to OWOB among children on Guam. With respect to OWOB prevention guidance, the study found evidence supporting previous studies' findings that traditional or low acculturation to be protective against obesity [39,59,60]. Healthy cultural behaviors, both unique to and shared across ethnic group(s), should be incorporated in future obesity interventions by highlighting healthy cultural values, practices and traditional foods. The obesogenic factors identified in the children in this study provide a basis for health promotion and obesity prevention guidance for children in Guam.

Author Contributions: R.T.L.G. led study concept, acquisition, analysis, and interpretation of data, and writing of manuscript; oversaw and had primary responsibility for final manuscript. L.R.B. assisted in study concept, interpretation of data, and writing of manuscript. M.P.H.-U. assisted in acquisition of data, and providing critical review of manuscript. M.A. assisted in acquisition and entry of data and providing critical review of manuscript. T.F.A. assisted in acquisition, entry and analysis of data, and writing of manuscript. Y.C.P. assisted in acquisition, entry and analysis of data, and writing of manuscript. L.R.W. participated in overall study design, contributed to statistical analysis, interpreted data, and writing of manuscript. R.N. initially assisted in the study concept, participated in design, interpreted data, and writing of manuscript. All authors provided critical review of the manuscript and gave final approval. All authors have read and agreed to the published version of the manuscript.

Acknowledgments: We would like to thank the parents and children who participated in the Children's Healthy Living Program (CHL), as well as our many community partners who assisted.

References

1. Ogden, C.L.; Carroll, M.D.; Kit, B.K.; Flegal, K.M. Prevalence of childhood and adult obesity in the United States, 2011–2012. *JAMA* **2014**, *311*, 806–814. [CrossRef] [PubMed]
2. Ogden, C.L.; Carroll, M.D.; Fryar, C.D.; Flegal, K.M. Prevalence of Obesity among Adults and Youth: United States, 2011–2014. *NCHS Data Brief* **2015**, *219*, 1–8.
3. Yang, L.; Colditz, G.A. Prevalence of Overweight and Obesity in the United States, 2007–2012. *JAMA Intern. Med.* **2015**, *175*, 1412–1413. [CrossRef] [PubMed]
4. Afshin, A.; Forouzanfar, M.H.; Reitsma, M.B.; Sur, P.; Estep, K.; Lee, A.; Marczak, L.; Mokdad, A.H.; Moradi-Lakeh, M.; Naghavi, M.; et al. Health Effects of Overweight and Obesity in 195 Countries over 25 Years. *N. Engl. J. Med.* **2017**, *377*, 13–27. [CrossRef]
5. Ng, M.; Fleming, T.; Robinson, M.; Thomson, B.; Graetz, N.; Margano, C.; Mullany, C.E.; Biryukov, S.; Abbafati, C.; Abera, F.S.; et al. Global, regional, and national prevalence of overweight and obesity in children and adults during 1980–2013: A systematic analysis for the Global Burden of Disease Study 2013. *Lancet* **2014**, *384*, 766–781. [CrossRef]
6. Novotny, R.; Fialkowski, M.K.; Li, F.; Paulino, Y.S.N.; Vargo, D.; Jim, R.; Coleman, P.; Bersamin, A.; Nigg, C.R.; Leon Guerrero, R.T.; et al. Systematic review of prevalence of young child overweight and obesity in the United States Affiliated Pacific region compared to the 48 contiguous states: A the Children's Health Living Program. *Am. J. Pub. Health* **2015**. [CrossRef]
7. Underwood, J. The native origins of the neo-Chamorros of the Mariana Islands. *Micronesia* **1976**, *12*, 203–209.
8. Vilar, M.G.; Chan, C.W.; Santos, D.R.; Lynch, D.; Spathis, R.; Garruto, R.M.; Lum, J.K. The origins and genetic distinctiveness of the Chamorros of the Marianas Islands: An mtDNA perspective. *Am. J. Hum. Biol.* **2013**, *25*, 116–122. [CrossRef]
9. Central Intelligence Agency: The World Factbook. Available online: https://www.cia.gov/library/publications/the-world-factbook/geos/gq.html (accessed on 30 June 2020).
10. *Asian and Pacific Islander American Health Forum Health Briefs: Chamorros in the United States*. Asian and Pacific Islander American Health Forum. 2006. Available online: https://www.apiahf.org/wp-content/uploads/2011/02/APIAHF_Healthbrief08j_2006-1.pdf (accessed on 25 June 2020).
11. Guerrero, R.T.L.; Paulino, Y.C.; Novotny, R.; Murphy, S.P. Diet and obesity among Chamorro and Filipino adults on Guam. *Asia Pac. J. Clin. Nutr.* **2008**, *17*, 216–222.
12. Hankin, J.; Reed, D.; Labarthe, D.; Nichaman, M.; Stallones, R. Dietary and Disease Patterns among Micronesians. *Am. J. Clin. Nutr.* **1970**, *23*, 346–357. [CrossRef]
13. Pollock, N. Food habits in Guam over 500 years. *Pac. Viewp.* **1986**, *27*, 120–143. [CrossRef]
14. Uncangco, A.; Badowski, G.; David, A.; Ehlert, M.; Haddock, R.; Paulino, Y. *First Guam BRFSS Report 2007–2010*; Guam Department of Public Health & Social Services: Mangilao, Guam, USA, 2012.
15. Singh, A.S.; Mulder, C.; Twisk, J.W.; van Mechelen, W.; Chinapaw, M.J. Tracking of childhood overweight into adulthood: A systematic review of the literature. *Obes. Rev.* **2008**, *9*, 474–488. [CrossRef] [PubMed]
16. Barker, D.J.; Osmond, C.; Forsen, T.J.; Kajantie, E.; Eriksson, J.G. Trajectories of growth among children who have coronary events as adults. *N. Engl. J. Med.* **2005**, *353*, 1802–1809. [CrossRef] [PubMed]
17. Wilken, L.R.; Novotny, R.; Fialkowski, M.K.; Boushey, C.J.; Nigg, C.; Paulino, Y.; Leon Guerrero, R.; Bersamin, A.; Vargo, D.; Kim, J.; et al. Children's Healthy Living (CHL) Program for remote underserved minority populations in the Pacific region: Rationale and design of a community randomized trial to prevent early childhood obesity. *BMC Pub. Health* **2013**, *13*, 944. [CrossRef] [PubMed]

18. Novotny, R.; Fialkowski, M.K.; Areta, A.A.; Bersamin, A.; Braun, K.; DeBaryshe, B.; Deenik, J.; Dunn, M.; Hollyer, J.; Kim, J.; et al. The Pacific Way to Child Wellness: The Children's Healthy Living Program for Remote Underserved Minority Populations of the Pacific Region (CHL). *Hawaii J. Med. Pub. Health* **2013**, *72*, 406–408.
19. McGreavey, J.A.; Donnan, P.T.; Pagliari, H.C.; Sullivan, F.M. The tayside children's sleep questionnaire: A simple tool to evaluate sleep problems in young children. *Child Care Health Dev.* **2005**, *31*, 539–544. [CrossRef]
20. Hirshkowitz, M.; Whiton, K.; Albert, S.M.; Alessi, C.; Bruni, O.; DonCarlos, L.; Hazen, N.; Herman, J.; Katz, E.S.; Kheirandish-Gozal, L.; et al. National Sleep Foundation's sleep time duration recommendations: Methodology and results summary. *Sleep Health* **2015**, *1*, 40–43. [CrossRef]
21. Coleman-Jensen, A.; Gregory, C.; Singh, A. *Household Food Security in the United States in 2013*; US Department of Agriculture, Economic Research Service, Ed.; USDA Economic Research Service: Washington, DC, USA, 2014.
22. Kaholokula, J.K.; Iwane, M.K.; Nacapoy, A.H. Effects of perceived racism and acculturation on hypertension in Native Hawaiians. *Hawaii Med. J.* **2010**, *69*, 11–15.
23. Li, F.; Wilkens, L.R.; Novotny, R.; Fialkowski, M.; Paulino, Y.C.; Nelson, R.; Bersamin, A.; Martin, U.; Deenik, J.; Boushey, C. Anthropometric Measurement Standardization in the US-Affiliated Pacific: Report from the Children's Healthy Living Program. *Am. J. Hum. Biol.* **2016**, *28*, 364–371. [CrossRef]
24. Cook, S.; Auinger, P.; Huang, T.T. Growth curves for cardio-metabolic risk factors in children and adolescents. *J. Pediatr.* **2009**, *155*, e15–e26. [CrossRef]
25. Barlow, S. Expert committee recommendations regarding the prevention, assessment, and treatment of child and adolescent overweight and obesity: Summary report. *Pediatrics* **2007**, *120* (Suppl. 4), S164–S192. [CrossRef] [PubMed]
26. *Centers for Disease Control and Prevention A SAS Program for the 2000 CDC Growth Charts (Ages 0 to <20 Years)*; Centers for Disease Control and Prevention; 2014. Available online: https://www.cdc.gov/nccdphp/dnpao/growthcharts/resources/sas.htm (accessed on 6 April 2020).
27. Zimmet, P.; Alberti, K.G.; Kaufman, F.; Tajima, N.; Silink, M.; Arslanian, S.; Wong, G.; Bennett, P.; Shaw, J.; Caprio, S.; et al. The metabolic syndrome in children and adolescents—An IDF consensus report. *Pediatr. Diabetes* **2007**, *8*, 299–306. [CrossRef] [PubMed]
28. Novotny, R.; Nigg, C.; McGlone, K.; Renda, G.; Jung, N.; Matsunaga, M.; Karanja, N. Pacific tracker 2—Expert system (PacTrac2-ES) behavioural assessment and intervention tool for the pacific kids DASH for health (PacDASH) study. *Food Chem.* **2013**, *140*, 471–477. [CrossRef] [PubMed]
29. Martin, C.L.; Murphy, S.P.; Leon Guerrero, R.T.; Davison, N.; Jung, Y.O.; Novotny, R. The Pacific Tracker (PacTrac): Development of a dietary assessment instrument for the Pacific. *J. Food Compost. Anal.* **2008**, *21*, S103–S108. [CrossRef] [PubMed]
30. Murphy, S.; Blitz, C.; Novotny, R. Pacific tracker (PacTrac): An interactive dietary assessment program at the CRCH website. *Hawaii Med. J.* **2006**, *65*, 175–178. [PubMed]
31. Rolland-Cachera, M.F.; Akrout, M.; Peneau, S. Nutrient Intakes in Early Life and Risk of Obesity. *Int. J. Environ. Res. Public Health* **2016**, *13*, 564. [CrossRef]
32. Weihrauch-Blüher, S.; Wiegand, S. Risk Factors and Implications of Childhood Obesity. *Curr. Obes. Rep.* **2018**, *7*, 254–259. [CrossRef]
33. 2015 Poverty Guidelines. Office of the Assistant Secretary for Planning and Evaluation. US Department of Public Health and Social Services. Available online: https://aspe.hhs.gov/2015-poverty-guidelines (accessed on 9 July 2020).
34. U.S. Department of Health and Human Services and U.S. Department of Agriculture. *2015–2020 Dietary Guidelines for Americans*, 8th ed.; December 2015. Available online: http://health.gov/dietaryguidelines/2015/guidelines/ (accessed on 22 April 2020).
35. Bowman, S.; Friday, J.; Moshfegh, A. *MyPyramid Equivalents Database, 2.0 for USDA Survey Foods, 2003–2004 [Online]*; Food Surveys Research Group, Beltsville Human Nutrition Research Center, Agricultural Research Service, U.S., Ed.; Department of Agriculture: Beltsville, MD, USA, 2008.
36. Friday, J.; Bowman, S. *MyPyramid Equivalents Database for USDA Survey Food Codes, 1994–2002 Version 1.0. [Online]*; USDA, Agricultural Research Service, Beltsville Human Nutrition Research Center, Ed.; Community Nutrition Research Group: Beltsville, MD, USA, 2006.
37. Popkin, B.M.; Armstrong, L.E.; Bray, G.M.; Caballero, B.; Frei, B.; Willett, W.C. A new proposed guidance system for beverage consumption in the United States. *Am. J. Clin. Nutr.* **2006**, *83*, 529–542. [CrossRef]

38. American Academy of Pediatrics. Children, adolescents, and television. *Pediatrics* **2001**, *107*, 423–426. [CrossRef]
39. Renzaho, A.M.; Swinburn, B.; Burns, C. Maintenance of traditional cultural orientation is associated with lower rates of obesity and sedentary behaviours among African migrant children to Australia. *Int. J. Obes.* **2008**, *32*, 594–600. [CrossRef]
40. Hixson, L.; Hepler, B.B.; Kim, M.O. *The Native Hawaiian and other Pacific Islander Population: 2010*; US Census Bureau, Ed.; US Census Bureau: Washington, DC, USA, 2012.
41. Wate, J. Chapter 2: The Obesity Pandemic in the Pacific. In *Wealthy but Unhealthy: Overweight and Obesity in Asia and the Pacific: Trends, Costs, and Policies for Better Health*; Helble, M., Sato, A., Eds.; Asian Development Bank Institute: Tokyo, Japan, 2018.
42. Skinner, A.C.; Ravanbakht, S.N.; Skelton, J.A.; Perrin, E.M.; Armstrong, S.C. Prevalence of obesity and severe obesity in US children, 1999–2016. *Pediatrics* **2018**. [CrossRef] [PubMed]
43. Paulino, Y.C.; Guerrero, R.T.; Uncangco, A.A.; Rosadino, M.G.; Quinene, J.C.; Natividad, Z.N. Overweight and obesity prevalence among public school children in Guam. *J. Health Care Poor Underserved* **2015**, *26* (Suppl. 2), 53–62. [CrossRef] [PubMed]
44. Minster, R.L.; Hawley, N.L.; Su, C.T.; Sun, G.; Kershaw, E.E.; Cheng, H.; Buhule, O.D.; Lin, J.; Reupena, M.S.; Viali, S.; et al. A thrifty variant in CREBRF strongly influences body mass index in Samoans. *Nat. Genet.* **2016**, *48*, 1049–1054. [CrossRef] [PubMed]
45. Furusawa, T.; Naka, I.; Yamauchi, T.; Natsuhara, K.; Kimura, R.; Nakazawa, M.; Ishida, T.; Inaoka, T.; Matsumura, Y.; Ataka, Y.; et al. The Q223R polymorphism in LEPR is associated with obesity in Pacific Islanders. *Hum. Genet.* **2010**, *127*, 287–294. [CrossRef]
46. Brambilla, P.; Bedogni, G.; Heo, M.; Pietrobelli, A. Waist circumference-to-height ratio predicts adiposity better than body mass index in children and adolescents. *Int. J. Obes.* **2013**, *37*, 943–946. [CrossRef]
47. Vieira, S.A.; Ribeiro, A.Q.; Hermsdorff, H.H.M.; Pereira, P.F.; Priore, S.E.; Franceschini, S. Waist-to-height ratio index or the prediction of overweight in children. *Rev. Paul. Pediatr.* **2018**, *36*, 7.
48. Rakić, R.; Pavlica, T.; Bjelanović, J.; Vasiljević, P. Predictive ability of waist-to-hip-ratio and waist-to-height-ratio in relation to overweight/obesity in adolescents from Vojvodina (the Republic of Serbia) predictive ability of waist-to-hip-ratio and waist-to-height-ratio: Predictive Ability of Waist-to-Hip-Ratio and Waist-to-Height-Ratio. *Prog. Nutr.* **2019**, *24*, 992–998.
49. Staiano, A.E.; Gupta, A.K.; Katzmarzyk, P.T. Cardiometabolic risk factors and fat distribution in children and adolescents. *J. Pediatr.* **2014**, *164*, 560–565. [CrossRef]
50. Freedman, D.S.; Dietz, W.H.; Srinivasan, S.R.; Berenson, G.S. The relation of overweight to cardiovascular risk factors among children and adolescents: The Bogalusa Heart Study. *Pediatrics* **1999**, *103 Pt 1*, 1175–1182. [CrossRef]
51. Kahn, H.S.; Imperatore, G.; Cheng, Y.J. A population-based comparison of BMI percentiles and waist-to-height ratio for identifying cardiovascular risk in youth. *J. Pediatr.* **2005**, *146*, 482–488. [CrossRef]
52. Dixon, B.; Peña, M.M.; Taveras, E.M. Lifecourse approach to racial/ethnic disparities in childhood obesity. *Adv. Nutr.* **2012**, *3*, 73–82. [CrossRef] [PubMed]
53. Epstein, L.H.; Myers, M.D.; Anderson, K. The association of maternal psychopathology and family socioeconomic status with psychological problems in obese children. *Obes. Res.* **1996**, *4*, 65–74. [CrossRef] [PubMed]
54. Davis, M.; Young, L.; Davis, S.P.; Moll, G. Parental depression, family functioning and obesity among African American children. *J. Cult. Divers.* **2008**, *15*, 61–65. [PubMed]
55. McConley, R.L.; Mrug, S.; Gilliland, M.J.; Lowry, R.; Elliott, M.N.; Schuster, M.A.; Bogart, L.M.; Franzini, L.; Escobar-Chaves, S.L.; Franklin, F.A. Mediators of maternal depression and family structure on child BMI: Parenting quality and risk factors for child overweight. *Obesity* **2011**, *19*, 345–352. [CrossRef]
56. Pacheco, S.R.; Miranda, A.M.; Coelho, R.; Monteiro, A.C.; Braganca, G.; Loureiro, H.C. Overweight in youth and sleep quality: Is there a link? *Arch. Endocrinol. Metab.* **2017**. [CrossRef]
57. Navarro-Solera, M.; Carrasco-Luna, J.; Pin-Arboledas, G.; Gonzalez-Carrascosa, R.; Soriano, J.M.; Codoner-Franch, P. Short Sleep Duration Is Related to Emerging Cardiovascular Risk Factors in Obese Children. *J. Pediatr. Gastroenterol. Nutr.* **2015**, *61*, 571–576. [CrossRef]

58. Sakamoto, N.; Gozal, D.; Smith, D.L.; Yang, L.; Morimoto, N.; Wada, H.; Maruyama, K.; Ikeda, A.; Suzuki, Y.; Nakayama, M.; et al. Sleep duration, snoring prevalence, obesity, and behavioral problems in a large cohort of primary school students in Japan. *Sleep* **2017**, *40*. [CrossRef]
59. Morrissey, B.; Allender, S.; Strugnell, C. Dietary and activity factors influence poor sleep and the sleep-obesity nexus among children. *Int. J. Environ. Res. Public Health* **2019**, *16*, 1778. [CrossRef]
60. Trinh, M.H.; Sundaram, R.; Robinson, S.L.; Lin, T.C.; Bell, E.M.; Ghassabian, A.; Yeung, E.H. Association of trajectory and covariates of children's screen media time. *JAMA Pediatr.* **2019**, *174*, 71–78. [CrossRef]
61. Twenge, J.M.; Hisler, G.C.; Krizan, Z. Associations between screen time and sleep duration are primarily driven by portable electronic devices: Evidence from a population-based study of U.S. children ages 0–17. *Sleep Med.* **2019**, *56*, 211–218. [CrossRef]
62. Guerrero, M.D.; Barnes, J.D.; Chaput, J.P.; Tremblay, M.S. Screen time and problem behaviors in children: Exploring the mediating role of sleep duration. *Int. J. Behav. Nutr. Phys. Act.* **2019**, *16*, 105. [CrossRef] [PubMed]
63. Aflague, T.; Boushey, C.; Leon Guerrero, R.; Ahmad, Z.; Kerr, D.; Delp, E. Feasibility and use of the mobile food record for capturing eating occasions among children ages 3–10 years in Guam. *Nutrients* **2015**, *7*, 4403–4415. [CrossRef] [PubMed]
64. Burt, C.H.; Simons, R.L.; Gibbons, F.X. Racial discrimination, ethnic-racial socialization, and crime: A micro-sociological model of risk and resilience. *Am. Sociol. Rev.* **2012**, *77*, 648–677. [CrossRef] [PubMed]
65. Delavari, M.; Sønderlund, A.L.; Swinburn, B.; Mellor, D.; Renzaho, A. Acculturation and obesity among migrant populations in high income countries—A systematic review. *BMC Public Health* **2013**, *13*, 458. [CrossRef] [PubMed]
66. Lind, C.; Mirchandani, G.G.; Castrucci, B.C.; Chávez, N.; Handler, A.; Hoelscher, D.M. The effects of acculturation on healthy lifestyle characteristics among Hispanic fourth-grade children in Texas public schools, 2004–2005. *J. School Health* **2012**, *82*, 166–174. [CrossRef] [PubMed]
67. Bolstad, A.L.; Bungum, T. Diet, acculturation, and BMI in Hispanics living in southern Nevada. *Am. J. Health Behav.* **2013**, *37*, 218–226. [CrossRef]
68. Lee, S.; Sobal, J.; Frongillo, E. Acculturation, food consumption, and diet-related factors among Korean Americans. *J. Nutr. Educ.* **1999**, *31*, 321–330. [CrossRef]
69. Pobocik, R.S.; Richer, J.J.; Hentges, D.L. Food sources of macronutrients in the diets of fifth grade children on Guam. *Asian Am. Pac. Isl. J. Health* **1999**, *7*, 25–37.
70. Pobocik, R.S.; Richer, J.J. Estimated intake and food sources of vitamin, A.; folate, vitamin, C.; vitamin, E.; calcium, iron, and zinc for Guamanian children aged 9 to 12. *Pac. Health Dialog* **2002**, *9*, 193–202.
71. LeonGuerrero, R.T.; Workman, R.L. Physical activity and nutritional status of adolescents on Guam. *Pac. Health Dialog* **2002**, *9*, 177–185.
72. Thomson, J.L.; Landry, A.S.; Tussing-Humphreys, L.M.; Goodman, M.H. Diet quality of children in the United States by body mass index and sociodemographic characteristics. *Obes. Sci. Pract.* **2020**, *6*, 84–98. [CrossRef] [PubMed]
73. Koletzko, B.; Godfrey, K.M.; Poston, L.; Szajewska, H.; van Goudoever, J.B.; de Waard, M.; Brands, B.; Grivell, R.M.; Deussen, A.R.; Dodd, J.M.; et al. Nutrition during pregnancy, lactation and early childhood and its implications for maternal and long-term child health: The early nutrition project recommendations. *Ann. Nutr. Metab.* **2019**, *74*, 93–106. [CrossRef] [PubMed]
74. Koletzko, B.; Brands, B.; Grote, V.; Kirchberg, F.F.; Prell, C.; Rzehak, P.; Uhl, O.; Weber, M. Long-term health impact of early nutrition: The power of programming. *Ann. Nutr. Metab.* **2017**, *70*, 161–169. [CrossRef] [PubMed]
75. Horta, B.L.; Loret de Mola, C.; Victora, C.G. Long-term consequences of breastfeeding on cholesterol, obesity, systolic blood pressure and type 2 diabetes: A systematic review and meta-analysis. *Acta. Paediatr.* **2015**, *104*, 30–37. [CrossRef]
76. Keller, A.; Bucher Della Torre, S. Sugar-sweetened beverages and obesity among children and adolescents: A review of systematic literature reviews. *Child. Obes.* **2015**, *11*, 338–346. [CrossRef]
77. Scharf, R.J.; DeBoer, M.D. Sugar-Sweetened Beverages and Children's Health. *Annu. Rev. Public Health* **2016**, *37*, 273–293. [CrossRef]

78. Frantsve-Hawley, J.; Bader, J.D.; Welsh, J.A.; Wright, J.T. A systematic review of the association between consumption of sugar-containing beverages and excess weight gain among children under age 12. *J. Public Health Dent.* **2017**, *77* (Suppl. 1), S43–S66. [CrossRef]
79. Laverty, A.A.; Magee, L.; Monteiro, C.A.; Saxena, S.; Millett, C. Sugar and artificially sweetened beverage consumption and adiposity changes: National longitudinal study. *Int. J. Behav. Nutr. Phys. Act.* **2015**, *12*, 137. [CrossRef]
80. Wojcicki, J.M.; Medrano, R.; Lin, J.; Epel, E. Increased cellular aging by 3 years of age in latino, preschool children who consume more sugar-sweetened beverages: A pilot study. *Child. Obes.* **2018**, *14*, 149–157. [CrossRef]
81. Macintyre, A.K.; Marryat, L.; Chambers, S. Exposure to liquid sweetness in early childhood: Artificially-sweetened and sugar-sweetened beverage consumption at 4–5 years and risk of overweight and obesity at 7–8 years. *Pediatr. Obes.* **2018**, *13*, 755–765. [CrossRef]
82. Dubois, L.; Farmer, A.; Girard, M.; Peterson, K. Regular sugar-sweetened beverage consumption between meals increases risk of overweight among preschool-aged children. *J. Am. Diet. Assoc.* **2007**, *107*, 924–934. [CrossRef] [PubMed]
83. Snowdon, W.; Raj, A.; Reeve, E.; Guerrero, R.; Fesaitu, J.; Cateine, K.; Guignet, C. Processed foods available in the Pacific Islands. *Glob. Health* **2013**, *9*, 53. [CrossRef] [PubMed]

4

Development of RisObIn.Com, a Screening Tool for Risk of Childhood Obesity in the Community

Ana Catarina Moreira [1,2,*], Patrícia Almeida Oliveira [1,3], Rute Borrego [1], Telma Nogueira [4,5], Raquel Ferreira [1,6] and Daniel Virella [7]

1 Escola Superior de Tecnologia da Saúde de Lisboa, Instituto Politécnico de Lisboa, 1990-096 Lisboa, Portugal; patricia.aao@gmail.com (P.A.O.); rute.borrego@estesl.ipl.pt (R.B.); raquel.ferreira@cm-sintra.pt (R.F.)
2 H &TRC—Health & Technology Research Center, 1990-096 Lisboa, Portugal
3 Faculdade de Medicina, Universidade de Lisboa, 1649-004 Lisboa, Portugal
4 Laboratório de Nutrição, Faculdade de Medicina, Universidade de Lisboa, 1649-028 Lisboa, Portugal; telmanogueira@medicina.ulisboa.pt
5 Instituto de Saúde Ambiental, Faculdade de Medicina, Universidade de Lisboa, 1649-028 Lisboa, Portugal
6 Núcleo de Educação e Qualidade Alimentar, Câmara Municipal de Sintra, 2710-307 Sintra, Portugal
7 Research Unit, Centro Hospitalar Universitário Lisboa Central, 1150-199 Lisboa, Portugal; danielvirella@chlc.min-saude.pt
* Correspondence: ana.moreira@estesl.ipl.pt

Abstract: The prevalence of childhood overweight has increased considerably in the past three decades and there is evidence that childhood obesity can persist into adulthood. A simple tool to identify relevant risk factors may alert families and prevent overweight and obesity. This study aims to develop a pre-school screening tool to assess the risk of childhood obesity. Child anthropometric measurements and several risk factors for childhood obesity factors were obtained. The effect of the variables on the outcome of obesity (defined as increased anthropometry-estimated adiposity) was assessed by binary logistic regression analyses. The identified variables were submitted for expert panel validation and combined for the tool development. A total of 304 children were included. Eight items were included in the tool. A higher score of the tool indicates a greater risk for obesity in childhood with the cutoff point set at 0. The tool sensitivity for obesity was 95%, specificity was 74.4%, the positive predictive value was 37.3%, and negative predictive value was 98.9%. The Risk of childhood Obesity In the Community (RisObIn.Com) tool is proposed to be a comprehensive tool to identify children at high risk for late childhood obesity at admission to primary school. Further studies are needed to assess the performance of the tool.

Keywords: childhood overweight; children; risk; community; screening; tool

1. Introduction

The prevalence of childhood overweight and obesity has increased considerably in the past decades, mostly in high-income countries but recently also rising in low- and middle-income countries. Although in high-income countries, a recent decrease has been observed [1], prevalence remains very high [2,3]. Obesity is defined as an abnormal fat accumulation that impairs health [4] but it has been shown that obesity defined by Body Mass Index (BMI) alone is a remarkably heterogeneous condition with varying cardiovascular and metabolic manifestations across individuals, which may differ according to age and gender [5]. This is a chronic disease that increases heavily the burden on citizens, health care systems, productivity, cities, and society and should be considered a top priority and main target to combat the increasing non-communicable diseases epidemic [6]. There is evidence that childhood obesity can persist into adulthood [7], lead to physical obesity-related complications, and affect psychological health and social and emotional well-being [8]. This emphasizes the importance of early intervention to prevent the onset of obesity in childhood. A comprehensive and proactive strategy to deal with the challenges imposed by the obesity epidemic is needed and requires the development and implementation of programs for prevention, early diagnosis, and treatment, especially in children [6]. However, interventions to reduce childhood obesity show limited effectiveness, particularly for weight-related outcomes [9].

Therefore, sustainable and effective interventions to prevent childhood obesity should target higher-risk children [10]. Obesity development involves a complex interplay between physiological environmental, psychological, social, and behavioral exposures [11,12]. There is evidence of epigenetic processes in utero that contribute to infant obesity, including DNA methylation, and gut microbiome alterations [13]. Breastfeeding is also associated with obesity protection [14,15]. Additional life course exposures include socio-economic status, food production and marketing, food insecurity, and obesogenic environments, that can promote unhealthy lifestyles. In this environment, some individuals are genetically more susceptible to develop obesity [16].

A simple tool to identify relevant obesity risk factors early in life may alert families and caretakers into positive changes, improving a child's weight trajectory and preventing overweight and obesity. Tools to identify children at risk for obesity have been published [17–19]. To our best knowledge, none of these include a large diversity of parameters known to affect weight gain trajectory; the broad variables related to obesity require a more comprehensive tool.

This study aims to develop a pre-school screening tool to assess the risk for childhood obesity based on a broad spectrum of risk factors considering peri-natal, anthropometric, sociodemographic, past eating habits, current eating habits, subjective anthropometry perception, subjective eating habits perception and physical activity, and sleeping habits, at a multivariable level.

2. Materials and Methods

Data from the community-based participatory research Sintra Grows Healthy (SGH) [20] was used for independent analysis, as a cross-sectional with nested case-control study. The study sample comprises schoolchildren aged 6–12 years attending the first to fourth grades of six public primary schools in Sintra municipality, Portugal. Anthropometric measurements of children were assessed and a wide set of data was obtained by the application of a questionnaire to the children's legal guardian, mainly their parents. For the purpose of the present study, an additional set of questions relevant for the study of obesity risk factors was collected by applying a second questionnaire to the children's legal guardian. Only children for whom both these questionnaires were filled, were selected for this study. Data were collected between 2017 and 2018. Written informed consent was obtained and the safety and confidentiality of all the collected and archived data were ensured. Approval was obtained from the National Commission of Data Protection and the Ethics Commission of Lisbon Academic Medical Center.

Anthropometric measurements were obtained directly by trained members of the SGH research team, using standardized anthropometric procedures [21]. Children were barefoot and wearing minimal clothing to assess height and weight. Height was assessed using a portable stadiometer to the nearest 0.1 cm (SECA 213®) in the vertical position, with feet together and the head in the Frankfort plane. Weight was assessed through a portable calibrated scale (SECA Robusta 813®, SECA Deutschland, Hamburg, Germany), expressed up to 0.1 kg. Body Mass Index (BMI) was calculated as weight (kg) divided by height squared (cm^2). BMI was classified according to age and gender z-scores of the World Health Organization for children aged 5 to 19 years old [22]. Waist circumference was directly measured on the skin to the nearest 0.1 cm according to the World Health Organization method with a non-extensible and flexible tape (SECA 201®, SECA Deutschland, Hamburg, Germany) [23]. Waist-to-Height Ratio (WtHR) was calculated as waist circumference (cm) divided by height (cm) and classified as an indicator for early health risk as ≤ 0.5 or >0.5 [24].

The set of questions specifically included for the present study were gathered and developed through a literature review regarding childhood obesity [11,12,16]. Children were asked to fill the questionnaire at home with their parents. To assure data confidentiality, each child was assigned a subject identification code. The questionnaires were collected by teachers and sent back to the SGH team. Data entry and revision was conducted through a standardized procedure. The information collected for the present analysis included (a) parental nationality; (b) parental level of education; (c) family type (nuclear/extended two-/one-parented); (d) number and age of siblings; (e) mean monthly income; (f) parental current employment status; (g) present parental weight and height (from which BMI was calculated and categorized into underweight, normal weight, overweight, or obese) and (h) father's and mother's body image perception. The caretakers were asked to recall peri-natal information: (a) maternal weight before and after pregnancy (from which BMI pre-pregnancy and adequacy of weight gain during pregnancy were calculated according to the Institute of Medicine recommendations [25]); (b) maternal tobacco consumption during pregnancy; (c) diagnosis of gestational diabetes and/or pre-eclampsia; (d) information given by the assistant physician during pregnancy on adequateness of the fetus for gestational age; and (e) the gestational age in complete weeks (to determine if the birth was pre-term or term). Information regarding anthropometric data throughout childhood was retrieved from the records in the child health bulletin: (a) birth weight and length [from which BMI was calculated through World Health Organization Anthro software for Windows, version 3.2.2. (World Health Organization—Department of Nutrition, Geneva, Switzerland), and classification into small for gestational age (SGA, < 10th percentile), appropriate for gestational age (10th–89th percentile), and large for gestational age (LGA, > 90th percentile) were obtained]; (b) weight and length at the ages of 12, 18, and 24 months and 3 and 5 years old [from which BMI z-score was calculated through the World Health Organization Anthro software for Windows, version 3.2.2. (World Health Organization—Department of Nutrition, Geneva, Switzerland)]. Overweight (including obesity) was defined according to age and sex z-scores (above 2) of the World Health Organization for children up to 5 years old [26]; since the medical visits from birth to 5-years-old may not have occurred at the exact dates selected to recall anthropometric data, the health record information closer to those ages and respective dates were collected to correctly assess z-scores. To classify anthropometric measurements at each visit, the exact age was calculated by the difference between birth date and the records visit date.

We collected data on child and family feeding patterns at two moments. We asked about breastfeeding (total and exclusive duration) and the introduction of solid foods (age, appetite, and type of meal first introduced). For present feeding pattern, we asked about: child's appetite, the Mediterranean diet pattern index of the child (KIDMED [27]) through adapted questions, and its family (PREDIMED [28]), and one question to both child and caretakers regarding child's intake when worried, irritated, or anxious, extracted from the from Child Eating Behaviour Questionnaire [29]. To assess the child's and caretaker's perception of the quantity of child usual intake, we used images of four meal plates with different portions of food (A to D, ascendingly). According to children's height-for-age, we determined the two images closer to their recommended portion (z-score ≤ 1 corresponded to images A and B; z-score > 1 corresponded to images B and C). Image D represented an excessive food portion for any children of our sample. We compared the adequacy of the caretaker's answers and classified them as adequate, excessive, or lower. Caretakers were asked to select an option regarding the child's nutritional status for age between "low weight," "adequate weight," or "excessive weight" and compared to the child's BMI. This perception was categorized as correct, underestimated, or overestimated.

Children and caretakers identified the child's body figure through body image scales [30]. We compared that perception with the corresponding child's BMI and categorized it as incorrect, relatively correct, or correct to child's BMI, as previously done [31]. The perceptions were additionally categorized as correct, underestimated, or overestimated. Caretakers also identified their own body figures through body image scales [32]. We compared that perception with the corresponding parental

BMI and categorized it as incorrect, relatively correct, or correct to child's BMI, as previously done [33]. The perceptions were additionally categorized as correct, underestimated, or overestimated.

We questioned about the physical activity and sedentary behaviors of the child, the frequency of consumption of meals in front of a screen, and the number of hours of sleep.

Variables were grouped into eight dimensions: peri-natal, anthropometric, sociodemographic, previous eating habits, current eating habits, subjective anthropometry (perception), subjective eating habits (perception), physical activity, and hours of sleep.

2.1. Development of the Risk Index Tool and Scoring

As the BMI, as a single measurement of obesity, does not reflect the whole complexity of the condition [6], the European Association for the Study of Obesity proposed to improve the diagnostic criteria for obesity with the inclusion of other dimensions, including the degree of adiposity [34]. Therefore, to increase the accuracy of the outcome measure, to reflect an adiposity-based condition, a composite variable was created using BMI and WtHr. Thus, the primary outcome measure in this study is increased adiposity, defined as overweight (including obesity) with WtHr > 0.5, while in primary school. To test the effect of the factors under investigation on the primary outcome, binary logistic regression analyses were performed. Exposures were tested within the aforementioned dimensions (dependent variable: overweight (including obesity) with WtHr > 0.5; factors: all risk factors by dimension).

The regression analysis was used to identify factors associated with the primary outcome on each of the eight dimensions. The studied risk factors that showed an association with our primary outcome were presented to an expert pediatric panel (nutrition, education, nursing, pediatrician, and exercise physiology experts) for external construct validation with the purpose of developing the proposed tool: RisObIn.Com (Risk of childhood Obesity In the Community).

The most agreed risk factor variables were then combined to develop the RisObIn.Com tool. At least one item from every considered dimension was included in the score if any of the items revealed significant statistical relevance. The Beta (β) values to a decimal case were used to generate the scoring system as an indicator of the association between each variable, and 0 and 1 scores were assigned to the response option regarding their association with the outcome variable (overweight including obesity with WtHr > 0.5). As an example, on the physical activity item, a score of 0 was assigned to the response option "plays regular and programmed physical activity," and a score of 1 to the response option "doesn't play regular and programmed physical activity." This score was then multiplied by 1.6 to obtain the item's score, as β was 1.642. The final score of the RisObIn.Com tool was obtained by the sum of all item scores and a correction factor was added to obtain zero as the cut-off value.

2.2. Statistical Analysis

All data were checked for entry errors. Statistical analysis was done using IBM SPSS Statistics for Windows, version 26 (IBM Corp, Armonk, NY, USA). OpenEpi Version 3.01 was used to calculate confidence intervals (CI) [35]. Continuous data were checked for normal distribution using the Kolmogorov-Smirnov test and graphically by evaluating histograms and expressed as mean and standard deviation. Non-normally distributed data were expressed as median (Min-Max). Comparisons between the participants studied and those not included were made by using *t*-tests for normally distributed continuous variables, Mann-Whitney rank-sum tests for non-normally distributed continuous variables, and $\chi 2$ tests for categorical variables.

Cutoff point analysis was performed to identify the optimal value that differentiates the risk of obesity from non-risk of obesity in children. The threshold was defined by the largest distance from the diagonal line of the receiver operating characteristic (ROC) curve (sensitivity × (1 − specificity)). Using the cutoff point obtained, both sensitivity and specificity and positive and negative predictive values were calculated, with their 95% CI. All *P* values reported were based on two-sided hypotheses and compared to a significance level of 5%.

3. Results

3.1. Study Sample Characteristics

Data was collected from 593 subjects. From those, 289 had incomplete data on crucial information to proceed with the analysis (for example, sex information) and therefore were excluded. The remain 304 gathered anthropometric measurements and data regarding our set of questions and therefore were included, despite some were not complete. In the portion of not included subjects, the children's median age was 8.0 (5.8–10.8) years old (missing 162), 7.8 (5.9–10.8) for girls, and 8.1 (5.8–10.4) for boys. The mother's median age was 39.0 (25.0–54.0) years old (missing 62), and father's was 41.0 (25.0–66.0) years old (missing 62). There were no significant differences between the child's age (U = 2371.0, $p = 0.166$), mother's age (U = 41,256.5, $p = 0.153$), child's BMI z-score (U = 23,156.0, $p = 0.204$), mother's (U = 38,080.0, $p = 0.240$) or father's nationality (U = 33,481.5, $p = 0.207$), parental current employment status (U = 30,097.5, $p = 0.308$), mean monthly income (U = 33,703.5, $p = 0.510$), and father's level of education (U = 36,689.0, $p = 0.939$) between the children included in the sample and those not included. The father's age (U = 33,362.5, $p = 0.021$) and the mother's level of education (U = 39,273.0, $p = 0.035$) was significantly different between the children included in the sample and those not included. The sociodemographic characteristics of the sample are presented in Table 1.

Table 1. Sociodemographic characteristics of the study sample.

Sample Characteristics			*n*	%	Girls	Boys
					n	*n*
Child	Age *n* = 300		Median 8.0 (5.9–10.2) years old			
	Sex *n* = 304	Girls	148	48.7	n/a	n/a
		Boys	156	51.3	n/a	n/a
	Body Mass Index *n* = 304	Underweight	4	1.3	1	3
		Normal weight	208	68.4	95	113
		Overweight	63	20.7	38	25
		Obesity	29	9.5	14	15
Caretakers	Mother's age *n* = 300		Median 38.0 (26.0–52.0)			
	Father's age *n* = 280		Median 40.0 (26.0–63.0)			
	Mother's Body Mass Index *n* = 288	Underweight	9	3.1	3	6
		Normal weight	165	57.3	82	83
		Overweight	84	29.2	43	41
		Obesity	30	10.4	14	16
	Father's Body Mass Index *n* = 275	Underweight	0	0	0	0
		Normal weight	104	37.8	57	47
		Overweight	132	48.0	55	77
		Obesity	39	14.2	22	17
	Mother's nationality *n* = 290	Portuguese	270	93.1	137	133
		Non-Portuguese	20	6.9	9	11
	Father's nationality *n* = 277	Portuguese	265	95.7	131	134
		Non-Portuguese	12	4.3	6	6

Table 1. *Cont.*

Sample Characteristics			*n*	%	Girls *n*	Boys *n*
Caretakers	Mother's education *n* = 297	Basic education or lower	62	20.9	32	30
		Higher secondary education or a professional course	119	40.1	68	51
		Graduation or bachelor's degree	99	33.3	44	55
		Master or doctoral degree	17	5.7	3	14
	Father's education *n* = 280	Basic education or lower	91	32.5	48	43
		Higher secondary education or a professional course	129	46.1	59	70
		Graduation or bachelor's degree	46	16.4	22	24
		Master or doctoral degree	14	5.0	6	8
	Professional situation *n* = 263	Both parents are employed	209	79.5	108	101
		Only one parent is employed	44	16.7	21	23
		Both parents are jobless	10	3.8	3	7
	Mean monthly household income *n* = 271	Less than €500	9	3.32	4	5
		€500–€1000	80	29.52	40	40
		€1000–€1500	80	29.52	36	44
		€1500–€2000	52	19.18	28	24
		€2000–€3000	41	15.12	17	24
		Above €3000	9	3.32	3	6

n/a—not applicable.

The overall prevalence estimates of underweight, normal weight, overweight, and obesity, and central adiposity are shown in Table 2. Overall, the prevalence rate was 20.7% for overweight and 9.5% for obesity. Most children (80.8%, $n = 244$) had WtHr ≤ 0.5. Combining BMI and WtHr, 16.8% [95% CI 13.0–21.4] ($n = 51$) children were overweight (including obesity) with WtHr > 0.5. Only seven children had a WtHr > 0.5 with a normal weight and four children had a WtHr ≤ 0.5 with obesity.

3.2. *Risk Factors for Overweight (Including Obesity) with WtHr > 0.5*

Risk estimation models for overweight (including obesity) with WtHr > 0.5 were explored within each dimension of variables. The significant risk factors on each of the eight dimensions are presented in Table 3 and Supplementary Table S1.

3.2.1. Peri-Natal Dimension

The only variable retained in the final peri-natal dimension estimation model was maternal pre-pregnancy BMI; being classified as overweight increases, in mean, 2.6-fold the risk of overweight (including obesity) with WtHr > 0.5, and being classified as obese increases, in mean, 4.1-fold the risk of overweight (including obesity) with WtHr > 0.5.

3.2.2. Anthropometric Dimension

For the anthropometric dimension, the retained variable was the BMI at 5 years old; being classified as overweight increases, in mean, 4.2-fold the risk of overweight (including obesity) with WtHr > 0.5.

Table 2. Characterization of anthropometric measurements and calculated indexes.

		Total				Girls				Boys			
		n	%	95% Confidence Interval		*n*	%	95% Confidence Interval		*n*	%	95% Confidence Interval	
				Lower Level	Upper Level			Lower Level	Upper Level			Lower Level	Upper Level
Body Mass Index z-Score								Median 0.36 (−2.77–3.89)					
Body Mass Index Class	**Underweight**	4	1.3	0.5	3.3	1	0.68	0.1	3.7	3	1.92	0.7	5.5
	Normal Weight	208	68.4	62.9	73.4	95	64.19	56.2	71.5	113	72.44	64.9	78.8
	Overweight	63	20.7	16.6	25.6	38	25.68	19.3	33.3	25	16.02	11.1	22.6
	Obesity	29	9.5	6.7	13.4	14	9.45	5.7	15.3	15	9.62	5.9	15.3
	***n* Total**	304	100.0	-	-	148	100.0	-	-	156	100.0	-	-
Waist Circumference								Median 58.5 (37.5–91.5)					
Waist-to-Height ratio								Median 0.46 (0.34–0.66)					
	≤0.5	244	80.8	75.9	84.8	110	74.8	67.2	81.2	134	86.5	80.2	90.9
	>0.5	58	19.2	15.5	24.4	37	25.2	18.9	32.8	21	13.5	9.0	19.8
	***n* Total**	302	100.0	-	-	147	100.0	-	-	155	100.0	-	-
Overweight (Including Obesity) with Waist-to-Height ratio	**>0.5**	51	16.8	13.0	21.4	31	20.9	15.3	28.4	20	12.8	8.5	18.9
	***n* Total**	304	-	-	-	148	-	-	-	156	-	-	-

Table 3. Variables retained in the statistical models.

Dimension	Variables		Exp(β) (95% Confidence Interval)	*p*-Value
Peri-natal	Pre-pregnancy Body Mass Index	Pre-pregnancy Body Mass Index of Overweight	2.591 (1.164–5.766)	0.020
		Pre-pregnancy Body Mass Index of Obesity	4.145 (0.925–8.570)	0.063
	Body Mass Index z-score 5-years-old		4.159 (2.404–8.497)	0.000
	Paternal Body Mass Index	Paternal Body Mass Index of Overweight	0.772 (0.252–2.364)	0.650
		Paternal Body Mass Index of Obesity	4.041 (1.271–12.844)	0.018
	Type of meal introduced in solid food introduction	Soup	0.401 (0.176–0.914)	0.030
Current eating habits	Child's appetite	Would eat only with insistence or frequently would not eat in totality; Would eat all and be satisfied	0.174 (0.050–0.603)	0.006
	Caretaker's perception of child's intake through image		1.489 (0.985–2.249)	0.059
	Family Mediterranean pattern (PREDIMED)	How many vegetable servings do you consume per day?	0.624 (0.389–0.999)	0.050
		How many servings of butter, margarine, or cream do you consume per day?	1.535 (0.976–2.413)	0.063
Subjective anthropometry perception	Adequacy of father's body image perception vs. actual Body Mass Index	Relatively correct	4.902 (1.116–21.536)	0.035
		Correct	2.597 (0.634–10.643)	0.185
	Adequacy of the caretaker's opinion on the child's nutritional status vs. child's Body Mass Index	Relatively correct	3.483 (0.882–13.753)	0.075
		Correct	31.605 (6.055–164.951)	0.000
Subjective eating habits perception	Caretaker's perception regarding child's intake when anxious	No	0.260 (0.056–1.204)	0.085
	Caretaker's perception of the adequacy of the child's food intake for age	Inferior or adequate	0.083 (0.024–0.286)	0.000
Physical activity and hours of sleep	Child's participation in programmed sport activity	Yes	0.194 (0.052–0.724)	0.015

3.2.3. Sociodemographic Dimension

The sociodemographic variable retained in the final estimation model was paternal BMI; paternal BMI reflecting overweight decreases, in mean, 33% the risk of overweight (including obesity) with WtHr > 0.5, and paternal BMI reflecting obesity increases, in mean, 4-fold the risk of overweight (including obesity) with WtHr > 0.5.

3.2.4. Past Eating Habits Dimension

For the past eating habits dimension, the only variable included in the final model was the type of meal used for solid foods introduction; if soup (rather than cereals) was the first solid food introduced, it decreases, in mean, 60% (the risk of overweight (including obesity) with WtHr > 0.5.

3.2.5. Current Eating Habits Dimension

For current eating habits, the variables child's appetite, the caretaker's perception of the child's intake through image, and the PREDIMED questions regarding vegetable daily intake and butter, margarine, and cream daily intake were included in the final model. The child's appetite decreases, in mean, 83% the risk of overweight (including obesity) with WtHr > 0.5. The caretaker's perception of the child's intake through image increases, in mean, 1.5-fold the risk of overweight (including obesity) with WtHr > 0.5. The PREDIMED question regarding vegetable daily intake decreases, in mean, 38% (the risk of overweight (including obesity) with WtHr > 0.5, and the PREDIMED question regarding butter, margarine, and cream daily intake increases, in mean, 1.5-fold the risk of overweight (including obesity) with WtHr > 0.5.

3.2.6. Subjective Anthropometry Perception Dimension

For subjective anthropometry perception, the two variables retained in the final model were (1) the adequacy of father's own body image perception in comparison to his real BMI; and (2) the adequacy of the caretaker's opinion regarding the child's nutritional status in comparison to the child's real BMI. The relatively correct adequacy of father's own body image perception compared to real BMI increases, in mean, 4.9-fold the risk of overweight (including obesity) with WtHr > 0.5, and the correct adequacy of father's own body image perception compared to real BMI increases, in mean, 2.6-fold the risk of overweight (including obesity) with WtHr > 0.5. Regarding the adequacy of the caretaker's opinion regarding the child's nutritional status compared to the child's real BMI, correct adequacy decreases, in mean, 31.6-fold the risk of overweight (including obesity) with WtHr > 0.5.

3.2.7. Subjective Eating Habits Perception Dimension

In the eating habits subjective data, the variables retained in the final estimation model were the caretaker's perception of child's food intake when worried, irritated, or anxious and the caretaker's perception of the adequacy of the child's food intake for age. The caretaker's perception that the child's food intake when worried, irritated, or anxious is not affected decreases, in mean, 74% the risk of overweight (including obesity) with WtHr > 0.5. The caretaker's perception that the child's food intake is inferior or adequate for age decreases, in mean, 92% the risk of overweight (including obesity) with WtHr > 0.5.

3.2.8. Physical Activity and Sleeping Habits Dimension

For physical activity and hours of sleep, the variables included in the final model were the child's participation in programmed sports activity, the number of sedentary hours in a weekday, the number of sedentary hours on a weekend day, and the total number of sedentary hours in a week. The child's participation in programmed sports activity decreases, in mean, 81% the risk of overweight (including obesity) with WtHr > 0.5.

3.3. Scoring and Risk Index

The set of 13 variables identified for the items of the screening tool were submitted to the pediatric expert panel.

The variable father's BMI from the sociodemographic dimension was excluded as two members of the panel did not agree with its inclusion in the tool, for lack of evidence of the variable impact in childhood obesity.

The current eating habits dimension variables for PREDIMED vegetable servings daily intake and butter, margarine, and cream servings daily intake, and the caretaker's perception of the child's intake through image were excluded. One member of the panel did not agree with the inclusion of the butter, margarine, and cream daily intake variable in the tool, for lack of evidence of the variable impact in childhood obesity.

The adequacy of the father's body image perception vs. BMI from the subjective anthropometry perception was excluded as two members of the panel did not agree with its inclusion in the tool, for lack of evidence of the variable impact in childhood obesity.

For the physical activity and sleep hours dimension, only the programmed physical activity practice variable was included. The remaining were excluded due to the observed lack of measurable effect.

Eight items were included in the tool and all dimensions except the sociodemographic were included. The items and respective scores are presented in Table 4.

Table 4. Items included in the Risk of childhood Obesity in the Community (RisObIn.Com) tool, categorization, and scoring.

Dimension	Item	Response Options and Scoring	Scoring
Anthropometric	Body Mass Index at 5 years old	0—Overweight	−2.3 (p = 0.031)
		1—Underweight, Normal weight	
Peri-natal	Mother's pre-pregnancy Body Mass Index	0—Obesity	−1.0 (p = 0.063)
		1—Underweight, Normal weight, Overweight	
Current eating habits	Child's appetite	0—Would eat only with insistence or frequently would not eat in totality; Would eat all and be satisfied	1.5 (p = 0.015)
		1—Would eat more than what is offered	
Previous eating habits	Type of meal introduced in solid food introduction	0—Soup	−0.9 (p = 0.030)
		1—Infant cereal	
Subjective eating habits perception	Caretaker's perception of the adequacy of the child's food intake for age	0—Less than adequate; Adequate	2.5 (p = 0.000)
		1—More than adequate	
	Caretaker's perception regarding the child's higher intake when worried, irritated, or anxious	0—No	1.4 (p = 0.085)
		1—Yes	
Subjective anthropometry perception	Adequacy of the caretaker's opinion on the child's nutritional status vs. child's Body Mass Index	0—Correct	3.4 (p = 0.000)
		1—Incorrect	
Physical activity and hours of sleep	Child's participation in programmed sport activity	0—Yes	1.6 (p = 0.015)
		1—No	

Applying the tool items to every child who gathered responses to all the tool items (n = 145), the sum of the items ranged from −4.20 to 4.60. Higher values of the tool indicated a greater risk of obesity in childhood. The area under the ROC curve was 0.897 [95%CI 0.825-0.968; $p < 0.001$] for girls and 0.779 [95%CI 0.612–0.947; $p = 0.016$]—Figure 1. The uncorrected optimal cutoff point of the RisObIn.Com tool was -1, thus, a correction factor (+1) was applied to obtain a cutoff point value of zero. The tool sensitivity, based on the optimal cutoff point, was 95.0%; that is, 95.0% of children who had overweight (including obesity) with WtHr > 0.5 while on primary school, got a score greater than 0 in the transition from pre-school to primary school had overweight (including obesity) with WtHr > 0.5 while on primary school. The specificity was 74.4%, meaning that 74.4% of children who did not have overweight (including obesity) with WtHr > 0.5 while on primary school, got a score equal or less than 0 in the transition from pre-school to primary school did not have overweight (including obesity) with WtHr > 0.5 while on primary school. The positive predictive value was 37.3%, meaning that among those who had a score greater than 0, the probability of having the condition was 37.3%. The negative predictive value was 98.9%, meaning that among those who had a score equal or less than 0, the probability of not having the condition was 98.9%.

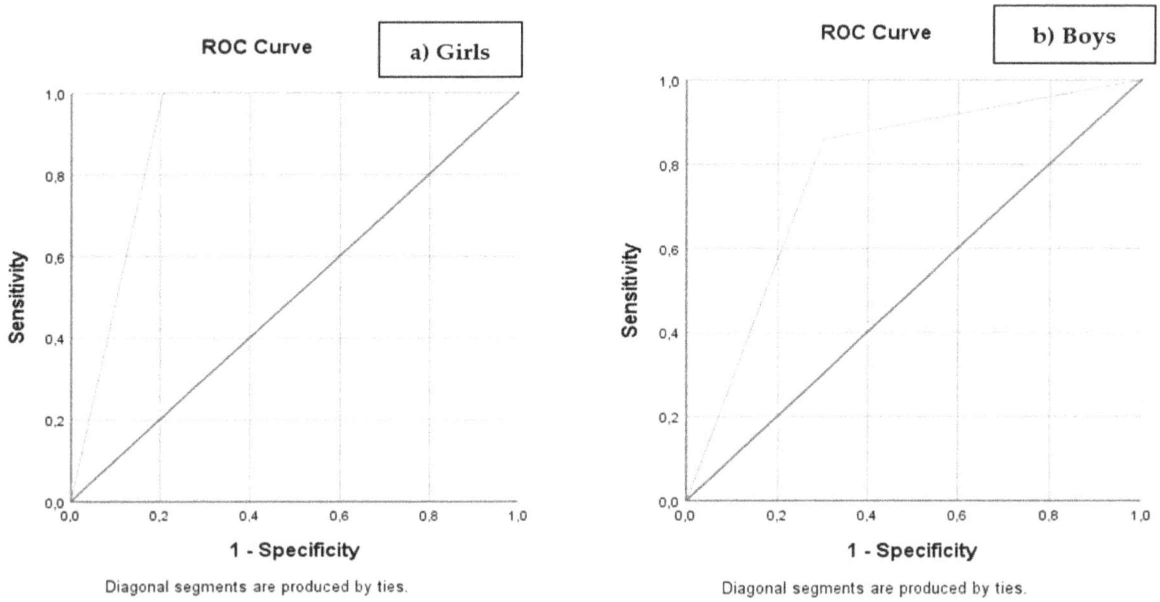

Figure 1. Performance of the proposed screening tool (RisObIn.Com) to identify girls (**a**) and boys (**b**) in the transition from pre-school to primary school that had overweight (including obesity) with WtHr > 0.5 while in primary school. The receiver operating characteristic (ROC) curves were calculated for the cutoff point value of zero. The area under the ROC curve was 0.897 (95%CI 0.825–0.968; $p < 0.001$) for girls; and the area under the ROC curve was 0.779 (95%CI 0.612–0.947; $p = 0.016$) for boys. CI: Confidence Interval; WtHr: Waist-to-Height Ratio.

4. Discussion

Preschool and primary school ages are among the most critical periods for determining obesity later in life [36]. A screening tool applied at this occasion will signal cases that will benefit from general and customized intervention, improving resources to prevent child obesity.

This new proposed tool combines elements that reflect the multifactor nature of obesity: maternal BMI before pregnancy; the child's own BMI at 5 years old; the first solid food introduced for diversification; the caretakers perception of the current appetite of the child; the parental opinion regarding the child's intake adequacy; the child's food intake when worried, irritated, or anxious; the parental perception of the child's nutritional status; and the regular practice of programmed physical activities. Through this weighted combination, RisObIn.Com provides a score that estimates the risk of obesity through school age.

To the best of our knowledge, this is the first screening tool to assess the risk of obesity in children at the entrance of primary school that includes a set of parameters from different dimensions and specific periods, acknowledged to affect weight gain trajectory. The development of this tool contrasts with other existing tools, which selected items through the opinion of experts [17] or literature review [37], focusing only on a specific period of childhood, such as the peri-natal period [18] or the present moment of assessment [19]; others attempted to associate a large number of variables to childhood obesity risk through data mining [38]. The inclusion of all these dimensions can justify the large areas under the ROC curve obtained by RisObIn.Com, larger than other tools [18,19,38]. We observed a difference between boys and girls regarding the ROC findings considering the sex variable, but we consider that it is not possible to infer this difference is maintained when the tool is applied in samples differ in dimension or population characteristics. RisObIn.Com achieves 95% sensitivity and 74.4% specificity despite the tool having been developed using a smaller sample than other studies.

4.1. Peri-Natal Dimension

Maternal pre-pregnancy BMI was the only variable retained in the final estimation model from the peri-natal dimension set. This variable has been shown to be positively associated with infant adiposity, as well as childhood obesity and overweight [12]. A recent meta-analysis identified significantly higher odds for childhood obesity with higher pre-pregnancy maternal BMI, 89% for the offspring of overweight women before pregnancy and 264% for those who were obese before pregnancy [39].

4.2. Anthropometric Dimension

On the anthropometric dimension, the retained variable was the BMI at 5 years of age. The growth patterns of BMI during childhood, particularly during critical periods, are closely related to adult obesity risk [40]. The second physiological rise in BMI occurs, in general, between 3 and 7 years [41]. Pei et al., in 2013, on the German birth cohorts GINIplus—The German Infant Study on the Influence of Nutrition Intervention plus Air pollution and Genetics on Allergy Development, and LISAplus—Influence of Life-style factors on Development of the Immune System and Allergies in East and West Germany plus Air Pollution and Genetics on Allergy Development, also found that BMI at 60–64 months of age was significantly associated with overweight at the age of 10 years [42]. Children with higher BMI at 5 years of age probably have already experienced an adiposity rebound, and early age at adiposity rebound is known to be a risk factor for later obesity [43].

4.3. Previous Eating Habits Dimension

Evidence shows that breastfeeding is a protective factor for obesity [14,15]. However, in this study, regarding previous eating habits, we found that only the type of first complementary solid food introduced was associated with overweight (including obesity) with WtHr > 0.5 while in primary school. Recent data does not support the hypothesis that the quality of complementary foods has a direct effect on the risk for later obesity [44]. Soup can be prepared using many different vegetables as ingredients; the quality and quantity of vegetables and fat used have a strong influence on its nutritional value. By opposition, infant cereals do not allow nutrient composition modifications, thus having a more constant energy value. In countries [45] such as Portugal, the traditional recommendation of the first complementary food to be introduced is infant cereals [46]. One can only speculate that, in infants that present a higher BMI or rapid weight gain [47], health professionals will recommend that the first food to introduce should be soup, since it allows to manipulate the amount of vegetables and fat content, in the attempt to reduce energy intake.

4.4. Current Eating Habits Dimension

In the current eating habits dimension, the parameters retained in the final model were the child's appetite and the caretaker's perception of high, low, or adequate appetite of the child. These measures relate to appetite and reflect self-regulation of energy intake. Biological regulation of appetite is very complex, engaging a number of tissues, organs, hormones, and neural circuits with several feedback pathways between the brain and peripheral tissues [48]. These mechanisms can be influenced and modulated by several factors, beyond the aim of the development of a screening tool. Adequate nutritional status children eat smaller portions at lunch/dinner and may eat more snacks throughout the day; the energy of those snacks is usually greater than the energy of lunch or dinner meals [49].

When parents perceive their child as having increased appetite, they may try to implement restrictive feeding practices. These practices can increase the preoccupation of the child with food and affect eating behaviors, eventually leading to paradoxical weight gain [50]. As both extremes of feeding practices could shape children's relation to food, we cannot exclude that, in the past, parents may have forced their children to eat after they are satisfied, promoting a dysregulation on this equilibrium, once the tendency to encourage children to clear their plate is reported to be associated with obesity [51].

The variables from the PREDIMED index, collected in the SGH study, while explored in the analysis, were excluded, because this Mediterranean diet assessment tool is not yet validated for Portugal; therefore, it may not be adapted to Portuguese food habits. The caretaker's perception of the child's intake through image was also excluded. We presented caretakers a set of four images of a lunch/dinner plate. By presenting an even number of options instead of an odd number, we avoid the tendency for the selection of the central option, improving the reliability of the answer. However, since the need to use images will be a challenge for the application of this tool and the removal of the item had a small effect in the final model, it was removed.

4.5. *Subjective Perception of Anthropometry Dimension*

Regarding the subjective perception of anthropometry, this study found a high proportion of parents that misclassified the nutritional status of their child. It has been speculated that the high prevalence of overweight and obesity in children in the last decades can influence the misinterpretation of the child's normal weight [52], leading to the perception of "normal" weight despite the BMI indication of overweight. If parents cannot recognize their child as overweight, they will not act to change behaviors and the situation can exacerbate, leading to obesity.

4.6. *Subjective Perception of Eating Habits Dimension*

Adequate dietary habits are important for health throughout life, but particularly during childhood, considering that the dietary habits during this specific period are potentially perpetuated into adulthood [53]. In the dimension related to the subjective perception of eating habits, the variables retained in the final estimation model were the caretaker's perception of the child's food intake while worried, irritated, or anxious and the caretaker's perception of the adequacy for age of the child's usual food intake. Previous studies have shown psychopathology to be associated with overweight in children [54,55]; validity data indicate that children as young as 4 years old can report on their own anxiety symptoms [56]. In reaction to anxiety, emotional eating acts as a biological response that provides temporary feelings of gratification/satisfaction [57]. The intervention approach for children with anxiety symptoms and emotional eating should be adapted to address the negative emotions underlying eating behaviors as well as teaching healthy coping strategies for these emotions [58]. Parents and their own perception of the child's dietary habits is one of the most important factors for the dietary habits of children [59]. Childhood obesity experts recommend that childhood overweight prevention should focus on parents, according to the growing evidence of the role of parental practices and family environment in promoting effective changes [11,12].

4.7. *Physical Activity and Sleeping Habits Dimension*

For the dimension concerning physical activity and sleeping habits, the variables included in the final model were the child's participation in programmed sports activity. The levels of physical inactivity are rising in many countries with major implications for general health and the prevalence of non-communicable diseases, such as obesity. The association had already been identified in a similar population living in Portugal's capital (Greater Lisbon) [60]. A recent multinational cross-sectional study demonstrated that low levels of moderate-to-vigorous physical activity or high sedentary levels during weekdays and weekends were associated with higher odds of obesity in 9–11-year-old children in 12 countries [61].

The RisObIn.Com tool seems to be a comprehensive tool to identify, at school entrance, 5-to-6-year-old children at higher risk for late childhood obesity. It was conceived to be applied either by the parents or by teachers or school health professionals, such as a school nurse, school nutritionist, or school social worker, with parental feedback and the child's health bulletin for easier recall of mother pre-pregnancy BMI and anthropometric measures at the age of 5 years. The tool carries a small and simple set of instructions for its effective use. A web-based tool allows a quick, simple, and automated form of application. RisObIn.Com is hosted in Health & Technology Research Center webpage available at https://htrc.estesl.ipl.pt/risobin-com/.

The synergy between the authors of this study and the SGH research team benefited from the logistics associated with data collection and allowed the enhancement and efficiency of resources. The methodology included direct anthropometric measurements, assessment of a set of variables identified as influent in obesity development (from peri-natal to the present moment, including sociodemographic, anthropometric, past and current eating habits, subjective anthropometry, and eating habits perception, and physical activity and hours of sleep) and had the endorsement of an expert panel group composed by skilled professionals from different areas. As a positive asset, the selected outcome measure reflects adiposity by the cumulative outcome of overweight (including obesity) with WtHr > 0.5, which allows both a better characterization of the nutritional status and better accuracy. On the other hand, the mixed design of case-control study nested on a cross-sectional study is a limitation, due to recollection bias, and causal inferences to be made, just epidemiologic and statistic associations. Another source of bias was related to maternal weight before and after pregnancy that was reported and not measured. The local nature of the sample and the differences observed between the children included and not included in the study do not allow immediate generalization of the findings to other populations; therefore, external validation of the screening tool and the study of its performance in different samples is required. Eventual ethnic differences were not explored, due to national ethical and legal restrictions related to data protection. The effective sample size was smaller than expected and it probably affected the ability to identify more exposure variables significantly associated with the study outcome; a larger sample would probably have improved the observed results. Longitudinal data analysis would allow evaluating the tool's ability to predict BMI change over time.

The RisObIn.Com screening tool is proposed to be routinely used by teachers and other school personnel with the participation of parents or caretakers for early identification of children who might benefit from preventive actions, but its use could also be extended to health care professionals such as nurses, family physicians, or pediatricians. The RisObIn.Com screening tool is a simple and inexpensive tool that can provide an evaluation of the risk factors for pediatric obesity and may identify those in need for healthy lifestyle changes.

5. Conclusions

The RisObIn.Com tool is proposed to be a comprehensive tool to identify children at high risk for late childhood obesity at admission to primary school, by the age of 5 to 6 years old. Further studies are needed to assess the external validity and the generalization of the findings, as well as to confirm both the performance of this tool to identify children with obesity risk at admission into primary school and the effect of the subsequent intervention to prevent obesity in children.

Author Contributions: Conceptualization, A.C.M.; methodology, A.C.M., R.F., T.N., P.A.O., and D.V.; software, D.V., and P.A.O.; formal analysis, D.V.; investigation, A.C.M. and R.B.; resources, R.F. and T.N.; data curation, T.N. and P.A.O.; writing—original draft preparation, P.A.O., A.C.M., and D.V.; writing—review and editing, P.A.O., A.C.M., and D.V.; supervision, A.C.M. All authors agreed on the submitted version of the manuscript.

Acknowledgments: We would like to acknowledge the members of the experts panel whose contribution was valuable for the development of the present tool (Bandola, L.; Barrigas, C.; Cunha, S.; Neves, C.; Sousa, J.). The present study is part of the MSc thesis in Clinical Nutrition of one of the authors (P.A.O.) (supervisor A.C.M.), from Faculty of Medicine of Lisbon and Lisbon School of Health Technology, Lisbon, Portugal. The authors are grateful to the SGH team and to its coordinator Joana Sousa, to whom we express our recognition. H&TRC authors gratefully acknowledge the FCT/MCTES national support through the UIDB/05608/2020 and UIDP/05608/2020.

References

1. Abarca-Gómez, L.; Abdeen, Z.A.; Hamid, Z.A.; Abu-Rmeileh, N.M.; Acosta-Cazares, B.; Acuin, C.; Adams, R.J.; Aekplakorn, W.; Afsana, K.; Aguilar-Salinas, C.A.; et al. Worldwide trends in body-mass index, underweight, overweight, and obesity from 1975 to 2016: A pooled analysis of 2416 population-based measurement studies in 128·9 million children, adolescents, and adults. *The Lancet* **2017**, *390*, 2627–2642. [CrossRef]
2. Wijnhoven, T.M.A.; Van Raaij, J.M.A.; Sjöberg, A.; Eldin, N.; Yngve, A.; Kunešová, M.; Starc, G.; Rito, A.I.; Duleva, V.; Hassapidou, M.; et al. WHO European childhood obesity surveillance initiative: School nutrition environment and body mass index in primary schools. *Int. J. Environ. Res. Public Health* **2014**, *11*, 11261–11285. [CrossRef]
3. Spinelli, A.; Buoncristiano, M.; Kovacs, V.A.; Yngve, A.; Spiroski, I.; Obreja, G.; Starc, G.; Pérez, N.; Rito, A.I.; Kunešová, M.; et al. Prevalence of Severe Obesity among Primary School Children in 21 European Countries. *Obes. Facts* **2019**, *12*, 244–258. [CrossRef]
4. WHO Consultation on Obesity. Diseases WHOD of N World Health Organization. In Proceedings of the Programme of Nutrition F and, R.H. Obesity: Preventing and Managing the Global Epidemic: Report of a WHO Consultation on Obesity, Geneva, Switzerland, 3–5 June 1997; World Health Organization: Geneva, Switzerland, 1997.
5. Neeland, I.J.; Poirier, P.; Després, J.P. Cardiovascular and Metabolic Heterogeneity of Obesity: Clinical Challenges and Implications for Management. *Circulation* **2018**, *137*, 1391–1406. [CrossRef] [PubMed]
6. Frühbeck, G.; Busetto, L.; Dicker, D.; Yumuk, V.; Goossens, G.H.; Hebebrand, J.; Halford, J.G.C.; Farpour-Lambert, N.J.; Blaak, E.E.; Woodward, E.; et al. The ABCD of obesity: An EASO position statement on a diagnostic term with clinical and scientific implications. *Obes. Facts* **2019**, *12*, 131–136. [CrossRef] [PubMed]
7. Simmonds, M.; Burch, J.; Llewellyn, A.; Griffiths, C.; Yang, H.; Owen, C.; Duffy, S.; Woolacott, N. The use of measures of obesity in childhood for predicting obesity and the development of obesity-related diseases in adulthood: A systematic review and meta-analysis. *Health Technol. Assess.* **2015**, *19*, 1–336. [CrossRef] [PubMed]
8. Bhadoria, A.; Sahoo, K.; Sahoo, B.; Choudhury, A.; Sufi, N.; Kumar, R. Childhood obesity: Causes and consequences. *J. Fam. Med. Prim. Care* **2015**, *4*, 187. [CrossRef]
9. van de Kolk, I.; Gerards, S.M.; Harms, L.S.E.; Kremers, S.P.J.; Gubbels, J.S. The effects of a comprehensive, integrated obesity prevention intervention approach (SuperFIT) on children's physical activity, sedentary behavior, and BMI z-score. *Int. J. Environ. Res. Public Health* **2019**, *16*, 5016. [CrossRef] [PubMed]
10. Lobstein, T.; Jackson-Leach, R.; Moodie, M.L.; Hall, K.D.; Gortmaker, S.L.; Swinburn, B.A.; James, W.P.T.; Wang, Y.; McPherson, K. Child and adolescent obesity: Part of a bigger picture. *Lancet* **2015**, *385*, 2510–2520. [CrossRef]
11. Birch, L.L.; Ventura, A.K. Preventing childhood obesity: What works? *Int. J. Obes.* **2009**, *33*, S74–S81. [CrossRef]
12. Davison, K.K.; Birch, L.L. Childhood overweight: A contextual model and recommendations for future research. *Obes. Rev.* **2001**, *2*, 159–171. [CrossRef] [PubMed]
13. Golab, B.P.; Santos, S.; Voerman, E.; Lawlor, D.A.; Jaddoe, V.W.; Gaillard, R.; Barros, H.; Bergström, A.; Charles, M.A.; Chatzi, L.; et al. Influence of maternal obesity on the association between common pregnancy complications and risk of childhood obesity: An individual participant data meta-analysis. *Lancet Child Adolesc. Health* **2018**, *2*, 812–821. [CrossRef]
14. Rito, A.I.; Buoncristiano, M.; Spinelli, A.; Salanave, B.; Kunešová, M.; Hejgaard, T.; Solano, M.G.; Fijałkowska, A.; Sturua, L.; Hyska, J.; et al. Association between Characteristics at Birth, Breastfeeding and Obesity in 22 Countries: The WHO European Childhood Obesity Surveillance Initiative–COSI 2015/2017. *Obes. Facts* **2019**, *12*, 226–243. [CrossRef] [PubMed]
15. Yan, J.; Liu, L.; Zhu, Y.; Huang, G.; Wang, P.P. The association between breastfeeding and childhood obesity: A meta-analysis. *BMC Public Health* **2014**, *14*, 1267. [CrossRef] [PubMed]
16. Schrempft, S.; Van Jaarsveld, C.H.M.; Fisher, A.; Herle, M.; Smith, A.D.; Fildes, A.; Llewellyn, C.H. Variation in the Heritability of Child Body Mass Index by Obesogenic Home Environment. *JAMA Pediatr.* **2018**, *172*, 1153–1160. [CrossRef]
17. Santos, M.; Cadieux, A.; Gray, J.; Ward, W. Pediatric Obesity in Early Childhood: A Physician Screening Tool. *Clin. Pediatr.* **2016**, *55*, 356–362. [CrossRef]

18. Manios, Y.; Birbilis, M.; Moschonis, G.; Birbilis, G.; Mougios, V.; Lionis, C.; Chrousos, G.P. Childhood Obesity Risk Evaluation based on perinatal factors and family sociodemographic characteristics: CORE Index. *Eur. J. Pediatr.* **2013**, *172*, 551–555. [CrossRef]
19. Simpson, J.R.; Keller, H.; Rysdale, L.; Beyers, J. Nutrition Screening Tool for Every Preschooler (NutriSTEP^{TM}): Validation and test-retest reliability of a parent-administered questionnaire assessing nutrition risk of preschoolers. *Eur. J. Clin. Nutr.* **2008**, *62*, 770–780. [CrossRef]
20. Sintra Cresce Saudável. Sintra Cresce Saudável [Internet]. Available online: http://crescesaudavel.sintra.pt/ (accessed on 26 September 2020).
21. World Health Organization. *Physical Status: The Use and Interpretation of Anthropometry*; WHO: Geneva, Switzerland, 1995.
22. de Onis, M.; Lobstein, T. Defining obesity risk status in the general childhood population: Which cut-offs should we use? *Int. J. Pediatr. Obes.* **2010**, *5*, 458–460. [CrossRef]
23. World Health Organization. *The WHO STEPwise Approach to Noncomunicable Disease Risk Factor Surveillance (STEPS)*; WHO: Geneva, Switzerland, 2017.
24. Taylor, R.W.; Williams, S.M.; Grant, A.M.; Taylor, B.J.; Goulding, A. Predictive Ability of Waist-to-Height in Relation to Adiposity in Children Is Not Improved With Age and Sex-Specific Values. *Obesity* **2011**, *19*, 1062–1068. [CrossRef]
25. Rasmussen, K.M.; Yaktine, A.L.; Institute of Medicine (U.S.). Committee to Reexamine IOM Pregnancy Weight Guidelines. In *Weight Gain during Pregnancy: Reexamining the Guidelines*; National Academies Press: Washington, DC, USA, 2009; p. 854.
26. World Health Organization. *Training Course on Child Growth Assessment: Interpreting Growth Indicators*; WHO: Geneva, Switzerland, 2008.
27. Serra-Majem, L.; Ribas, L.; Ngo, J.; Ortega, R.M.; García, A.; Pérez-Rodrigo, C.; Aranceta, J. Food, youth and the Mediterranean diet in Spain. Development of KIDMED, Mediterranean Diet Quality Index in children and adolescents. *Public Health Nutr.* **2004**, *7*, 931–935. [CrossRef] [PubMed]
28. Martínez-González, M.A.; García-Arellano, A.; Toledo, E.; Salas-Salvadó, J.; Buil-Cosiales, P.; Corella, D.; Covas, M.I.; Schröder, H.; Arós, F.; Gómez-Gracia, E.; et al. A 14-item Mediterranean diet assessment tool and obesity indexes among high-risk subjects: The PREDIMED trial. *PLoS ONE* **2012**, *7*, e43134. [CrossRef] [PubMed]
29. Viana, V.; Sinde, S.; Saxton, J. Questionário do Comportamento Alimentar da Criança (CEBQ). In *Instrumentos e Contextos de Avaliação Psicológica*; Almedina: Lisbon, Portugal, 2011.
30. Collins, M.E. Body figure perceptions and preferences among preadolescent children. *Int. J. Eat. Disord.* **1991**, *10*, 199–203. [CrossRef]
31. Daraganova, G. Data and measurement. In *The Longitudinal Study of Australian Children Annual Statistical Report 2013*; Australian Institute of Family Studies: Melbourne, Australia, 2014.
32. Stunkard, A.J.; Sørensen, T.I.A.; Schulsinger, F. Use of the Danish Adoption Register for the study of obesity and thinness. *Res. Publ. Assoc. Res. Nerv. Ment. Dis.* **1983**, *60*, 115–120.
33. Freedman, D.S.; Khan, L.K.; Serdula, M.K.; Dietz, W.H.; Srinivasan, S.R.; Berenson, G.S. Inter-relationships among childhood, B.M.I.; childhood height, and adult obesity: The Bogalusa Heart Study. *Int. J. Obes.* **2004**, *28*, 10–16. [CrossRef]
34. Hebebrand, J.; Holm, J.C.; Woodward, E.; Baker, J.L.; Blaak, E.; Durrer Schutz, D.; Farpour-Lambert, N.J.; Frühbeck, G.; Halford, J.G.C.; Lissner, L.; et al. A Proposal of the European Association for the Study of Obesity to Improve the ICD-11 Diagnostic Criteria for Obesity Based on the Three Dimensions Etiology, Degree of Adiposity and Health Risk. *Obes Facts* **2017**, *10*, 284–307. [CrossRef]
35. Dean, A.; Sullivan, K.; Soe, M. OpenEpi: Open Source Epidemiologic Statistics for Public Health, Version 3.01. Updated 2013/04/06 [Internet]. Available online: www.OpenEpi.com (accessed on 26 September 2020).
36. Toschke, A.M.; Grote, V.; Koletzko, B.; Von Kries, R. Identifying Children at High Risk for Overweight at School Entry by Weight Gain during the First 2 Years. *Arch. Pediatr. Adolesc. Med.* **2004**, *158*, 449–452. [CrossRef]
37. Avis, J.L.S.; Holt, N.L.; Maximova, K.; van Mierlo, T.; Fournier, R.; Padwal, R.; Cave, A.L.; Martz, P.; Ball, G.D.C. The Development and Refinement of an e-Health Screening, Brief Intervention, and Referral to Treatment for Parents to Prevent Childhood Obesity in Primary Care. *Telemed. e-Health* **2016**, *22*, 385–394. [CrossRef]

38. Hammond, R.; Athanasiadou, R.; Curado, S.; Aphinyanaphongs, Y.; Abrams, C.; Messito, M.J.; Gross, R.; Katzow, M.; Jay, M.; Razavian, N.; et al. Predicting childhood obesity using electronic health records and publicly available data. *PLoS ONE* **2019**, *14*, e0215571. [CrossRef]
39. Heslehurst, N.; Vieira, R.; Akhter, Z.; Bailey, H.; Slack, E.; Ngongalah, L.; Pemu, A.; Rankin, J. The association between maternal body mass index and child obesity: A systematic review and meta-analysis. *PLoS Med.* **2019**, *16*, e1002817. [CrossRef]
40. Zhang, T.; Whelton, P.K.; Xi, B.; Krousel-Wood, M.; Bazzano, L.; He, J.; Chen, W.; Li, S. Rate of change in body mass index at different ages during childhood and adult obesity risk. *Pediatr. Obes.* **2019**, *14*, e12513. [CrossRef] [PubMed]
41. Cole, T.J. Children grow and horses race: Is the adiposity rebound a critical period for later obesity? *BMC Pediatr.* **2004**, *4*, 6. [CrossRef]
42. Pei, Z.; Flexeder, C.; Fuertes, E.; Thiering, E.; Koletzko, B.; Cramer, C.; Berdel, D.; Lehmann, I.; Bauer, C.-P.; Heinrich, J.; et al. Early life risk factors of being overweight at 10 years of age: Results of the German birth cohorts GINIplus and LISAplus. *Eur. J. Clin. Nutr.* **2013**, *67*, 855–862. [CrossRef] [PubMed]
43. Williams, S.M.; Goulding, A. Patterns of gowth associated with the timing of adiposity rebound. *Obesity* **2009**, *17*, 335–341. [CrossRef]
44. Grote, V.; Theurich, M.; Koletzko, B. Do complementary feeding practices predict the later risk of obesity? Vol. 15, Current Opinion in Clinical Nutrition and Metabolic Care. *Curr. Opin. Clin. Nutr. Metab. Care* **2012**, *15*, 293–297. [CrossRef] [PubMed]
45. Miles, G.; Siega-Riz, A.M. Trends in food and beverage consumption among infants and toddlers: 2005–2012. *Pediatr. Am. Acad. Pediatr.* **2017**, *139*, e20163290. [CrossRef]
46. Rêgo, C.; Lopes, C.; Durão, C.; Pinto, E.; Mansilha, H.; Pereira da Silva, L.; Nazareth, M.; Graça, P.; Ferreira, R.; Lima, R.M.; et al. *Alimentação Saudável dos 0 aos 6 anos–Linhas De Orientação Para Profissionais E Educadores*; Direção-Geral da Saúde: Lisbon, Portugal, 2019.
47. Zheng, M.; Lamb, K.E.; Grimes, C.; Laws, R.; Bolton, K.; Ong, K.K.; Campbell, K. Rapid weight gain during infancy and subsequent adiposity: A systematic review and meta-analysis of evidence. *Obes. Rev.* **2018**, *19*, 321–332. [CrossRef]
48. MacLean, P.S.; Blundell, J.E.; Mennella, J.A.; Batterham, R.L. Biological control of appetite: A daunting complexity. *Obesity* **2017**, *25* (Suppl. 1), S8–S16. [CrossRef]
49. Santos, T.; Moreira, A.C. Alimentação em contexto pré-escolar: Relação com estado nutricional e local de residência. *Acta Port. Nutr.* **2017**, *8*, 34–37. [CrossRef]
50. Eagleton, S.G.; Brown, C.L.; Moses, M.J.; Skelton, J.A. Restrictive feeding and excessive hunger in young children with obesity: A case series. *Clin. Case Rep.* **2019**, *7*, 1962–1967. [CrossRef]
51. Robinson, E.; Aveyard, P.; Jebb, S.A. Is plate clearing a risk factor for obesity? A cross-sectional study of self-reported data in US adults. *Obesity* **2015**, *23*, 301–304. [CrossRef] [PubMed]
52. Robinson, E. Overweight but unseen: A review of the underestimation of weight status and a visual normalization theory. *Obes. Rev.* **2017**, *18*, 1200–1209. [CrossRef]
53. Klesges, R.C.; Stein, R.J.; Eck, L.H.; Isbell, T.R.; Klesges, L.M. Parental influence on food selection in young children and its relationships to childhood obesity. *Am. J. Clin. Nutr.* **1991**, *53*, 859–864. [CrossRef] [PubMed]
54. Pinto, I.; Wilkinson, S.; Virella, D.; Alves, M.; Calhau, C.; Coelho, R. Anxiety, family functioning and neuroendocrine biomarkers in obese children. *Acta Med. Port.* **2017**, *30*, 273–280. [CrossRef]
55. Pinto, I.; Wilkinson, S.; Virella, D.; Alves, M.; Calhau, C.; Coelho, R. Attachment Strategies and Neuroendocrine Biomarkers in Obese Children. *Acta Med. Port.* **2016**, *29*, 332–339. [CrossRef]
56. Luby, J.L.; Belden, A.; Sullivan, J.; Spitznagel, E. Preschoolers' Contribution to their Diagnosis of Depression and Anxiety: Uses and Limitations of Young Child Self-Report of Symptoms. *Child Psychiatry Hum. Dev.* **2007**, *38*, 321–338. [CrossRef]
57. Fox, C.K.; Gross, A.C.; Rudser, K.D.; Foy, A.M.H.; Kelly, A.S. Depression, Anxiety, and Severity of Obesity in Adolescents. *Clin. Pediatr.* **2016**, *55*, 1120–1125. [CrossRef]
58. Sheinbein, D.H.; Stein, R.I.; Hayes, J.F.; Brown, M.L.; Balantekin, K.N.; Conlon, R.P.K.; Saelens, B.E.; Perri, M.G.; Welch, R.R.; Schechtman, K.B.; et al. Factors associated with depression and anxiety symptoms among children seeking treatment for obesity: A social-ecological approach. *Pediatr. Obes.* **2019**, *14*, e12518. [CrossRef] [PubMed]

59. Rodgers, R.F.; Paxton, S.J.; Massey, R.; Campbell, K.J.; Wertheim, E.H.; Skouteris, H.; Gibbons, K. Maternal feeding practices predict weight gain and obesogenic eating behaviors in young children: A prospective study. *Int. J. Behav. Nutr. Phys. Act.* **2013**, *10*, 24. [CrossRef]
60. Gouveia, C.; Pereira-da-Silva, L.; Silva, P.; Virella, D.; Videira-Amaral, J. [Physical activity and sedentarism in adolescent students in Lisbon] Actividade física e sedentarismo em adolescentes escolarizados do Concelho de Lisboa. *Acta Pediatr. Port.* **2007**, *38*, 7–12.
61. Li, N.; Zhao, P.; Diao, C.; Qiao, Y.; Katzmarzyk, P.T.; Chaput, J.P.; Fogelholm, M.; Kuriyan, R.; Kurpad, A.; Lambert, E.V.; et al. Joint associations between weekday and weekend physical activity or sedentary time and childhood obesity. *Int. J. Obes.* **2019**, *43*, 691–700. [CrossRef] [PubMed]

Promoting Healthy Eating among Young People—A Review of the Evidence of the Impact of School-Based Interventions

Abina Chaudhary [1], František Sudzina [2,3,*] and Bent Egberg Mikkelsen [4]

[1] Independent Researcher, Kastrupvej 79, 2300 Copenhagen, Denmark; abinachaudhary@yahoo.com
[2] Department of Materials and Production, Faculty of Engineering and Science, Aalborg University, A. C. Meyers Vænge 15, 2450 Copenhagen, Denmark
[3] Department of Systems Analysis, Faculty of Informatics and Statistics, University of Economics, nám. W. Churchilla 1938/4, 130 67 Prague, Czech Republic
[4] Department of Geosciences and Natural Resource Management, Faculty of Science, University of Copenhagen, Rolighedsvej 23, 1958 Frederiksberg C, Denmark; bemi@ign.ku.dk
* Correspondence: sudzina@business.aau.dk or frantisek.sudzina@vse.cz

Abstract: Intro: Globally, the prevalence of overweight and obesity is increasing among children and younger adults and is associated with unhealthy dietary habits and lack of physical activity. School food is increasingly brought forward as a policy to address the unhealthy eating patterns among young people. Aim: This study investigated the evidence for the effectiveness of school-based food and nutrition interventions on health outcomes by reviewing scientific evidence-based intervention studies amongst children at the international level. Methods: This study was based on a systematic review using the PRISMA guidelines. Three electronic databases were systematically searched, reference lists were screened for studies evaluating school-based food and nutrition interventions that promoted children's dietary behaviour and health aiming changes in the body composition among children. Articles dating from 2014 to 2019 were selected and reported effects on anthropometry, dietary behaviour, nutritional knowledge, and attitude. Results: The review showed that school-based interventions in general were able to affect attitudes, knowledge, behaviour and anthropometry, but that the design of the intervention affects the size of the effect. In general, food focused interventions taking an environmental approach seemed to be most effective. Conclusions: School-based interventions (including multicomponent interventions) can be an effective and promising means for promoting healthy eating, improving dietary behaviour, attitude and anthropometry among young children. Thus, schools as a system have the potential to make lasting improvements, ensuring healthy school environment around the globe for the betterment of children's short- and long-term health.

Keywords: school children; food and nutrition; intervention; healthy eating

1. Introduction

Childhood is one of the critical periods for good health and development in human life [1,2]. During this age, the physiological need for nutrients increases and the consumption of a diet high in nutritional quality is particularly important. Evidence suggests that lifestyle, behaviour patterns and eating habits adopted during this age persist throughout adulthood and can have a significant influence on health and wellbeing in later life [3,4]. Furthermore, the transition from childhood into adolescence is often associated with unhealthy dietary changes. Thus, it is important to establish healthful eating behaviours early in life and specially focus on the childhood transition period. A healthy diet during the primary age of children reduces the risk of immediate nutrition-related health problems of primary concern to school children, namely, obesity, dental caries and lack of physical activity [5–7].

Furthermore, young people adopting these healthy habits during childhood are more likely to maintain their health and thus be at reduced risk of chronic ailments in later life [7–9]. Thus, healthy behaviours learnt at a young age might be instrumental in reaching the goals of good health and wellbeing of the 2030 Sustainability Agenda which has implications at the global level.

Globally, the prevalence of overweight and obesity rose by 47.1% for children and 27.5% for adults between 1980 and 2013 [10]. A recent WHO (World Health Organization) Commission report [10] stated that if these same trends were to continue, then by 2025, 70 million children are predicted to be affected [11]. Hence, the increased prevalence might negatively affect child and adult morbidity and mortality around the world [12,13]. Worldwide the dietary recommendations for healthy diets recommend the consumption of at least five portions of fruits and vegetables a day, reduced intake of saturated fat and salt and increased consumption of complex carbohydrates and fibres [14]. However, studies show that most children and adolescent do not meet these guidelines [15,16] and, thus, as a result, childhood and adolescent obesity are alarming nearly everywhere [17]. Recent figures show that the prevalence has tripled in many countries, making it the major public health issue in the 21st century [18–21]. According to WHO [4], 1 in 3 children aged 6–9 were overweight and obese in 2010, up from 1 in 4 children of the same age in 2008.

The increased prevalence of overweight and obesity has fuelled efforts to counteract the development, as seen for instance in the action plan on childhood obesity [17]. Increasingly policy makers have been turning their interest to the school setting as a well-suited arena for the promotion of healthier environments [18]. As a result, schools have been the target of increased attention from the research community to develop interventions and to examine the school environment to promote healthful behaviours including healthy eating habits.

Globally, interventions in the school environment to promote healthier nutrition among young people have received considerable attention from researchers over the past years. But there is far from a consensus on what are the most effective ways to make the most out of schools' potential to contribute to better health through food-based actions. Is it the environment that makes a difference? Is it the education or is it the overall attention given to food and eating that plays the biggest role? School food and nutrition intervention strategies have witnessed a gradual change from knowledge orientation to behavioural orientation [22] and from a focus on the individual to the food environment. Research evidence has shown that adequate nutrition knowledge and positive attitudes towards nutrition do not necessarily translate to good dietary practices. Similarly, research has shown that the food environment plays a far bigger role in behaviour than originally believed [23,24].

School-based interventions can a priori be considered as an effective method for promoting better eating at the population level. Schools reach a large number of participants across diverse ethnic groups. It not only reaches children, but school staffs, family members as well as community members [8,25]. Schools can be considered a protected place where certain rules apply and where policies of public priority can be deployed relatively easily. In addition, schools are professional spaces in which learning and formation is at the heart of activities and guided by a skilled and professional staff. Schools, as such, represent a powerful social environment that hold the potential to promote and provide healthy nutrition and education. Besides the potential to create health and healthy behaviours, good nutrition at school has, according to more studies, the potential to add to educational outcomes and academic performance [26–28].

However, taking the growth in research studies and papers in the field into account, it is difficult for both the research community and for policy makers to stay up to date on how successful school-based interventions have been in improving dietary behaviours, nutritional knowledge and anthropometry among children. Also, the knowledge and insights into how it is possible to intervene in the different corners of the school food environment has developed which obviously has influenced over recent decades how programs and interventions can be designed. It has also become clear that food at school is more than just the food taken but includes curricular and school policy components. The findings from school-based studies on the relationship between school, family as well as community-based interventions and health impact suggest that health impacts are dependent on the context in which they have been carried out as well as the methodology. Thus, an updated overview as well as a more detailed analysis of initiatives is needed in order to develop our understanding of the nature of the mechanisms through which the school can contribute to the shaping of healthier dietary behaviour among children and adolescents before more precise policy instruments can be developed. Our study attempted to fill the need for better insight into which of the many intervention components works best. It attempted to look at school food and nutrition interventions reported in the literature that have been looking at healthy eating programmes, projects, interventions or initiatives.

School-based interventions in the Western world are traditionally targeted at addressing obesity and over-nutrition, but school food interventions are also addressing under nutrition and, as such, their role in a double burden of disease perspective should not be underestimated. Many studies have reported on micronutrient malnutrition among school-aged children in developing countries (for instance [29–31]) but it has also been reported in the context of developed countries [32]. Against this backdrop, the aim of this study was to provide an analysis of the evidence of the effectiveness of school-based food interventions by reviewing recent scientific, evidence-based intervention studies on healthy eating promotion at school. The specific objectives of the study were to identify which interventions had an effect on primary outcomes, such as BMI, or on secondary outcomes such as dietary behaviour, nutritional knowledge and attitude.

2. Materials and Methods

The functional unit of the review were healthy eating programmes, projects or initiatives that have been performed using the school as a setting. We included only programmes, projects or initiatives that were studied in a research context, in the sense that they were planned by researchers, carried out under controlled settings using a research protocol, and reported in the literature. School-based programmes, projects, interventions or initiatives are, per definition, cluster samples where a number of schools first were chosen for intervention followed by performing an outcome measurement before and after the intervention and, in most cases, also in one or more control schools. The outcome measurement in the studies reviewed was performed on a sample of students that was drawn from each school (cluster).For this, the systematic review and meta-analysis (PRISMA) guidelines and the standardised quality assessment tool "effective public health practice project (EPHPP) quality assessment tool for quantitative studies" were used for analysing the quality assessment of the included studies [33]. This EPHPP instrument can be used to assess the quality of quantitative studies with a variety of study designs.

2.1. Literature Search

The literature review involved searches in PubMed, Web of Science and Cochrane Library database. The search strategy was designed to be inclusive and focused on three key elements: population (e.g., children); intervention (e.g., school-based); outcome (e.g., diet and nutrition, knowledge, attitude and anthropometrics). The search terms used in PubMed database were: "effectiveness of school food AND nutrition AND primary school children", "effectiveness of school food AND nutrition AND interventions OR programs AND among primary school children AND increase healthy consumption", "primary school children and education and food interventions", "Effectiveness of school-based food interventions among primary school", "effectiveness of school-based nutrition and food interventions", "primary school interventions and its effectiveness", and "obesity prevention intervention among Primary schools". Search terms such as: "effectiveness of school-based food interventions among primary school", "effectiveness of school based food and nutrition interventions", "primary school interventions and its effectiveness" and "obesity prevention interventions", were used in the Web of Science database. Lastly, search terms such as: "nutrition interventions in primary schools" and "Nutrition education interventions in school" were used in the Cochrane Library database to find the articles. In addition, reference lists of all retrieved articles and review articles [34] were screened for potentially eligible articles. The search strategy was initially developed in PubMed and adapted for use in other databases. In addition, snowballing of the reference list of the selected articles was conducted.

2.2. *Inclusion Criteria*

Studies selected for the inclusion were studies which investigated the effectiveness of a school-based interventions targeting food and nutrition behaviour, healthy eating and nutrition education as a primary focus during the intervention. Also, to be included in this review, only articles from 2014 to 2019 were selected and of those inclusion criteria included articles targeting primary school children aged between 5 and 14 years. Participants included both boys and girls without considering their socio-economic background. Study design included randomized controlled trial "RCT", cluster randomized controlled trial "RCCT", controlled trial "CT", pre-test/post-test with and without control "PP", experimental design "Quasi". Studies which did not meet the intervention components/exposures, such as information and teaching (mostly for the target group and parents were additional), family focus on social support and food focus (which mainly focuses on the availability of free foods including food availability from school gardening), were excluded. Systematic review papers and studies written in different language except for English were excluded as well. Studies which met the intervention criteria but had after school programs were excluded.

2.3. *Age Range*

Since the review covers a broad range of different countries and since school systems are quite different, the sampling principle had to include some simplification and standardisation. The goal of the review was to cover elementary (primary) and secondary education and, as a result, the age range of 5–14 was chosen to be the best fit, although it should be noted that secondary education in some countries also covers those 15–18 years of age. In most countries, elementary education/primary education is the first—and normally obligatory—phase of formal education. It begins at approximately age 5 to 7 and ends at about age 11 to 13 and in some countries 14. In the United Kingdom and some other countries, the term primary is used instead of elementary. In the United States the term primary refers to only the first three years of elementary education, i.e., grades 1 to 3. Elementary education is, in most countries, preceded by some kind of kindergarten/preschool for children aged 3 to 5 or 6 and normally followed by secondary education.

2.4. *Assessment of Study Eligibility*

For the selection of the relevant studies, all the titles and abstracts generated from the searches were examined. The articles were rejected on initial screening if the title and abstract did not meet the inclusion criteria or met the exclusion criteria. If abstracts did not provide enough exclusion information or were not available, then the full text was obtained for evaluation. The evaluation of full text was done to refine the results using the aforementioned inclusion and exclusion criteria. Thus, those studies that met predefined inclusion criteria were selected for this study.

2.5. *Analytical Approach*

The first step of data collection was aimed at organizing all studies with their key information. In the second step, we created coded columns. A coded column served as a basis for being able to do further statistical analysis. In other words, in a coded column we added a new construct not originally found in the papers as a kind of dummy variable that standardized otherwise non-standardized information, allowing us to treat otherwise un-calculable data statistically. For the impact columns, we used the following approach to construct codes where impacts where put on a 1–4-point Likert scale with 1 being "ineffective", 2 "partially effective", 3 "effective" and 4 "very effective".

For the design column, the following approach was adopted as illustrated in the Table 1. Quasi experimental/pre–post studies were labelled QED and were considered to always include a baseline and follow-up outcome measurement. As the simplest design with no comparison but just a pre/post study of the same group, we constructed a power column and assigned 1 to this for a QED design. For the controlled trial (CT), we assigned the power 2. A controlled trial is the same as QED but with a comparison/control in which no interventions are made and with no randomization. We considered a study to be of that kind if some kind of controls were made which could be, for instance, matching. All CTs in our study included 2 types of comparisons: pre and post (baseline and follow-up) as well as a comparison between intervention/no intervention. For the RCT/RCCT—a trial that is controlled through the randomization—we assigned the power 3. This "top of hierarchy" design includes the case (intervention) and a control (no intervention) and normally two types of comparisons (pre and post) as well as an intervention/no intervention. For the context of this study, we did not differentiate between RCTs and RCCTs. The latter is sometimes used to stress the fact that the school (or the class) is the sampling unit from which the subjects are recruited. But since in the context of schools RCCT is simply a variation of RCT, we coded them in the same class of power. We simply assumed that when authors spoke about an RCT, they in fact meant an RCCT since they could not have been sampling subjects without using the school as the unit.

Table 1. Coding table for study designs. The table shows the types of studies examined in the review and the power assigned to them.

Code	Design	Power
PP	Pre-Test/Post-Test	1
OBS	Observational	1
CT	Controlled Trial	2
RCT	Randomized Controlled Trial	3
RCCT	Randomized Controlled Cluster Trial	3

Codes and categorization were used to standardize the information found in the papers for our statistical analysis. Categorisation of the age/class level, such as EA—Early age, EML—Early middle late, EL—Early late, was used.

For the intervention components ("what was done") we translated all studies into three columns: information and teaching, family and social support and environmental components, food provision and availability. The latter was further expanded into three columns labelled as: focus on and provisioning of F & V; free food availability through school gardening and availability of food and healthier food environment. Our inclusion criteria were that studies should contain at least one of these components. For the environmental component—food provision and availability intervention components—we identified 2 distinct types: either a broad healthier eating focus or a narrow and more targeted fruit and vegetable focus. After the coding, we started to ask questions about the data. Most importantly, we were interested in knowing whether there existed a relationship between "what was done" and "what was the impact". In other words, we were interested in knowing more whether there was a pattern in the way the studies intervened and the outcomes.

2.6. Queries Made

We performed queries for each intervention component (the independent variable in columns K, L and M) for each single outcome measure.

Is there a relationship between age and outcome? We used the coded column (EA, EML, etc.) to study that relationship.

In addition, we made queries regarding the relationship among study designs. For instance, would the duration of studies influence whether an effect could be found or not? Would more powerful designs result in more impact?

Furthermore, we made queries on the relationship between one intervention and a multi-interventional component and their effect on the outcome measure. Also, the queries on target groups were made. Codes such as S and NS (refer Table 4) in the column were used to study the relationship. In our analysis a distinction was made between "standard" and "extreme" (special cases). From the reviewed papers, it was clear that some studies put little emphasis on the school selected. We classified those as standard (S). However, a few papers used a stratification approach and case/cluster selection that can be classified as an "extreme" or non-standard case. We coded these as non-standard (NS). For instance, studies could be targeted to include only refugees or subjects of low socio-economic status. It can be speculated that being a "special case" or extreme case could have an influence. As a result, we reserved a code for these cases, although it became clear that they represented only a minority.

In our study, availability plays a central role, since it is used in many food-at-school intervention studies. Availability signals that food is "pushed" as opposed to being used in the "pull" mode, where individuals are expected to request food in the sense that is the behaviour of the individual that becomes the driving force rather than the "out thereness". Availability is in most studies used in combination with the idea of a food environment. The literature shows that availability can be of two types. One is when food is made available for the individual to take where visibility, salience, product placement, etc., are used as factors. The other type of availability is when it is made free and the individual as a result does not have to pay. Free availability has been studied extensively in intervention studies but for obvious reason it is difficult to implement "post-study" since there needs to be a permanent financing present. The only exceptions to this are the collective meal models found in countries such as Sweden, Finland, Estonia and Brazil as well as in the EU scheme where the EU subsidizes the fruit.

Study design and other characteristics are provided in Table 2, and their findings are provided in Table 3.

Table 2. The review sample: study design/characteristics. The table shows the 43 studies of the review Illustrating study design and study characteristics of the included studies.

Author	Year	Title/Reference	Main Aim (from Abstract)	Main Aim in Brief	Program Name	Location & Country	Study Design	Study Design Coded	Power	Intervention Components			
											Food Focus		
					Acronym		Column I	RCT, PP, CT, RCCT, Quasi		Information and Teaching	Environmental/Food Focus on Healthy Meal Availability	Environmental/Food Focus through School Gardening	Family/Social Support
Harake et al. [35]	2018	Impact of pilot school-based nutrition intervention on dietary knowledge, attitudes, behaviours and nutritional status of Syrian refugee children in the Bekaa, Lebanon	This study aimed to evaluate the impact of a six-month pilot school-based nutrition intervention on changes in dietary knowledge, attitude, and behavior of Syrian refugee children enrolled in informal primary schools located in the rural region of the Bekaa in Lebanon. A secondary objective of the study was to explore the effect of the intervention on the dietary intake and nutritional status of children.	Nutritional knowledge, attitude, HE & FV	GHATA	Bekaa Lebanon	Quasi experimental	QED	1	x		x	
Adab P, et al. [36]	2018	Effectiveness of a childhood obesity prevention programme delivered through schools, targeting >6 (more than 6 years) and 7 years old cluster randomised controlled trial (WAVES study)	To assess the effectiveness of a school and family based healthy lifestyle programme (WAVES intervention) compare with usual practice, in preventing childhood obesity.	Anthropometry, HE & FV	WAVES	UK primary schools from the West Midlands within 35 miles of the study centre	Randomized Controlled Cluster Trials	RCCT	3	x			
Harley A, et al. [37]	2018	Youth Chef Academy: Pilot Results From a Plant-Based Culinary and Nutrition Literacy Program for Sixth and Seventh Graders	The study aim was to examine the effectiveness of Youth Chef Academy (YCA), a classroom-based experiential culinary and nutrition literacy intervention for sixth and seventh graders (11- to 13-year-old) designed to impact healthy eating.	HE & FV, Nutritional knowledge	YCA	US (exact location is missing)	Controlled Trial (CT)	CT	2	x			
Hermans R.C.J. et al. [38]	2018	Feed the Alien! The Effects of a Nutrition Instruction Game on Children's Nutritional Knowledge and Food Intake	The aim of this study was to test the short-term effectiveness of the Alien Health Game, a videogame designed to teach elementary school children about nutrition and healthy food choices.	HE & FV, Nutritional knowledge	AHG	Dutch, Netherland	Pre-test post-test, experimental study design	QED	1	x			

Table 2. *Cont.*

Author	Year	Title/Reference	Main Aim (from Abstract)	Main Aim in Brief	Program Name	Location & Country	Study Design	Study Design Coded	Power	Intervention Components			
											Food Focus		
					Acronym		Column I	RCT, PP, CT, RCCT, Quasi		Information and Teaching	Environmental/Food Focus on Healthy Meal Availability	Environmental/Food Focus through School Gardening	Family/Social Support
Piana N., et al. [39]	2017	An innovative school-based intervention to promote healthy lifestyles	To describe an innovative school-based intervention to promote healthy lifestyles. To evaluate its effects on children's food habits and to highlight the key components which contribute most to the beneficial effects obtained from children's, teachers' and parents' perspectives.	HE & FV, Nutritional knowledge, Physical activity	Kidmed test	Spoleto, Umbria	Pre-test post-test	PP	1	x			x
Battjes-Fries M.C.E., et al. [40]	2017	Effectiveness of Taste Lessons with and without additional experiential learning activities on children's willingness to taste vegetables	The aim of this study was to assess the effect of Taste Lessons with and without extra experiential learning activities on children's willingness to taste unfamiliar vegetables, food neophobia, and vegetable consumption.	HE & FV, attitude	TLVM	Dutch province of Gelderland	Quasi experimental design	QED	1	x			
Bogart L.M., et al. [41]	2014	A Randomized Controlled Trial of Students for Nutrition and eXercise (SNaX): A Community-Based Participatory Research Study	To conduct a randomized controlled trial of Students for Nutrition and eXercise (SNaX), a 5-week middle-school-based obesity-prevention intervention combining school-wide environmental changes, multimedia, encouragement to eat healthy school cafeteria foods, and peer-led education.	HE & FV, Nutritional knowledge	SNaX	Los Angeles Unified School District	Randomized Controlled Trial	RCT	3	x			
Shriqui V.K., et al. [42]	2016	Effects of a School-Based Intervention on Nutritional Knowledge and Habits of Low-Socioeconomic School Children in Israel: A Cluster Randomized Controlled Trial	Examining the effect of a school-based comprehensive intervention on nutrition knowledge, eating habits, and behaviours among low socioeconomic status (LSES) school-aged children was performed	Anthropometry, HE & FV, Nutritional knowledge	NRI & PA	Beer Sheva, a big metropolis in southern Israel	Randomized Controlled Cluster Trial	RCCT	3	x			x

Table 2. *Cont.*

Author	Year	Title/Reference	Main Aim (from Abstract)	Main Aim in Brief	Program Name	Location & Country	Study Design	Study Design Coded	Power	Intervention Components			
											Food Focus		
					Acronym		Column I	RCT, PP, CT, RCCT, Quasi		Information and Teaching	Environmental/Food Focus on Healthy Meal Availability	Environmental/Food Focus through School Gardening	Family/Social Support
Sharma S.V. et al. [43]	2016	Evaluating a school-based fruit and vegetable co-op in low-income children: A quasi-experimental study	The purpose of this study was to evaluate the effectiveness of a new school-based food co-op program, Brighter Bites (BB), to increase fruit and vegetable intake, and home nutrition environment among low-income 1st graders and their parents.	HE & FV, Nutritional knowledge	BB	Houston, Texas	Quasi-experimental non-randomized controlled study	QED	1	x		x	x
Lawlor A.D. et al. [44]	2016	The Active for Life Year 5 (AFLY5) school-based cluster randomised controlled trial: effect on potential mediators	To determine the effect of the intervention on potential mediators	Anthropometry, HE & FV	AFLY5	South East of England	Cluster RCT	RCCT	3	x			x
Steyn P.N. et al. [45]	2016	Did Health kick, a randomised controlled trial primary school nutrition intervention improve dietary quality of children in low-income settings in South Africa?	To promote healthy eating habits and regular physical activity in learners, parents and educators by means of an action planning process	HE & FV, PA	HK	Western Cape (WC) Province	Cluster RCT	RCCT	3	x			
Jones M. et al. [46]	2017	Association between Food for Life, a Whole Setting Healthy and Sustinable Food Programme, and Primary School Children's Consumption of Fruit and Vegetables: A cross Sectional Study in England	The aim of the study was to examine the association between primary school engagement in the Food for Life programme and the consumption of fruit and vegetables by children aged 8–10 years.	HE & FV, Nutritional knowledge	FLP	England	Cross sectional school matched comparison approach	Cross-sectional study design	1	x		x	
Larsen L.A. et al. [47]	2015	RE-AIM analysis of a randomized school-based nutrition intervention among fourth-grade classrooms in California	To promote healthy eating behaviours and attitudes in children	HE & FV, Nutritional knowledge, Attitude	NPP	California	RCT with pre-, post-, and follow-up assessments	RCT	3	x			x

Table 2. *Cont.*

Author	Year	Title/Reference	Main Aim (from Abstract)	Main Aim in Brief	Program Name	Location & Country	Study Design	Study Design Coded	Power	Intervention Components			
											Food Focus		
					Acronym		Column I	RCT, PP, CT, RCCT, Quasi		Information and Teaching	Environmental/Food Focus on Healthy Meal Availability	Environmental/Food Focus through School Gardening	Family/Social Support
Shen, Hu and Sun [48]	2015	Assessment of School-Based Quasi-Experimental Nutrition and Food Safety Health Education for Primary School Students in Two Poverty-Stricken Counties of West China	Aimed to assess the reliability of the knowledge, attitude and behaviour of nutrition and food safety questionnaire for primary school students (Grade 4 to 6) in poverty-stricken counties of China, and evaluate the effectiveness of health education through a quasi experiment, in order to promote policy establishment for child and adolescent health in the future	HE & FV, Nutritional knowledge, Attitude	NFSE	West China (Shaanxi and Yunnan provinces)	Quasi-experimental design	QED	1	x			
Gallotta C.M. et al. [21]	2016	Effects of combined physical education and nutritional programs on schoolchildren's healthy habits	To evaluate the efficacy of three 5-month combined physical education (PE) and nutritional interventions on body composition, physical activity (PA) level, sedentary time and eating habits of schoolchildren	Anthropometry, HE & FV, Nutritional knowledge, PA	ESFS	Rome (Italy)	Randomised Controlled Cluster Trial	RCCT	3	x			x
Fairclough J.S. et al. [49]	2013	Promoting healthy weight in primary school children through physical activity and nutrition education: a pragmatic evaluation of the CHANGE! randomised intervention study	To assess the effectiveness of the CHANGE! intervention on measures of body size, PA and food intake	Anthropometry, HE & FV, PA	CHANGE	Wigan Borough in northwest England, UK	Cluster randomised intervention	RCCT	3	x			
Cunha B.D. et al. [50]	2013	Effectiveness of a randomized school-based intervention involving families and teachers to prevent excessive weight gain among Adolescents in Brazil	To evaluate the effectiveness of a school-based intervention involving the families and teachers that aimed to promote healthy eating habits in adolescents; the ultimate aim of the intervention was to reduce the increase in body mass index (BMI) of the students	Anthropometry, HE & FV, PA	PAPPAS	Duque de Caxias, Rio de Janeiro, Brazil	Paired cluster randomized school-based trial	RCCT	3	x			

Table 2. *Cont.*

Author	Year	Title/Reference	Main Aim (from Abstract)	Main Aim in Brief	Program Name	Location & Country	Study Design	Study Design Coded	Power	Intervention Components			
											Food Focus		
					Acronym		Column I	RCT, PP, CT, RCCT, Quasi		Information and Teaching	Environmental/Food Focus on Healthy Meal Availability	Environmental/Food Focus through School Gardening	Family/Social Support
Aviles O.A. et al. [51]	2017	A school-based intervention improved dietary intake outcomes and reduced waist circumference in adolescents: a cluster randomized controlled trial	The program aimed at improving the nutritional value of dietary intake, physical activity (primary outcomes), body mass index, waist circumference and blood pressure (secondary outcomes)	Anthropometry, HE & FV, PA	ACTIVITAL	Urban area of Cuenca, Ecuador	Pair-matched cluster randomized controlled trial	RCCT	3	x			x
Muros J.J. et al. [52]	2013	Results of a seven-week school-based physical activity and nutrition pilot program on health-related parameters in primary school children in Southern Spain	To determine the effect of nutrition education combined with sessions of vigorous extracurricular physical activity (VEPA) on the improvement of health-related parameters in children in primary education	Anthropometry, HE & FV, PA	VEPA	Southern Spain	Pilot study, PP	QED	1	x			
Moss A et al. [53]	2013	Farm to School and Nutrition Education: Positively Affecting Elementary School-Aged Children's Nutrition Knowledge and Consumption Behavior	To introduce the CATCH nutrition curriculum and Farm to School program to assess nutrition knowledge of 3rd grade students, and increase their fruit and vegetable consumption behavior	HE & FV, Nutritional knowledge	CATCH	Southern Illinois	Quasi-experimental design	QED	1	x			
Zota D. et al. [54]	2016	Promotion of healthy nutrition among students participating in a school food aid program: a randomized trial	To evaluate the potential benefits on students' eating habits, of incorporating healthy nutrition education as part of a school food aid program	Anthropometry, HE & FV	DIATROFI	Greece	Randomised Controlled Trial with the aspects of pre and post intervention questionnarie	RCT	3	x		x	x
Gold A. et al. [55]	2017	Classroom Nutrition Education Combined With Fruit and Vegetable Taste Testing Improves Children's Dietary Intake	To test the classroom curriculum, go wild with fruits & veggies! (GWWFV) effectiveness to increase FV intake of third graders in rural and urban communities in North Dakota	HE & VF	GWWFV	North Dakota	Intervention study with RCT aspects (the schools were randomized to control and intervention school)	RCT, Intervention study	3	x			
Mbhatsani H.V., et al. [56]	2017	Development and Implementation of Nutrition Education on Dietary Diversification for Primary School Children	To ensure that people consume a variety of foods that, together, provide adequate quantities of all the essential micronutrients necessary for health	HE & FV, Nutritional knowledge	NET & HBoIF	Vhembe District of Limpopo Province in South Africa	Quasi-experimental, with a one-group pre-test/post-test intervention	QED	1	x			

Table 2. *Cont.*

Author	Year	Title/Reference	Main Aim (from Abstract)	Main Aim in Brief	Program Name	Location & Country	Study Design	Study Design Coded	Power	Intervention Components			
											Food Focus		
					Acronym		Column I	RCT, PP, CT, RCCT, Quasi		Information and Teaching	Environmental/Food Focus on Healthy Meal Availability	Environmental/Food Focus through School Gardening	Family/Social Support
Hutchinson J. et al. [57]	2015	Evaluation of the impact of school gardening interventions on children's knowledge of and attitudes towards fruit and vegetables. A cluster randomised controlled trial	To evaluate whether ongoing gardening advice and gardening involvement from the Royal Horticultural Society (RHS) gardening specialists was associated with better fruit and vegetable outcomes in children than those at teacherled schools that obtained standard advice from the RHS Campaign for School Gardening	Nutritional knowledge, Attitude	CPSG	London boroughs, Wandsworth, Tower Hamlets, Greenwich and Sutton	Randomised Controlled Cluster Trial	RCCT	3	x	x		
Viggiano A et al. [58]	2018	Healthy lifestyle promotion in primary schools through the board game Kaledo: a pilot cluster randomized trial	The board game Kaledo seems to improve knowledge in nutrition and helps to promote a healthy lifestyle in children attending middle and high schools. So, this study was conducted to investigate whether similar effects of Kaledo could be found in younger children in primary school.	Anthropometry, HE & FV, Nutritional knowledge	Kaledo	Campania, Italy	Pilot cluster randomized trial	RCCT	3	x			
Waters E. et al. [59]	2017	Cluster randomised trial of a school-community child health promotion and obesity prevention intervention: findings from the evaluation of fun 'n healthy in Moreland!	Fun 'n healthy in Moreland! aimed to improve child adiposity, school policies and environments, parent engagement, health behaviours and child wellbeing	Anthropometry, HE & FV	FHM	Victoria, Australia	Randomised Controlled Cluster Trial	RCCT	3	x			
Xu F et al. [60]	2015	Effectiveness of a Randomized Controlled Lifestyle Intervention to Prevent Obesity among Chinese Primary School Students: CLICK-Obesity Study	To evaluate whether the lifestyle intervention was able to reduce obesity risk and increase healthy behaviors and knowledge	Anthropometry, Nutritional knowledge	CLICK-Obesity	Mainland China	Randomised Controlled Cluster Trial	RCCT	3	x			x
Jung et al. [61]	2018	Influence of school-based nutrition education program on healthy eating literacy and healthy food choice among primary school children	To examine the effectiveness of a school-based healthy eating intervention program, the Healthy Highway Program, for improving healthy eating knowledge and healthy food choice behavior among elementary school students	Nutritional knowledge, HE & FV	Healthy highway program	Oswego County, New York State	Pre-/post-test	QED	1	x			

Table 2. *Cont.*

Author	Year	Title/Reference	Main Aim (from Abstract)	Main Aim in Brief	Program Name	Location & Country	Study Design	Study Design Coded	Power	Intervention Components			
											Food Focus		
					Acronym		Column I	RCT, PP, CT, RCCT, Quasi		Information and Teaching	Environmental/Food Focus on Healthy Meal Availability	Environmental/Food Focus through School Gardening	Family/Social Support
Jhou W et al. [62]	2014	Effectiveness of a school-based nutrition and food safety education program among primary and junior high school students in Chongqing, China	To examine the effectiveness of a school-based nutrition and food safety education program among primary and junior high school students in China	Nutritional knowledge, attitude	school-based nutrition and food safety education	Chongqing, China	Pre-/post-test	QED	1	x			
Anderson EL, et al. [63]	2016	Long-term effects of the Active for Life Year 5 (AFLY5) school-based cluster-randomised controlled trial	To investigate the long-term effectiveness of a school-based intervention to improve physical activity and diet in children.	HE & FV, PA	AFLY5	Southwest of England	Randomised Controlled Cluster Trial	RCCT	3	x			
Griffin T.L. et al. [64]	2015	A Brief Educational Intervention Increases Knowledge of the Sugar Content of Foods and Drinks but Does Not Decrease Intakes in Scottish Children Aged 10–12 Years	To assess the effectiveness of an educational intervention to improve children's knowledge of the sugar content of food and beverages	Nutritional knowledge, attitude	NEMS	Aberdeen, Scotland	Randomised Controlled Cluster Trial	RCCT	3	x			
Kipping R.R. et al. [65]	2014	Effect of intervention aimed at increasing physical activity, reducing sedentary behaviour, and increasing fruit and vegetable consumption in children: Active for Life Year 5 (AFLY5) school-based cluster randomised controlled trial	To investigate the effectiveness of a school-based intervention to increase physical activity, reduce sedentary behaviour, and increase fruit and vegetable consumption in children	HE & FV, PA	AFLY5	South west of England	Randomised Controlled Cluster Trial	RCCT	3	x			
Gaar V.M. et al. [66]	2014	Effects of an intervention aimed at reducing the intake of sugar-sweetened beverages in primary school children: a controlled trial	Aimed at reducing children's SSB consumption by promoting the intake of water	Nutritional knowledge, attitude	Water campaign	Rotterdam, Netherland	Controlled trial	CT	2	x			
Moore GF et al. [67]	2014	Impacts of the Primary School Free Breakfast Initiative on socio-economic inequalities in breakfast consumption among 9–11-year-old schoolchildren in Wales	To examine the impacts of the Primary School Free Breakfast Initiative in Wales on inequalities in children's dietary behaviours and cognitive functioning	HE & FV	FSM	Wales, UK	Randomised Controlled Cluster Trial	RCCT	3			x	

Table 2. *Cont.*

Author	Year	Title/Reference	Main Aim (from Abstract)	Main Aim in Brief	Program Name	Location & Country	Study Design	Study Design Coded	Power	Intervention Components			
											Food Focus		
					Acronym		Column I	RCT, PP, CT, RCCT, Quasi		Information and Teaching	Environmental/Food Focus on Healthy Meal Availability	Environmental/Food Focus through School Gardening	Family/Social Support
Nyberg G. et al. [68]	2016	Effectiveness of a universal parental support programme to promote health behaviours and prevent overweight and obesity in 6-year-old children in disadvantaged areas, the Healthy School Start Study II, a cluster-randomised controlled trial	To develop and evaluate the effectiveness of a parental support programme to promote healthy dietary and physical activity habits and to prevent overweight and obesity in six-year-old children in disadvantaged areas	Anthropometry, HE & FV	A Healthy School Start	Stockholm, Sweden	Randomised Controlled Cluster Trial	RCCT	3	x			
Mittmann S., Austel A., and Ellrott T. [69]	2016	Behavioural effects of a short school-based fruit and vegetable promotion programme: 5-a-Day for kids	To evaluate the acceptance of the scheme as well as the short- and intermediate-term effects of the German "5-a-day for kids" project	HE & FV	5-a-day for kids	Hannover, Germany	Pre-/post-test	PP	1	x		x	
Huys N. et al. [70]	2019	Effect and process evaluation of a real-world school garden program on vegetable consumption and its determinants in primary schoolchildren	To investigate the effectiveness of a school garden program on children's vegetable consumption and determinants and to gain insight into the process of the program	HE & FV, Nutritional knowledge	Taste Garden	Ghent, Belgium	Non-equivalent pre-test. Post–test control group design	PP	1	x	x		
Weber K.S. et al. [71]	2017	Positive effects of promoting physical activity and balanced diet in a primary school setting with a high proportion of migrant school children	To evaluate the effects of a school-based intervention offering additional hours of supervised physical activity and dietary education for 3rd and 4th graders in primary schools	HE & FV, Nutritional knowledge	'Be smart. Join in. Be fit.'	Düsseldorf, Germany	Controlled trial	CT	2	x			
Llargue's E. et al. [72]	2016	Four-year outcomes of an educational intervention in healthy habits in schoolchildren: the Avall 3 Trial	To investigate the impact of the intervention on physical activity, BMI and prevalence of overweight and obesity after 4 years	Anthropometry	The Avall project	Granollers, Spain	Randomised Controlled Cluster Trial	RCCT	3	x			
Martins M.L. et al. [73]	2015	Strategies to reduce plate waste in primary schools—experimental evaluation	To determine and compare the effect of two interventions in reducing the plate waste of school lunches	Nutritional Knowledge	Reduce plate waste	City of Porto, Portugal	Controlled trial	CT	2	x		x	

Table 2. *Cont.*

Author	Year	Title/Reference	Main Aim (from Abstract)	Main Aim in Brief	Program Name	Location & Country	Study Design	Study Design Coded	Power	Intervention Components			
											Food Focus		
					Acronym		Column I	RCT, PP, CT, RCCT, Quasi		Information and Teaching	Environmental/Food Focus on Healthy Meal Availability	Environmental/Food Focus through School Gardening	Family/Social Support
Rosario R. et al. [74]	2016	Impact of a school-based intervention to promote fruit intake: a cluster randomized controlled trial	To examine the effects of a six-month dietary education intervention programme, delivered and taught by trained teachers, on the consumption of fruit as a dessert in children aged 6–12 years	HE & FV	Dietary education intervention programme	City in north of Portugal	Randomised Controlled Cluser Trial	RCCT	3	x			
Zafiropulos V. et al. [75]	2015	Preliminary results of a dietary intervention among primary school children	To evaluate the effectiveness of the dietary intervention by measuring body composition and dietary behavior of children prior to and after the intervention	Anthropometry, HE & FV	WBDI	central/eastern Crete Greece	RCT with the aspects of pre and post intervention	RCT	3	x			

Table 3. The review sample-findings. The table shows the findings from the 43 studies of the review.

Author	Year	Age	Age Coded			Sample Size, n	Time Duration/Month	Outcome Measures				Effectiveness Among Children				Target Group	Target Group Coded	
		Years	EA	EML	EL			Anthropometry	HE/FV	Nutritional Knowledge	Attitude	Anthropometry	HE/FV	Nutritional Knowledge	Attitude		S	NS
Harake et al. [35]	2018	6–14 years	x	x	x	183	6	x	x	x	x	3	3	4	2	Syrian refugee children in grade 4 to 6 from three informal primary schools (2 intervention and one control)		x
Adab P, et al. [36]	2018	6–7 years	x			1392	12	x	x			1	1			UK primary schools	x	
Harley A, et al. [37]	2018	11–13 years			x	248	1 and half		x	x			4	4		8 public kindergarten		x
Hermans R.C.J. et al. [38]	2018	10–13 years		x	x	108	N.A.		x	x			1	1		Dutch children (elementary school children)—3 primary school in the souther part of Netherland	x	
Piana N., et al. [39]	2017	7–9 years	x	x		190	4		x	x			4	4		11 primary school classes in five schools	x	
Battjes-Fries M.C.E., et al. [40]	2017	10–11 years		x	x	1010	3		X		X		1		1	children of 34 elementary school grade 6 and 7	x	
Bogart L.M., et al. [41]	2014	N.A.				2997	41		x	x			4	4		10 schools	x	
Shriqui V.K., et al. [42]	2016	4–7 years	x			240	10	x	x	x		2	4	4		Children attending LSES school classes	x	

Table 3. *Cont.*

Author	Year	Age	Age Coded			Sample Size, n	Time Duration/Month	Outcome Measures				Effectiveness Among Children				Target Group	Target Group Coded	
		Years	EA	EML	EL			Anthropometry	HE/FV	Nutritional Knowledge	Attitude	Anthropometry	HE/FV	Nutritional Knowledge	Attitude		S	NS
Sharma S.V. et al. [43]	2016	N.A. (first grade students)	x			172	24		x	x			3	3		Public or charter schools 1st grade students and their family members		x
Lawlor A.D. et al. [44]	2016	9–10 years		x		2221 (valid data for the 10 mediators were available for 87% to 96% of participants	36	x	x			1	1			primary school children	x	
Steyn P.N. et al. [45]	2016	Mean age 9.9 years	x			500 intervention and 498 control	36		x				1			primary school children from low income settings	x	
Jones M. et al. [46]	2017	8–10 years		x		2411	24		x	x			4	4		schools engaged with the Food for Life programme	x	
Larsen L.A. et al. [47]	2015	(fourth grade students) average 9 years	x			1713	2		x	x	x		4	4	3	47 fourth-grade California classrooms	x	
Shen, Hu and Sun [48]	2015	10.80 ± 1.14		x		478	8		x	x	x		4	4	1	Twelve primary schools in west China	x	
Gallotta C.M. et al. [21]	2016	8–11 years		x	x	230	5	x	x	x		3	4	3		three primary schools in the rural area in the north of the city of Rome (Italy)	x	
Fairclough J.S. et al. [49]	2013	10–11 years		x	x	318	6	x	x			3	1			12 primary schools	x	
Cunha B.D. et al. [50]	2013	10–11 years		x	x	574	9	x		x		1		3		20 schools with fifth grade classes	x	
Aviles O.A. et al. [51]	2017	12–14 years			x	1430	28	x	x			2	3			20 schools	x	
Muros J.J. et al. [52]	2013	10–11 years		x	x	54	2	x	x			2	2			2 schools from rular environment with same socio economic status	x	
Moss A et al. [53]	2013	N.A. 3rd grade students				65	1		x	x			3	4		3rd grade students	x	
Zota D. et al. [54]	2016	4–11 years	x	x	x	21261	12	x	x	x		3	4	3		students attending both elementary and secondary schools in areas of low socioeconomic status (SES)	x	

Table 3. *Cont.*

Author	Year	Age	Age Coded			Sample Size, n	Time Duration/Month	Outcome Measures				Effectiveness Among Children				Target Group	Target Group Coded	
		Years	EA	EML	EL			Anthropometry	HE/FV	Nutritional Knowledge	Attitude	Anthropometry	HE/FV	Nutritional Knowledge	Attitude		S	NS
Gold A. et al. [55]	2017	8–9 years		x		662	12		x				4			3rd grade children from 26 schools	x	
Mbhatsani H.V., et al. [74]	2017	9–14 years		x	x	172	6		x	x			3	3		2 rural primary schools with similar socioeconomic backgrounds	x	
Hutchinson J. et al. [57]	2015	7–10 years	x	x		1256	12		x	x	x		3	3	2	21 London schools	x	
Viggiano A et al. [58]	2018	7–11 years	x	x	x	1313	2.5	x	x	x		2	3	3		10 primary schools	x	
Waters E. et al. [59]	2017	5–12 years	x	x	x	2965	42	x	x	x		1	3	3		24 schools of Moreland municipality	x	
Xu F et al. [60]	2015	Mean age 10.2		x		1182	10	x		x		2		3		4th grade students from 8 schools of Nanjing, China	x	
Jung et al. [61]	2018	NA (elementry school-kindergarden, 2nd, 3rd, 4th, 5th and 6th graders)	x	x	x	646	12		x	x	x		2	3	2	2 elementary schools	x	

The information from abstracts were organized in a table with the following information:

Column A: Authors. The column lists the researchers/authors conducting the study.

Column B: Year. The column shows the year of the publication of the article.

Column C: Title/Reference. The column lists the title of the article.

Column D: Main aim. The column lists the main aim presented by authors in the abstract of each article.

Column E: Main aim in brief. This column is a constructed variable that refers to the main aim of each study. The idea was to give in brief the study idea and which outcome measures was focused on in the study.

Column F: Program name. The column gives the name of the project, program or intervention reported in in the article.

Column G: Location and Country. The column lists the specific place or location where the study was performed.

Column H: Study design. The column shows research design of the study according to authors.

Column I: Study design coded. This column is a constructed variable to capture the research design of the study and used to make an analysis of power possible, see Column J.

Column J: Power. The column was constructed to express the strength of the design. It is a dummy variable that was assigned a numerical value that allowed for a quantitative analytical approach.

Column K, L and M: Intervention components. The column shows which intervention components that was used in the study. We used a model that categorizes components into three different mechanisms of influence: cognitive (K), environmental (L, M, N) and social (O).

The environmental component includes actions where availability of meals—or fruit and vegetable (F & V)—were increased. Either through passive provision (F & V and meals) or through active participation such as gardening. The social category included actions where families and/or peers were actively influencing the participants. The cognitive category included teaching and learning.

Column L: Environmental/food focus on F & V. In this column, interventions which were targeted towards fruits and vegetables were flagged. This includes interventions whose focus was providing cooking lessons and maintaining healthy cafeterias during the intervention periods. Also, maintaining healthy cafeteria here refers to school canteens providing healthy options to its menu where children's while buying food have healthier options to choose.

Column M: Environmental/food focus on increasing availability through school gardening. In this column, interventions which provided free foods among participants through gardening within the school were listed.

Column N: Environmental/food interventions focused on healthy meal availability. Interventions which provided healthy meals, breakfast, snacks during the school hours and distributed fresh fruits among the participants were listed in this column.

Column O: Family/social support. In this column interventions that included social components were flagged. These interventions included peer and family influence mechanisms.

Column P: Age. The column lists the age of the targeted groups of the intervention expressed in years according to the primary article data provided by authors.

Column Q: Age construct EA. This column shows a constructed variable for the age categorization based on the primary data given by authors. The constructed code was made to make statistical analyses possible. The construct Early Age (EA) was assigned if intervention were carried out in early school.

Column R: Age construct EML. This column shows a constructed variable for the age categorization based on the primary data given by authors. The code Early Middle Late (EML) was assigned if intervention was targeted all age groups.

Column S: Age construct EL. This column shows a constructed variable for the age categorization based on the primary data given by authors. The code EL refers to Early late and was assigned if the intervention was targeted early and early and late school.

Column T: Sample size. The number of young people enrolled in the intervention was listed in this column.

Column U: Time duration. This column shows the length of the intervention expressed in months. It is a constructed variable based on the primary data given by authors and was made to standardize duration and make it ready for cross study analysis.

Columns V, W, X, Y: Outcome measures. In Columns T, U, V, W, the outcome measures named as Anthropometry, HE/FV (healthy eating fruits and vegetables), Nutritional knowledge, and Attitude, respectively, were listed according to our outcome model shown in Figure 1. Only a few include all outcome measures, but all studies included at least one of them.

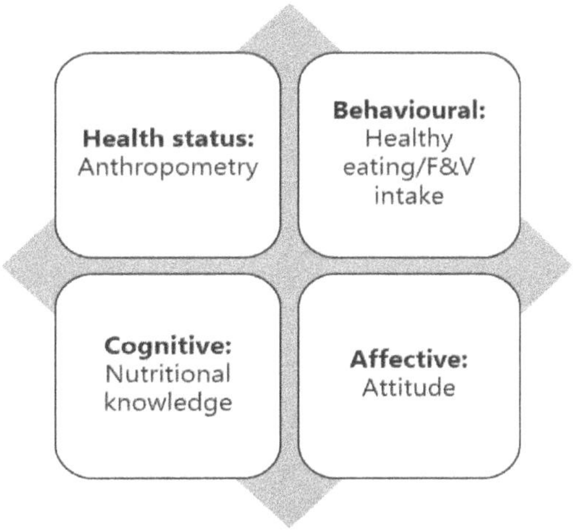

Figure 1. Outcome measures model. The figure illustrates the four types of outcome measures found in the interventions.

Columns X, AA, AB, AC: Effectiveness. The effectiveness as measured by the outcomes measured are listed in this column. Each outcome measure was rated using a Likert scale from 0–4. The effectiveness of outcome measures among participants as measured by the measures in our model (Figure 1): attitude, anthropometry, HE/FV, nutritional knowledge and attitude were listed in the Columns X, Y, Z, AA, respectively.

Column AD: Target group. This column provides information on the target group of interventions such as information on grades of subjects and municipalities.

Columns AE, AF: Target group. This column is a constructed variable created to capture if the intervention had a special ethnic or socio-economic focus. Columns AC and AD consisted of coded target group named as Standard (S) and Non-Standard (NS). The "NS" here represents the target group either from refugees or immigrants or lower socio-economic classes.

Column AG: Keywords. This column lists the keywords found in the interventions.

Ordinary least squares regression was applied in this study; specifically, we used the linear regression function in IBM SPSS 22. We opted for a multi-variate approach; i.e., multiple linear regression was used. Anthropometry, behaviour (healthy eating and food focus), attitude and nutritional knowledge were used as dependent variables. In order to better account for control variables, such as sample size and study length, a dummy variable was introduced for study length of one year and more; and a logarithm of the sample size was used instead of the actual sample size to eliminate scaling effects. We grouped countries by continents (while splitting Europe into North and South as there were enough studies and no countries in between) and introduced related dummy variables. The remaining variables were used as independent variables without any additional manipulations.

Since the aim was to create models consisting only of independent variables that significantly influence the dependent variables, we used the backwards function. Because there were too many independent variables for the backwards function for the attitude model (with only eight observations), the stepwise function was used instead.

Information and teaching was present in all but one study. Free food was found only in two studies and focus on fruit and vegetables in three studies. Therefore, it is not surprising that neither of the three variables were found to be significant in any of the models.

2.7. Study Sample

The search strategy resulted in 1826 titles which were screened for duplicates and potential relevance. After this initial screening, 345 titles and abstracts were assessed against the inclusion and exclusion criteria. Articles that studied school interventions after school hours were excluded. In addition, articles which studied interventions among children in out of school context such as at community level were excluded. The justification is that both "after school" and "out of school" since can be regarded as non-typical school environments. We aimed to study the "school" as an artefact that can be considered as a "standard" across countries despite some national differences. For both "after school" and "out of school", we argue that there are considerable differences among countries and that an inclusion of such studies would negatively influence our analytical approach. In total, 42 articles were identified as relevant and full papers were obtained as the final sample. Figure 2 below illustrates the search terms and selection process of articles.

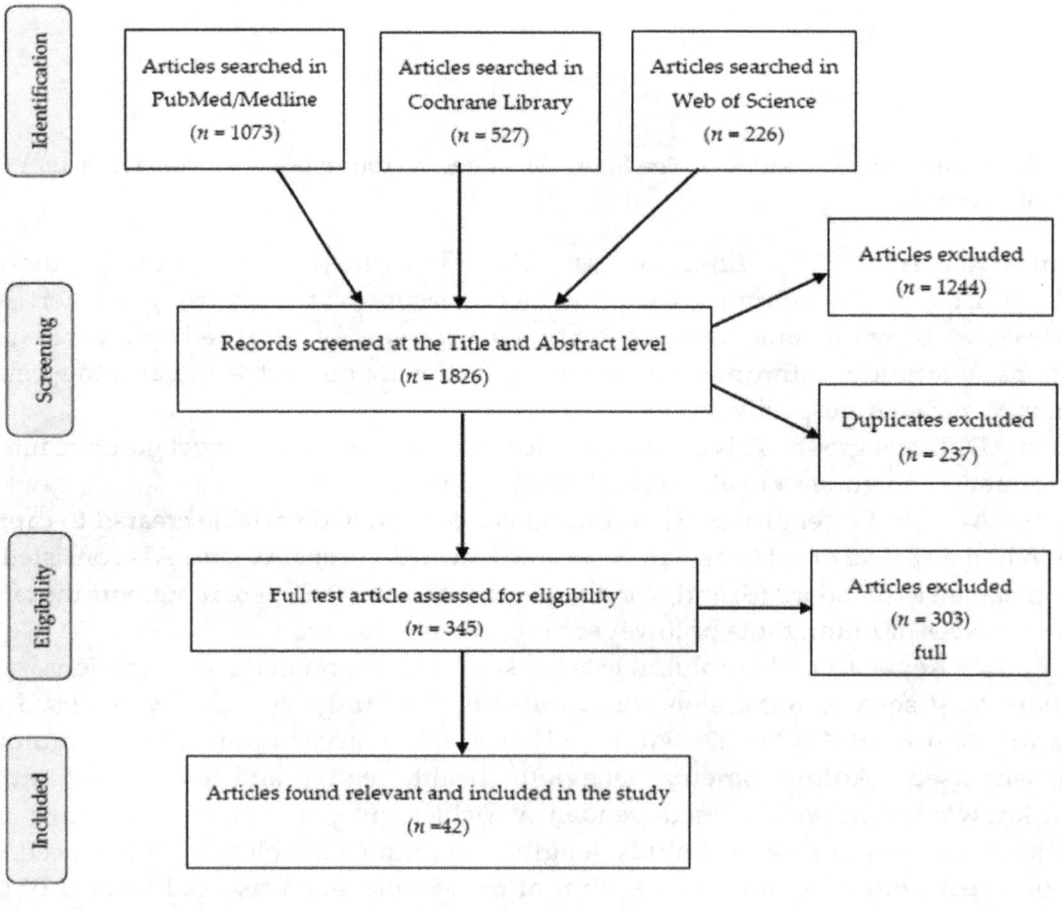

Figure 2. Review flow chart. The figure shows the progress of the literature review process following the PRISMA 2009 approach.

2.8. Intervention Study Characteristics

For all 43 items in our sample, Table 2 provides the information about the study, intervention methodologies, characteristics strategies, etc. In our extract of studies, the sample size ranged from 65-2997 subjects/participants, and the intervention duration ranged from 1 and half month to 36 months. The systematic review locations identified by the author were: 26 from Europe [21,36,38–40,44,46,49,52,54,57,58,63–75], six from Asia [35,42,48,59,60,62], 10 from America [37,41,43,45,47,50,51,53,55,61] and one from Africa [56]. We categorized all interventions according to their intervention components. To this end, we had constructed three classes: Information and Teaching, Food Focus and Family/Social support as illustrated. The interventions characteristics of each included study are shown in Table 2.

Of the total study sample, the majority of studies (n = 41) involved "Information and Teaching" components consisting mainly of classroom-based activities (e.g., an adapted curriculum and distribution of educational materials, health and nutrition education program). Another 12 studies along with "Information and Teaching" involved a food focus and availability component. These food and availability components which consisted mainly of supervised school gardening, environmental modifications to stimulate a more healthful diet, such as increased availability and accessibility of healthy foods, distributions free food programmes, school provided free breakfast, school lunch modifications and incentives. Only two studies combined all the three intervention components of this study. Family/social support intervention was clearly focused on in nine study. In other studies, even though their interventions were not primarily or secondarily focused on family/social support component, they indirectly acknowledged the importance of parents and included them in their studies.

All of the reviewed studies included intervention components that were delivered in school settings and within school hours. Our sample showed that consumption of fruit and vegetables was the most used intervention component and was include in more than half of the interventions. Most studies were designed and carried in a way where a research assistant was trained by senior researchers/co-authors to ensure that each members of the research team followed same procedures for data collection. Since all studies were "in situ" studies included a close researcher/school staff cooperation component. In most of the listed studies, teachers being the responsible person to implement the interventions were trained beforehand.

2.9. *Types of Interventions*

Table 2 shows an overview of the programmes and their intervention components. From the table, it can be seen that studies differed according to how broadly they intervened. Some studies have included a narrow intervention (i.e., only one intervention components which targeted behavioural components), whereas others included multicomponent approaches where all three intervention components were used in the study.

3. Results

Finding the right approach to intervening for healthier eating at school is a major challenge. In other words, which interventions create which impacts and how should the public best invest in new policies, strategies, and practices at school if long term health is the intended end point?

The purpose of this review was to compile the evidence regarding the effectiveness of successful school-based interventions in improving dietary behaviours, nutritional knowledge, attitudes and anthropometry among children. The analysis of the data showed a number of relationships between outcome effect and a number of other characteristics of the intervention (i.e., age, location/region, intervention type, duration). Descriptive statistics are provided in Table 4.

Table 4. Descriptive statistics.

	N	Minimum	Maximum	Mean	Standard Deviation
Power	42	1.00	3.00	2.2619	0.91223
InfoAndTeach	42	0.00	1.00	0.9762	0.15430
FandV	42	0.00	1.00	0.0714	0.26066
FreeFood	42	0.00	1.00	0.0476	0.21554
AvailFood	42	0.00	1.00	0.1667	0.37720
FamilySocialSupport	42	0.00	1.00	0.2143	0.41530
EA—early age	42	0.00	1.00	0.3810	0.49151
EML—early middle late age	42	0.00	1.00	0.7381	0.44500
EL—early late age	42	0.00	1.00	0.5476	0.50376
SampleSize	42	54.00	21261.00	1464.2619	3277.18184
log10SampleSize	42	1.73	4.33	2.7904	0.54986
Months	41	1.00	112.00	14.6585	19.00245
YearOrMore01	41	0.00	1.00	0.4390	0.50243
AnthropometryScale	18	0.00	4.00	2.0000	1.13759
HEFVScale	36	1.00	4.00	2.5556	1.27491
NutritionalKnowledgeScale	26	1.00	4.00	3.1923	0.89529
AttitudeScale	9	1.00	3.00	1.7778	0.66667

The linear regression models carried out for each intervention component is added in the text and the tables have been referred to each associated result. Out of 42 studies, 36 studies reported the outcome on HE/FV behaviour scale while anthropometry and attitude impacts were observed in 18 and six studies, respectively. The item one of the results in this article presents the most general finding from the literature review, item two describes the variable found significant in two cases, while the remaining variables were significant in once case each. Additionally, item four, five and six are related "design" phenomena effects in the sense that they are not related to intervention components but to the study was designed your study. The rest is related to (intervention components rather than designs. In Table 5, the outcome measures for which an effect could be seen has been listed. The linear regression model describing what influences the attitude is provided in Table 6.

Table 5. Linear regression model for attitude.

Model	Unstandardized Coefficients		Standardized Coefficients	t	Significance
	B	SE	Beta		
(Constant)	1.250	0.177		7.071	0.000
FamilySocialSupport	1.000	0.395	0.500	2.530	0.045
EA—early age	0.750	0.250	0.593	3.000	0.024

Table 6. Linear regression model for anthropometry.

Model	Unstandardized Coefficients		Standardized Coefficients	t	Significance
	B	SE	Beta		
(Constant)	4.140	1.008		4.109	0.001
Power	1.511	0.468	0.859	3.231	0.007
AvailFood	3.432	0.804	0.976	4.267	0.001
YearOrMore	0.870	0.403	0.384	2.161	0.050
log10SampleSize	−2.437	0.503	−1.267	−4.846	0.000

With regards to the explanatory power of the model, $R^2 = 0.789$, R^2 adj. $= 0.719$, and significance $= 0.009$. The linear regression model describing what influences the anthropometry is provided in Table 6. With regards to the explanatory power of the model, $R^2 = 0.683$, R^2 adj. $= 0.586$, and significance $= 0.003$. The linear regression model describing what influences the behaviour is provided in Table 7.

Table 7. Linear regression model for behaviour.

Model	Unstandardized Coefficients		Standardized Coefficients		t	Significance
	B	SE	Beta			
(Constant)	2.321	0.229		10.131	0.000	
FamilySocialSupport	1.054	0.486	0.348	2.168	0.037	

With regards to the explanatory power of the model, $R^2 = 0.121$, R^2 adj. $= 0.096$, and significance = 0.037.

An alternative linear regression model describing what influences the behaviour is provided in Table 8.

Table 8. Alternative linear regression model for behaviour.

Model	Unstandardized Coefficients		Standardized Coefficients	t	Significance
	B	SE	Beta		
(Constant)	3.227	0.205		15.761	0.000
Neurope	−1.727	0.328	−0.670	−5.260	0.000

With regards to the explanatory power of the model, $R^2 = 0.449$, R^2 adj. $= 0.432$, and significance < 0.001.

3.1. School-Based Interventions in General Create Impact

Looking across the whole study sample, it can be seen that in general the interventions created an impact in one or more ways either on knowledge, intentions, eating habits and/or anthropometry. In other words, it was hard to find studies that created no impact. This finding adds to the body of evidence that suggests that food-based interventions are a well-suited and effective policy tool when it comes to promoting healthier eating among young people.

3.2. Family Support Affects Healthier Eating Behaviour and Attitude

Out of all the included studies, nine studies focused on family support as an intervention component. But out of those, our analysis showed that the family involvement was impactful among participants when it comes to promoting healthier food choices. Parents being influencers and role models in the family in these studies seemed to help to influence children's dietary habits. Studies which involved participants' parents in the intervention and provided them with nutritional knowledge and healthy cooking skills (i.e., knowledge about the importance of healthy food and nutrition during the early age of their children), seemed to be able to help young people prepare more healthy and nutritious food at home. As studies showed, this seemed to increase children's intentions towards eating more fruits and vegetables and eventually resulted in consumption of more healthy foods. However, this did not seem to be the case for all ages. Intention to eat more fruits and vegetables was seen among early age participants (EA) either alone or with family support. It should be noted that the regression models did not include interactions, since the number of analysed studies was only ~40. It was not possible to include age as a continuous variable in the models because (as it can be seen in Table 5) age was a range, and sometimes even a wide range, e.g., 8–11 or 4–11. Family support increases the outcome measure by approximately 1 in both cases. Please refer to Tables 5 and 7 for detailed linear regression model used for attitude and behaviour.

3.3. Interventions Done in Northern Europe (7 Studies) Had a Smaller Impact on Behaviour than the Studies Conducted in the Rest of the World (22 Studies)

The results from the models which was created to measure the efficiency of HE/FV highlighted the fact that HE/FV scale depends only on region where the intervention was done. The behaviour outcome for Northern Europe was on average 1.5 while the average for the rest was 3.2 (please refer to Table 8).

3.4. Effect of Anthropometry Measures Increases with Study Power

The results suggested that the design of the study plays a role when it comes to be able to show impact of interventions. From the findings, it was clear that the anthropometry measured among the participants were increasing with the power of the study. That is, the stronger the design the greater the likelihood of being able to measure impact on anthropometric outcomes—a unit increase in the design power is associated with an outcome increase of approximately 1.5 (please refer to Table 6). To examine the influence of study design we used the score that was constructed for the purpose (please refer to Table 1). This score assigns a higher power to randomized designs than non-randomized ones.

3.5. Study Duration Impacts Anthropometric Outcomes

It was also clear that the intervention duration does have impact on the outcome, i.e., the longer the duration better the anthropometric results among the children. Interventions that lasted a year or more, had the outcome measure on average almost one unit higher than shorter studies (please refer to Table 6).

3.6. Larger Samples Impacts Anthropometry Measures

Results showed that anthropometric outcome decreased within the sample size. Increasing the sample size by a factor of 10, from approximately 100 to 1000, decreased the outcome measure by almost 2.5 (please refer to Table 6). Thus, bigger the sample size a reverse effect on outcome was obtained. The studies whose intervention was done for long period of time (i.e., couple of months or year and among small participants) were found to be effective in the outcome. It might be the case that it was hard to administer the same thing to large sample size post intervention and thus could have decreased the anthropometry outcome among the participants.

3.7. Food Availability Interventions Influence Anthropometric Outcomes

Our analyses showed that a food focus, specifically healthy meal availability had an impact on the children's anthropometric outcomes—increasing it by almost 3.5 on average (please refer to Table 6).

3.8. Interventions among Younger Students Influence Attitude Among Participants

Results showed that the younger the study subjects were, the more influence interventions had on attitudes (the outcome was on average 0.75 higher than for other age groups). Thus, the result suggests that the participants' attitude increases when they are in their early age (EA) i.e., 4–7 years old. Furthermore, results suggest that increased family support associated with participants' attitude towards healthy eating helps in changing the behaviour among them. Early age (EA) and family support seemed to impact positively both alone and together. Meaning that the intervention had positive impacts on participants (i.e., EA participants) attitudes towards healthy eating either with the involvement of their family support or without the involvement of family support. Please refer to Table 5 for detail linear regression model for attitude.

3.9. No Effect of School Based Interventions on Nutritional Knowledge

Findings showed that nutritional knowledge among participants (i.e., of all age group) does not depend on school-based interventions. Thus, none of the collected variables have influences on nutritional knowledge.

4. Discussion

4.1. Discussion of Results of This Review in Relation to Others

In the discussion we aim to relate our findings with what has been found in previous studies, discuss our methodological approach and reflect on what are the policy implications. Since the discussion on how to counteract the unhealthy eating pattern and the worrying increase in nutrition related disorders among young people is attracting much attention and since the discussion on how the school could contribute we aim to give policy makers and practitioners an up to date insight into the potentials of the school to act as a hub for promotion of healthier eating and provide inspiration for the development of new types of school-based interventions and strategies.

The huge interest in using the infrastructure of the school to initiate and promote healthier eating among young people has resulted in a large number of interventions studies over the past decades. This research interest per definition as the same time creates a need for syntheses of the findings in order to make them feed into the public health and school policy cycle and to "send the results to work". Taken the huge investment that better food at school strategies at school will cost for states it is worth appreciating that the Evidence-Informs-Policy pathway seems to be working. At the same time the conceptual approaches and the understanding of what intervention components might work better than others, which age groups might benefit the most etc. as developed considerably which again adds to the rationale for synthesis of intervention study findings. Most recent reviews by Julie et al. [76], Noguera el al. [77], Evans et al. [78], Cauwenberghe et al. [34] and Brown et al. [79] has created a time gap of almost five years. Covering the last five years of research our review makes a needed contribution and in addition we argue it makes a needed contribution to a standardization and conceptualization of both sampling and intervention design methodologies.

Overall, the findings from this review suggest that school-based interventions that include intervention components such as information and teaching, food focus and family support are effective in improving the HE/FV, anthropometric measurements and attitude towards healthy dietary behaviour among the participants. On the other hand, nutritional knowledge among participants did not seem to be influenced much by any of the intervention components used.

Impacts on HE/FV behaviours were observed, but mostly among early age children revealing a distinct age pattern in the findings. Thus, age was seen as a significant factor in determining effectiveness in several study [35,37,39,42]. Impact was greater on young children in the 4–7 year old age range, suggesting that dietary influences may vary with age.

Multicomponent approaches that includes good quality instruction and programs, a supportive social environment both at school and home, family support has been effective in addressing childhood related diseases through focusing on diet and physical activity. Most of the studies in this review implemented with combination of school staff and intervention specialists provide evidence for the effectiveness of the program. Thus, evidence supports that family involvement and nutrition education curriculum delivered by the teacher under supervision of intervention specialists can alter the intake of fruit and vegetables while impacting positively on anthropometric measurements. Teacher led interventions have been effective and can be the most sustainable approach for long term impact of the program. The same conclusion was found in a review done in investigating the effectiveness of school-based interventions in Europe which provided the effectiveness of multicomponent intervention promoting a healthy diet in school aged children in Europe [34].Studies with a food focus in their intervention approaches showed significant improvements in BMI [35,54,58]. Significant improvements in BMI here refers to the studies whose probability value was less or equal to 0.05. This means that the interventions in that case showed reduction in body mass of participants. We looked at studies whose aim was to focus on interventions of obesity prevention or reduction among primary school children's. Thus, search term such as: "obesity prevention intervention among primary schools", was used as explained in the methods section. When performing the search for school-based interventions we did not encounter any studies that were focusing on underweight. Making the options for healthy choices of food in the school cafeterias and having the option of free food from the school gardens decreases the sugar sweetened beverages and junk options among the children's and thus resulting in improvements in BMI. This review evidence further highlights that duration of the intervention, i.e., a year or more has an impact on anthropometric measurements. This is in contrast to reviews of Julie et al. [76] and Cauwenberghe et al. [34] review that found that making the better options of food choices and duration of the studies were effective in reducing the sedentary behaviour and noting improvements in BMI. This study also found that larger sample sizes reverse the outcome of anthropometric measurements (i.e., sample size negatively influences the outcome). This might be the case because it might be harder to administer the same thing to more individual. Thus, more studies are needed to examine the effects of bigger sample sizes.

Our study is far from being the first to create overview of the large number of studies that are studying interventions that can promote healthier eating habits and that can counteract the worrying increase in obesity and overweight among young people the general. The huge interest is reflected in the number of studies trying to assess the impact and effectiveness of school-based interventions as well as in the number of reviews aiming to synthesize the findings from the growing body of evidence of the effect of school-based food interventions into actionable school food policies. Our study adds to this body of knowledge and fills a gap since our study looks at the most recent studies.

Comparing our review with others we find that the majority of the studies on school food-based interventions have been conducted in high income countries. This is also the case in our study and this fact is important to keep in mind since it introduces a bias in the insight created from school food effectiveness reviews. It is also important to keep in mind that studies—and as a result also reviews-covers different types of school food cultures. These cultures can roughly be divided in collective, semi collective and non-collective types. In the collective type found in countries such as Sweden, Finland, Estonia and Brazil school food provision is an integrated—and mainly free—part of the school day. In semi-collective approaches food is in most cases traditionally a part of what is offered at school, but due to payment. In the non-collective approach found in countries such as Denmark, Norway and the Netherlands there is little infrastructure and tradition for school organized foodservice. In this approach parents organized lunch boxes as well as competitive foods traditionally play a bigger role.

A further important note to make is the distinction between narrow F & V approaches and broader healthier eating intervention approaches. This classification can also be seen in previous studies and in more recent reviews. The first type of interventions that follow the six-a-day tradition that to some extent has been fuelled by the European School Fruit program introduced by the EU in 2009 was reviewed by Noguera et al. [77] and by Evans et al. [78]. In a study by Noguera el al. [77] a meta-analysis on F&V interventions was done but limited to educational interventions in the sense that it only looked at computer-based interventions and covering mostly European research. The study showed that this targeted but narrowed approach was effective in increasing FV consumption but that broader multicomponent types of interventions including free/subsidized FV interventions were not effective. In the review paper from 2012 by Evans et al. [78] examined studies done in United Kingdom, United States, Canada, Denmark, New Zealand, Norway and the Netherlands. Evans and co-workers [78] found that school-based interventions were able to moderately improve fruit intake but that they had only minimal impact on vegetable intake. These reviews and previous ones generally conclude that F&V targeted interventions are able to improve young people's eating patterns towards higher intake of fruit.

In the category of reviews taking a broader approach to healthier lifestyle promotion we find studies and reviews that looks at promotion of healthier eating in general—and that in some cases include physical activity. A review by Julie et al. [76] covered studies from United States, United Kingdom, Australia, Spain and the Netherlands. This review also included physical activity as part of broader school-based obesity prevention interventions. In particular, interventions should focus on extending physical education classes, incorporating activity breaks, and reducing sedentary behaviours to improve anthropometric measures. Julie et al. concluded that interventions taking a broader approach should include employing a combination of school staff and intervention specialists to implement programs; that they should include psychosocial/psychoeducational components; involve peer leaders; use incentives to increase fruit and vegetable consumption and should involve family. In a study by Cauwenberghe et al. [34] intervention studies done in a European union studies were reviewed. This review—as our study do—made an age distinction in the sense that a categorization was done between children and adolescents. Among children the authors found a strong evidence of effect for multicomponent interventions on fruit and vegetable intake. For educational type of interventions Cauwenberghe et al. [34] found limited evidence of effect as found when looking at behaviour and fruit and vegetable intakes. The study found limited evidence on effectiveness of interventions that specifically targeted children from lower socio-economic status groups. For adolescents Cauwenberghe et al. [34] found moderate evidence of effect was found for educational interventions on behaviour and limited evidence of effect for multicomponent programmes on behaviour. In the same way as our review authors distinguished between behaviour and anthropometrics and found that effects on anthropometrics were often not measured in their sample. Therefore, evidence was lacking and resulted in inconclusive evidence. Cauwenberghe et al. [34] concluded that there was evidence was found for the effectiveness of especially multicomponent interventions promoting a healthy diet but that evidence for effectiveness on anthropometrical obesity-related measures was lacking. In a review by Brown et al. [79] studies mostly from Europe but also covering United States, New Zealand, Canada and Chile it was found that intervention components most likely to influence BMI positively included increased physical activity, decreased sugar sweetened beverages intake, and increased fruit intake.

Our review adds to the increasing support for the idea that school should play a role in promoting healthier eating habits among young people. As such the school can be seen as an important actor when it comes to the promotion of human rights. In particular; the right to adequate food, the right to the highest attainable standard of health and right to the education, school plays an integral part which has also been highlighted in the "United Nations System Standing Committee on Nutrition" new statement for school-based and nutrition interventions [25]. Furthermore, Mikkelsen and colleagues [80] in their study have also suggested the fact that the international framework of human rights should invoke its strategies, policies, and regulations in the context of school and that national, regional, and local level actors has important roles to play. Additionally, they have highlighted that ensuring healthy eating in school environment can be a good investment in children short- and long-term health and education achievements. Thus, schools, as a system have the potential to make lasting improvements in students nutrition both in terms of quality and quantity and simultaneously contribute to realization of human rights around the globe [25].

4.2. *Discussion of Methods*

Strengths and Limitations

All attempts to reduce complexity of research studies in a research field suffers from in built weaknesses. Standardising the work of others in attempts to make generalizations is always difficult. As per definition a review includes attempts to standardize its study material in order to create an overview of "what works" and what "this that works" depends on. For obvious reasons research protocols depends very much on the context of the study: What is doable in one study setting on one country might not work on other settings. Additionally, reporting procedures vary among authors. The aim of a review is to standardize this heterogeneity to something that is homogenous and computable. So, in our case our constructs represent an attempt to make different studies with similar but slightly different approaches and methodologies comparable by making them computable. This has obviously some disadvantages.

Another limitation is that our review restricted itself to cover only published English language articles. Therefore, publication bias cannot be excluded, as it is possible that the inclusion of unpublished articles written in other languages than English will have affected the results of this review. Second, most of the studies included in the present were carried out in countries from Southern and Northern parts of Europe. This raises questions about the generalisability of these results to other countries in Europe, especially because contextual variables were often lacking in the included studies. And the same questions about the generalisability could be raise in other parts of the world i.e., in Latin America, North America, Asia and Africa, as very few studies were reported from this part of the world.

On the other hand, large dropouts were reported in many listed studies and the study follow up were reported in few studies and was for short time period. Among these studies which did follow up, was right after the end of the intervention period and thus this could have affected the effectiveness among this study outcomes. Long-term follows-up post-interventions would help to study the retention of behaviour change and effect on the body composition among the participants. Thus, long terms studies post interventions are needed to draw the conclusion about the sustainability of an intervention. Additionally, in future studies to improve the quality of the evidence of effectiveness in this kind of interventions, studies with high quality, rigorous design, appropriate sample size, post interventions long term follow up, assessment of implementation issues and cost effectiveness of the intervention should be executed.

On the strength side the standardisation approach helps to find patterns and to create overview of a large material within a given field of research. The strength of this study is that it provides a broad up to date overview of what is known about the relationship between school-based intervention and policies and healthy eating outcomes among children and that it contributes to the deeper understanding of the fact that current research findings are quite limited. This is among the very few recent reviews which evaluated the effect of school-based food at nutrition interventions among children only. A systematic review approach of this study attempted efficiently to integrate existing information and provide data for researchers' rationale in the decision making of future research. Furthermore, the applied explicit methods used in this limited bias and, contributed to improved reliability and accuracy of drawn conclusions. Other advantages are that this study looks specifically at the evidence available in Northern and Southern Europe. Statistical analyses of pooled data have facilitated a more through synthesis of the result is one of the biggest strengths of this study.

4.3. Policy Implications

The evidence of the impact of school intervention derived from our review suggests several topics to be dealt with in future research not only in Europe but also the other part of the world. First, this review highlights the need for researchers to recognize the importance of further investigations on the measures of anthropometrics, nutritional knowledge, and attitude. Among these 42 studies carried out in different regions very few looked upon the effects on participants' attitudes and anthropometrics measures. And of those showed positive impact if family support was provided, if started at early age and lastly if food focus was part of the intervention. Additionally, most of the included studies were not aiming to contribute to obesity prevention. Thus, it is highly recommendable that there is urgent need for more studies to be done that includes more measures of efficiency of participants' attitude towards the healthy behaviour and healthy lifestyle and measures for anthropometrics. Second, to increase the comparability between studies and to facilitate the assessment of effectiveness, more agreement is needed for best measures of the diet and questionnaires. Third, more research is needed to be done among specific groups like low socio-economic group, immigrants or minorities. As mention earlier, only few listed studies included this specific group in their studies. Furthermore, evidence suggest that health inequalities such as prevalence of overweight are as a result of dietary habits and ethnicity and socio-economic status are identified as determinants of health eating. Thus, future research should not exclude these specific groups as European countries have become ethnically diverse.

To improve or decrease childhood diseases such as overweight and obesity and other aspects of health, many policy documents have been calling for the development of the effective strategies among children's and adolescents. Even though the limited to moderate impact and evidence was found among these school-based interventions, it should be noted that interventions were not primarily targeting obesity prevention but, in many cases, had a broader scope. Thus, in order to deliver these evidence-based recommendations to policy makers factors such as sustainability of intervention, context and cost effectiveness should be considered. Additionally, the policy makers should ensure school policies and the environment that encourage physical activity and a healthy diet.

5. Conclusions

Findings from this systematised review suggest that applying multicomponent interventions (environmental, educational, and physical strategies) along with parental involvement and of long-term initiatives may be promising for improving dietary habits and other childhood related diseases among primary school children. Despite being challenging to find experimental studies done in related fields, those studies found showed positive trend. Thus, to conclude, evidence of the effect was found among school-based food and nutrition initiatives among primary school children. However, to strengthen the perspectives of this study, further systematic review targeting the more long-term studies assessing the long-term sustainability of the interventions should be considered. Also, studies with goal to increase efficiency of anthropometric measurements in their future school-based interventions could include increasing PA, increasing fruit and vegetable intake and decreasing sedentary behaviour. This study has provided fundamentals background on which further research could be done in this area of school-based food and nutrition interventions. Thus, the findings from this systematic review can be used as guidelines for future interventions in school settings related to food and nutrition. Also, the categorization of intervention components we see as useful for the planning of future interventions.

Author Contributions: Conceptualization, B.E.M. and A.C.; methodology, B.E.M., A.C. and F.S.; validation B.E.M.; formal analysis, F.S.; investigation, A.C.; resources B.E.M. and A.C.; data curation, A.C. and F.S.; writing—original draft preparation, B.E.M., A.C. and F.S.; writing—review and editing, B.E.M., A.C. and F.S.; project administration, B.E.M. All authors have read and agreed to the published version of the manuscript.

References

1. Micha, R.; Karageorgou, D.; Bakogianni, I.; Trichia, E.; Whitsel, L.P.; Story, M.; Penalvo, J.L.; Mozaffarian, D. Effectiveness of school food environment policies on children's dietary behaviors: A systematic review and meta-analysis. *PLoS ONE* **2018**, *13*, e0194555. [CrossRef]
2. WHO Europe. *Food and Nutrition Policy for Schools Copenhagen, Security PfNaF*; WHO: Geneva, Switzerland, 2006.
3. EU Commission. *EU Action Plan on Childhood Obesity 2014–2020*; EU Commission: Brussels, Belgium, 2014.
4. Lytle, L.A.; Kubik, M.Y. Nutritional issues for adolescents. *Best Pract. Res. Clin. Endocrinol. Metab.* **2003**, *17*, 177–189. [CrossRef]
5. WHO. Obesity and Overweight 2020. Available online: https://www.who.int/news-room/fact-sheets/detail/obesity-and-overweight (accessed on 20 July 2020).
6. WHO. *Diet, Nutrition and The Prevention of Chronic Diseases*; Contract No.: WHO Technical Report Series 916; WHO: Geneva, Switzerland, 2003.
7. Serra-Paya, N.; Ensenyat, A.; Castro-Vinuales, I.; Real, J.; Sinfreu-Bergues, X.; Zapata, A.; Mur, J.M.; Galindo-Ortego, G.; Solé-Mir, E.; Teixido, C. Effectiveness of a Multi-Component Intervention for Overweight and Obese Children (Nereu Program): A Randomized Controlled Trial. *PLoS ONE* **2015**, *10*, e0144502. [CrossRef] [PubMed]
8. Hruby, A.; Hu, F.B. The Epidemiology of Obesity: A Big Picture. *Pharmacoeconomics* **2015**, *33*, 673–689. [CrossRef] [PubMed]
9. WHO. *Interim Report of the Commission on Ending Childhood Obesity*; WHO: Geneva, Switzerland, 2015.
10. Aceves-Martins, M.; Llauradó, E.; Tarro, L.; Moreno-García, C.F.; Trujillo Escobar, T.G.; Sola, R.; Giralt, M. Effectiveness of social marketing strategies to reduce youth obesity in European school-based interventions: A systematic review and meta-analysis. *Nutr. Rev.* **2016**, *74*, 337–351. [CrossRef] [PubMed]

11. Cali, A.M.G.; Caprio, S. Obesity in children and adolescents. *J. Clin. Endocrinol. Metab.* **2008**, *93*, S31–S36. [CrossRef]
12. Abdelaal, M.; le Roux, C.W.; Docherty, N.G. Morbidity and mortality associated with obesity. *Ann. Transl. Med.* **2017**, *5*, 161. [CrossRef] [PubMed]
13. WHO. Child and Adolescent Health Copenhagen: UN City 2019. Available online: http://www.euro.who.int/en/health-topics/Life-stages/child-and-adolescent-health/child-and-adolescent-health (accessed on 20 July 2020).
14. Lynch, C.; Kristjansdottir, A.G.; Te Velde, S.J.; Lien, N.; Roos, E.; Thorsdottir, I.; Krawinkel, M.; de Almeida, M.D.V.; Papadaki, A.; Ribic, C.H.; et al. Fruit and vegetable consumption in a sample of 11-year-old children in ten European countries—The PRO GREENS cross-sectional survey. *Public Health Nutr.* **2014**, *17*, 2436–2444. [CrossRef] [PubMed]
15. Rippin, H.L.; Hutchinson, J.; Jewell, J.; Breda, J.J.; Cade, J.E. Child and adolescent nutrient intakes from current national dietary surveys of European populations. *Nutr. Res. Rev.* **2019**, *32*, 38–69. [CrossRef]
16. EU Science Hub. Childhood Obesity: Local Data Feeds Local Solutions 2018. Available online: https://ec.europa.eu/jrc/en/news/childhood-obesity-local-data-feeds-local-solutions (accessed on 21 July 2020).
17. Stefan, S.G.B.; Joao, B.; Sandra, C.; Michael, N.; Jan, W. School Food and Nutrition in Europe: Policies, Interventions and Their Impact: EU Science Hub. 2019. Available online: https://ec.europa.eu/jrc/en/publication/eur-scientific-and-technical-research-reports/school-food-and-nutrition-europe-policies-interventions-and-their-impact (accessed on 20 July 2020).
18. WHO. Obesity UN City Marmorvej 51 DK-2100 Copenhagen Ø: WHO Regional Office for Europe. 2018. Available online: http://www.euro.who.int/en/health-topics/noncommunicable-diseases/obesity/obesity (accessed on 21 July 2020).
19. ROfE WHO. *WHO European Childhood Obesity Surveillance Initiative (COSI): UN City*; Marmorvej 51 DK-2100; ROfE WHO: Copenhagen, Denmark, 2014; Available online: http://www.euro.who.int/en/health-topics/disease-prevention/nutrition/activities/who-european-childhood-obesity-surveillance-initiative-cosi (accessed on 21 July 2020).
20. Gallotta, M.C.; Iazzoni, S.; Emerenziani, G.P.; Meucci, M.; Migliaccio, S.; Guidetti, L.; Baldari, C. Effects of combined physical education and nutritional programs on schoolchildren's healthy habits. *PeerJ* **2016**, *4*, e1880. [CrossRef]
21. Contento, I.R. Nutrition education: Linking research, theory, and practice. *Asia Pac. J. Clin. Nutr.* **2008**, *17*, 176–179. [PubMed]
22. Glanz, K. Measuring Food Environments: A Historical Perspective. *Am. J. Prev. Med.* **2009**, *36*, S93–S98. [CrossRef] [PubMed]
23. Vereecken, C.; Haerens, L.; De Bourdeaudhuij, I.; Maes, L. The relationship between children's home food environment and dietary patterns in childhood and adolescence. *Public Health Nutr.* **2010**, *13*, 1729–1735. [CrossRef] [PubMed]
24. Nutrition UNSSCo. *Schools as a System to Improve Nutrition*; UNSCN: Geneva, Switzerland, 2017; p. 64.
25. Hollar, D.; Messiah, S.E.; Lopez-Mitnik, G.; Hollar, T.L.; Almon, M.; Agatston, A.S. Effect of a Two-Year Obesity Prevention Intervention on Percentile Changes in Body Mass Index and Academic Performance in Low-Income Elementary School Children. *Am. J. Public Health* **2010**, *100*, 646–653. [CrossRef]
26. Florence, M.D.; Asbridge, M.; Veugelers, P.J. Diet Quality and Academic Performance. *J. Sch. Health* **2008**, *78*, 209–215. [CrossRef]
27. Anderson, M.L.; Gallagher, J.; Ritchie, E.R. School meal quality and academic performance. *J. Public Econ.* **2018**, *168*, 81–93. [CrossRef]
28. Amare, B.; Moges, B.; Fantahun, B.; Tafess, K.; Woldeyohannes, D.; Yismaw, G.; Ayane, T.; Yabutani, T.; Mulu, A.; Ota, F.; et al. Micronutrient levels and nutritional status of school children living in Northwest Ethiopia. *Nutr. J.* **2012**, *11*, 108. [CrossRef]
29. Herrador, Z.; Sordo, L.; Gadisa, E.; Buño, A.; Gómez-Rioja, R.; Iturzaeta, J.M.; Armas, L.F.D.; Benito, A.; Aseffa, A.; Moreno, J.; et al. Micronutrient Deficiencies and Related Factors in School-Aged Children in Ethiopia: A Cross-Sectional Study in Libo Kemkem and Fogera Districts, Amhara Regional State. *PLoS ONE* **2014**, *9*, e112858. [CrossRef]
30. Christian, P.; Murray-Kolb, L.E.; Khatry, S.K.; Katz, J.; Schaefer, B.A.; Cole, P.M.; Leclerq, S.C.; Tielsch, J.M.

Prenatal Micronutrient Supplementation and Intellectual and Motor Function in Early School-aged Children in Nepal. *JAMA* **2010**, *304*, 2716–2723. [CrossRef]

31. The NEMO Study Group. Effect of a 12-mo micronutrient intervention on learning and memory in well-nourished and marginally nourished school-aged children: 2 parallel, randomized, placebo-controlled studies in Australia and Indonesia. *Am. J. Clin. Nutr.* **2007**, *86*, 1082–1093. [CrossRef]
32. Effective Public Health Practice Project. Available online: https://merst.ca/ephpp/ (accessed on 21 July 2020).
33. Van Cauwenberghe, E.; Maes, L.; Spittaels, H.; van Lenthe, F.J.; Brug, J.; Oppert, J.M.; De Bourdeaudhuij, I. Effectiveness of school-based interventions in Europe to promote healthy nutrition in children and adolescents: Systematic review of published and 'grey' literature. *Br. J. Nutr.* **2010**, *103*, 781–797. [CrossRef] [PubMed]
34. El Harake, M.D.; Kharroubi, S.; Hamadeh, S.K.; Jomaa, L. Impact of a Pilot School-Based Nutrition Intervention on Dietary Knowledge, Attitudes, Behavior and Nutritional Status of Syrian Refugee Children in the Bekaa, Lebanon. *Nutrients* **2018**, *10*, 913. [CrossRef] [PubMed]
35. Adab, P.; Pallan, M.J.; Lancashire, E.R.; Hemming, K.; Frew, E.; Barrett, T.; Bhopal, R.; Cade, J.E.; Canaway, A.; Clarke, J.L.; et al. Effectiveness of a childhood obesity prevention programme delivered through schools, targeting 6 and 7 year olds: Cluster randomised controlled trial (WAVES study). *BMJ* **2018**, *360*, k211. [CrossRef] [PubMed]
36. Harley, A.; Lemke, M.; Brazauskas, R.; Carnegie, N.B.; Bokowy, L.; Kingery, L. Youth Chef Academy: Pilot Results From a Plant-Based Culinary and Nutrition Literacy Program for Sixth and Seventh Graders. *J. Sch. Health* **2018**, *88*, 893–902. [CrossRef]
37. Hermans, R.C.; van den Broek, N.; Nederkoorn, C.; Otten, R.; Ruiter, E.L.; Johnson-Glenberg, M.C. Feed the Alien! The Effects of a Nutrition Instruction Game on Children's Nutritional Knowledge and Food Intake. *Games Health J.* **2018**, *7*, 164–174. [CrossRef]
38. Piana, N.; Ranucci, C.; Buratta, L.; Foglia, E.; Fabi, M.; Novelli, F.; Casucci, S.; Reginato, E.; Pippi, R.; Aiello, C.; et al. An innovative school-based intervention to promote healthy lifestyles. *Health Educ. J.* **2017**, *76*, 716–729. [CrossRef]
39. Battjes-Fries, M.C.; Haveman-Nies, A.; Zeinstra, G.G.; van Dongen, E.J.; Meester, H.J.; van den Top-Pullen, R.; van't Veer, P.; de Graaf, K. Effectiveness of Taste Lessons with and without additional experiential learning activities on children's willingness to taste vegetables. *Appetite* **2017**, *109*, 201–208. [CrossRef]
40. Bogart, L.M.; Cowgill, B.O.; Elliott, M.N.; Klein, D.J.; Dawson, J.H.; Uyeda, K.; Elijah, J.; Binkle, D.G.; Schuster, M.A. A randomized controlled trial of students for nutrition and eXercise: A community-based participatory research study. *J. Adolesc. Health* **2014**, *55*, 415–422. [CrossRef]
41. Kaufman-Shriqui, V.; Fraser, D.; Friger, M.; Geva, D.; Bilenko, N.; Vardi, H.; Elhadad, N.; Mor, K.; Feine, Z.; Shahar, D.R. Effect of a School-Based Intervention on Nutritional Knowledge and Habits of Low-Socioeconomic School Children in Israel: A Cluster-Randomized Controlled Trial. *Nutrients* **2016**, *8*, 234. [CrossRef]
42. Sharma, S.V.; Markham, C.; Chow, J.; Ranjit, N.; Pomeroy, M.; Raber, M. Evaluating a school-based fruit and vegetable co-op in low-income children: A quasi-experimental study. *Prev. Med.* **2016**, *91*, 8–17. [CrossRef]
43. Lawlor, D.A.; Jago, R.; Noble, S.M.; Chittleborough, C.R.; Campbell, R.; Mytton, J.; Howe, L.D.; Peters, T.J.; Kipping, R.R. The Active for Life Year 5 (AFLY5) school-based cluster randomised controlled trial: Effect on potential mediators. *BMC Public Health* **2016**, *16*, 68. [CrossRef] [PubMed]
44. Steyn, N.P.; Villiers, A.D.; Gwebushe, N.; Draper, C.E.; Hill, J.; Waal, M.D.; Dalais, L.; Abrahams, Z.; Lombard, C.; Lambert, E.V. Did HealthKick, a randomised controlled trial primary school nutrition intervention improve dietary quality of children in low-income settings in South Africa? *BMC Public Health* **2015**, *15*, 948. [CrossRef]
45. Jones, M.; Pitt, H.; Oxford, L.; Bray, I.; Kimberlee, R.; Orme, J. Association between Food for Life, a Whole Setting Healthy and Sustainable Food Programme, and Primary School Children's Consumption of Fruit and Vegetables: A Cross-Sectional Study in England. *Int. J. Environ. Res. Public Health* **2017**, *14*, 639. [CrossRef] [PubMed]
46. Larsen, A.L.; Robertson, T.; Dunton, G. RE-AIM analysis of a randomized school-based nutrition intervention among fourth-grade classrooms in California. *Transl. Behav. Med.* **2015**, *5*, 315–326. [CrossRef] [PubMed]
47. Shen, M.; Hu, M.; Sun, Z. Assessment of School-Based Quasi-Experimental Nutrition and Food Safety Health Education for Primary School Students in Two Poverty-Stricken Counties of West China. *PLoS ONE* **2015**, *10*, e0145090. [CrossRef]

48. Fairclough, S.J.; Hackett, A.F.; Davies, I.G.; Gobbi, R.; Mackintosh, K.A.; Warburton, G.L.; Stratton, G.; van Sluijs, E.M.; Boddy, L.M. Promoting healthy weight in primary school children through physical activity and nutrition education: A pragmatic evaluation of the CHANGE! randomised intervention study. *BMC Public Health* **2013**, *13*, 626. [CrossRef]
49. Cunha, D.B.; de Souza, B.d.S.N.; Pereira, R.A.; Sichieri, R. Effectiveness of a randomized school-based intervention involving families and teachers to prevent excessive weight gain among adolescents in Brazil. *PLoS ONE* **2013**, *8*, e57498. [CrossRef]
50. Ochoa-Avilés, A.; Verstraeten, R.; Huybregts, L.; Andrade, S.; Camp, J.V.; Donoso, S.; Ramirez, P.L.; Lachat, C.; Maes, L.; Kolsteren, P. A school-based intervention improved dietary intake outcomes and reduced waist circumference in adolescents: A cluster randomized controlled trial. *Nutr. J.* **2017**, *16*, 79. [CrossRef]
51. Muros, J.J.; Zabala, M.; Oliveras-López, M.J.; Ocaña-Lara, F.A.; de la Serra, H.L.G. Results of a 7-Week School-Based Physical Activity and Nutrition Pilot Program on Health-Related Parameters in Primary School Children in Southern Spain. *Pediatr. Exerc. Sci.* **2013**, *25*, 248–261. [CrossRef]
52. Moss, A.; Smith, S.; Null, D.; Long, R.S.; Tragoudas, U. Farm to School and Nutrition Education: Positively Affecting Elementary School-Aged Children's Nutrition Knowledge and Consumption Behavior. *Child Obes.* **2013**, *9*, 51–56. [CrossRef]
53. Zota, D.; Dalma, A.; Petralias, A.; Lykou, A.; Kastorini, C.M.; Yannakoulia, M.; Karnaki, P.; Belogianni, K.; Veloudaki, A.; Riza, E.; et al. Promotion of healthy nutrition among students participating in a school food aid program: A randomized trial. *Int. J. Public Health* **2016**, *61*, 583–592. [CrossRef] [PubMed]
54. Gold, A.; Larson, M.; Tucker, J.; Strang, M. Classroom Nutrition Education Combined With Fruit and Vegetable Taste Testing Improves Children's Dietary Intake. *J. Sch. Health* **2017**, *87*, 106–113. [CrossRef] [PubMed]
55. Mbhatsani, V.H.; Mbhenyane, X.G.; Mabapa, S.N. Development and Implementation of Nutrition Education on Dietary Diversification for Primary School Children. *Ecol. Food Nutr.* **2017**, *56*, 449–561. [CrossRef] [PubMed]
56. Hutchinson, J.; Christian, M.S.; Evans, C.E.L.; Nykjaer, C.; Hancock, N.; Cade, J.E. Evaluation of the impact of school gardening interventions on children's knowledge of and attitudes towards fruit and vegetables. A cluster randomised controlled trial. *Appetite* **2015**, *91*, 405–414. [CrossRef] [PubMed]
57. Viggiano, E.; Viggiano, A.; Costanzo, A.D.; Viggiano, A.; Viggiano, A.; Andreozzi, E.; Romano, V.; Vicidomini, C.; Tuoro, D.D.; Gargano, G.; et al. Healthy lifestyle promotion in primary schools through the board game Kaledo: A pilot cluster randomized trial. *Eur. J. Pediatr.* **2018**, *177*, 1371–1375. [CrossRef] [PubMed]
58. Waters, E.; Gibbs, L.; Tadic, M.; Ukoumunne, O.C.; Magarey, A.; Okely, A.D.; Silva, A.D.; Armit, C.; Green, J.; O'Connor, T.; et al. Cluster randomised trial of a school-community child health promotion and obesity prevention intervention: Findings from the evaluation of fun 'n healthy in Moreland! *BMC Public Health* **2017**, *18*, 92. [CrossRef] [PubMed]
59. Xu, F.; Ware, R.S.; Leslie, E.; Tse, L.A.; Wang, Z.; Li, J.; Wang, Y. Effectiveness of a Randomized Controlled Lifestyle Intervention to Prevent Obesity among Chinese Primary School Students: CLICK-Obesity Study. *PLoS ONE* **2015**, *10*, e0141421. [CrossRef]
60. Jung, T.; Huang, J.; Eagan, L.; Oldenburg, D. Influence of school-based nutrition education program on healthy eating literacy and healthy food choice among primary school children. *Int. J. Health Promot. Educ.* **2019**, *57*, 67–81. [CrossRef]
61. Zhou, W.-J.; Xu, X.; Li, G.; Sharma, M.; Qie, Y.-L.; Zhao, Y. Effectiveness of a school-based nutrition and food safety education program among primary and junior high school students in Chongqing, China. *Glob. Health Promot.* **2014**, *23*, 37–49. [CrossRef]
62. Anderson, E.L.; Howe, L.D.; Kipping, R.R.; Campbell, R.; Jago, R.; Noble, S.M.; Wells, S.; Chittleborough, C.; Peters, T.J.; Lawlor, D.A. Long-term effects of the Active for Life Year 5 (AFLY5) school-based cluster-randomised controlled trial. *BMJ Open* **2016**, *6*, e010957. [CrossRef]
63. Griffin, T.L.; Jackson, D.M.; McNeill, G.; Aucott, L.S.; Macdiarmid, J.I. A Brief Educational Intervention Increases Knowledge of the Sugar Content of Foods and Drinks but Does Not Decrease Intakes in Scottish Children Aged 10–12 Years. *J. Nutr. Educ. Behav.* **2015**, *47*, 367–373.e1. [CrossRef]
64. Kipping, R.R.; Howe, L.D.; Jago, R.; Campbell, R.; Wells, S.; Chittleborough, C.R.; Mytton, J.; Noble, S.M.;

Peters, T.J.; Lawlor, D.A. Effect of intervention aimed at increasing physical activity, reducing sedentary behaviour, and increasing fruit and vegetable consumption in children: Active for Life Year 5 (AFLY5) school based cluster randomised controlled trial. *BMJ Br. Med J.* **2014**, *348*, g3256. [CrossRef]

65. Van de Gaar, V.M.; Jansen, W.; Grieken, A.V.; Borsboom, G.J.J.M.; Kremers, S.; Raat, H. Effects of an intervention aimed at reducing the intake of sugar-sweetened beverages in primary school children: A controlled trial. *Int. J. Behav. Nutr. Phys. Act.* **2014**, *11*, 98. [CrossRef]
66. Moore, G.F.; Murphy, S.; Chaplin, K.; Lyons, R.A.; Atkinson, M.; Moore, L. Impacts of the Primary School Free Breakfast Initiative on socio-economic inequalities in breakfast consumption among 9-11-year-old schoolchildren in Wales. *Public Health Nutr.* **2014**, *17*, 1280–1299. [CrossRef]
67. Nyberg, G.; Norman, Å.; Sundblom, E.; Zeebari, Z.; Elinder, L.S. Effectiveness of a universal parental support programme to promote health behaviours and prevent overweight and obesity in 6-year-old children in disadvantaged areas, the Healthy School Start Study II, a cluster-randomised controlled trial. *Int. J. Behav. Nutr. Phys. Act.* **2016**, *13*, 4. [CrossRef]
68. Mittmann, S.; Austel, A.; Ellrott, T. Behavioural effects of a short school-based fruit and vegetable promotion programme: 5-a-Day for kids. *Health Educ.* **2016**, *116*, 222–237. [CrossRef]
69. Huys, N.; Cardon, G.; Craemer, D.M.; Hermans, N.; Renard, S.; Roesbeke, M.; Stevens, W.; Lepeleere, S.D.; Deforche, B. Effect and process evaluation of a real-world school garden program on vegetable consumption and its determinants in primary schoolchildren. *PLoS ONE* **2019**, *14*, e0214320. [CrossRef]
70. Weber, K.S.; Spörkel, O.; Mertens, M.; Freese, A.; Strassburger, K.; Kemper, B.; Bachmann, C.; Diehlmann, K.; Stemper, T.; Buyken, A.E.; et al. Positive Effects of Promoting Physical Activity and Balanced Diets in a Primary School Setting with a High Proportion of Migrant School Children. *Exp. Clin. Endocrinol. Diabetes* **2017**, *125*, 554–562. [CrossRef]
71. Llargués, E.; Recasens, M.A.; Manresa, J.-M.; Jensen, B.B.; Franco, R.; Nadal, A.; Vila, M.; Recasens, I.; Perez, M.J.; Castel, C. Four-year outcomes of an educational intervention in healthy habits in schoolchildren: The Avall 3 Trial. *Eur. J. Public Health* **2016**, *27*, 42–47. [CrossRef]
72. Liz Martins, M.; Rodrigues, S.S.P.; Cunha, L.M.; Rocha, A. Strategies to reduce plate waste in primary schools–experimental evaluation. *Public Health Nutr.* **2016**, *19*, 1517–1525. [CrossRef]
73. Rosário, R.; Araújo, A.; Padrão, P.; Lopes, O.; Moreira, A.; Abreu, S.; Vale, S.; Pereira, B.; Moreira, P. Impact of a school-based intervention to promote fruit intake: A cluster randomized controlled trial. *Public Health* **2016**, *136*, 94–100. [CrossRef] [PubMed]
74. Zafiropulos, V.; Chatzi, V.; Petros, D.; Markaki, A.; Zacharias, F.; Nikolaos, T. Preliminary Results of A Dietary Intervention among Primary-School Children. In Proceedings of the European Congress on Obesity, Prague, Czech Republic, 6–9 May 2015.
75. Charlebois, J.; Gowrinathan, Y.; Waddell, P. A Review of the Evidence: School-based Interventions to Address Obesity Prevention in Children 6–12 Years of Age. *Tor. Public Health* **2012**, *48*, 102.
76. Delgado-Noguera, M.; Tort, S.; Martínez-Zapata, M.J.; Bonfill, X. Primary school interventions to promote fruit and vegetable consumption: A systematic review and meta-analysis. *Prev. Med.* **2011**, *53*, 3–9. [CrossRef] [PubMed]
77. Evans, C.E.; Christian, M.S.; Cleghorn, C.L.; Greenwood, D.C.; Cade, J.E. Systematic review and meta-analysis of school-based interventions to improve daily fruit and vegetable intake in children aged 5 to 12 y. *Am. J. Clin. Nutr.* **2012**, *96*, 889–901. [CrossRef]
78. Brown, E.C.; Buchan, D.S.; Baker, J.S.; Wyatt, F.B.; Bocalini, D.S.; Kilgore, L. A Systematised Review of Primary School Whole Class Child Obesity Interventions: Effectiveness, Characteristics, and Strategies. *BioMed Res. Int.* **2016**, *2016*, 4902714. [CrossRef]
79. Mikkelsen, B.E.; Kngesveen, K.; Afflerbach, T.; Barnekow, V. The human rights framework, the school and healthier eating among young people a European perspective. *Public Health Nutr.* **2016**, *19*, 15–25. [CrossRef]
80. Rashid, V.; Engberink, M.F.; Eijsden, M.V.; Nicolaou, M.; Dekker, L.H.; Verhoeff, A.P.; Weijs, P.J.M. Ethnicity and socioeconomic status are related to dietary patterns at age 5 in the Amsterdam born children and their development (ABCD) cohort. *BMC Public Health* **2018**, *18*, 115. [CrossRef]

6

How Minority Parents could Help Children Develop Healthy Eating Behaviors

Chishinga Callender [1], Denisse Velazquez [1], Meheret Adera [1], Jayna M. Dave [1], Norma Olvera [2], Tzu-An Chen [3], Shana Alford [4] and Debbe Thompson [1,*]

1 USDA/ARS Children's Nutrition Research Center, Department of Pediatrics, Baylor College of Medicine, 1100 Bates Street, Houston, TX 77030, USA; Chishinga.Callender@bcm.edu (C.C.); himedenisse@gmail.com (D.V.); msa8@rice.edu (M.A.); jmdave@bcm.edu (J.M.D.)

2 Psychological, Health, and Learning Sciences Department, University of Houston, 3657 Cullen Boulevard Room 491, Houston, TX 77204, USA; nolvera@central.uh.edu

3 HEALTH Research Institute, University of Houston, 4849 Calhoun Road, Houston, TX 77204, USA; ann0516@gmail.com

4 Common Threads, 222 W. Merchandise Mart Plaza, Suite 1212, Chicago, IL 60654, USA; salford@commonthreads.org

* Correspondence: dit@bcm.edu.

Abstract: Minority children and children living in under-resourced households are at the greatest risk for obesity and diet-related disparities. Identifying effective strategies to reduce these risks is an important step in child obesity prevention. Parents influence the home environment and play a critical role in child obesity prevention. Eighteen parent–child dyads living in under-resourced Houston area communities participated in a mixed methods study (online surveys, telephone interviews). The purpose of the research reported here was to conduct a secondary analysis of the qualitative data to explore Black/African American and Hispanic parent and child perspectives of the ways in which parents could help their children make healthy food choices. Descriptive statistics were calculated for parent and child demographic characteristics; hybrid thematic analysis was used to code and analyze the interview transcripts. Frequencies were calculated for children's interview responses to rating scales and the grade they gave their eating habits. Mothers' responses were grouped into two broad categories: facilitators (modeling, availability, and teaching) as ways parents could help their child eat healthy, and barriers (lack of time, cost of healthy foods, and lack of knowledge) to helping their child eat healthy. Alternatively, child responses focused on ways in which parents could provide support: environmental support (home availability, home cooking, and introducing new foods) and personal support (providing child choice, teaching, and encouragement). Most children reported that eating healthy was easy, and most rated their personal eating habits as an A or B. These findings suggest that understanding the perspectives of Black/African American and Hispanic parent–child dyads can provide insight into the development of culturally and economically relevant healthy eating strategies and interventions for families living in under-resourced communities.

Keywords: minority; parents; children; obesity; prevention; diet; nutrition promotion; Black/African American; Hispanic; qualitative

---

1. Introduction

The high prevalence of child obesity in the United States is a significant public health issue [1], with the highest prevalence among Black/African American and Hispanic children [2,3] and children living in low-income households [4]. Identifying effective strategies to reduce the risk of child obesity and related disparities is an important step in child obesity prevention [5].

Several factors influence child obesity risk, including diet, physical activity, and sedentary behavior [6,7]. Through excessive caloric intake, diet plays a significant role in obesity risk [6,7]. Several factors influence dietary intake, including the home food environment [8], parenting styles [9], family meals [9], personal food preferences [10], and household income [11]. Furthermore, the diet quality of children in the United States falls below the national dietary recommendations [12].

Similar to obesity-related disparities, diet-related disparities exist, and it is imperative to address them as well. Racial and ethnic minorities (i.e., Black/African American, Hispanic) experience diet-related disparities and tend to have poorer diet quality compared to their white counterparts [13]. In addition, these disparities exist in low-income populations, as poor diet quality is associated with socioeconomic status [14]. For example, a study found that lower-income individuals ate lower-quality foods than their higher-income counterparts [14]. Families living in under-resourced communities are more likely to be exposed to advertising of less healthy foods and beverages [15], have more access to fast food restaurants [16], and less access to stores with affordable healthy foods [17]. Thus, minority, under-resourced families may be at the greatest risk for experiencing diet-related disparities. Understanding how these factors influence child dietary behaviors is essential in developing effective interventions to reduce poor diet quality for children.

Parents exert a strong influence on the home food environment [9,18]. Therefore, they play an important role in child obesity prevention. It is critical for parents to encourage children to engage in healthy dietary behaviors at an early age to reduce children's risk of obesity and related diseases and to help them develop and maintain a healthy lifestyle into adulthood. Previous research identifies the challenges that families living in under-resourced communities experience accessing healthy foods [11,19]. In addition, previous studies have identified parents' perspectives on strategies to promote healthy eating behaviors [20–23]. However, few studies have explored perspectives of racial and ethnic minority parent–child dyads regarding ways parents can help their children practice healthy eating behaviors. The perspectives of parents and children in minority and under-resourced communities are essential for developing effective, culturally appropriate, and acceptable obesity prevention and nutrition promotion interventions. Thus, the purpose of this research was to expand the voices of minority families in the literature by investigating both parent and child perspectives of the ways in which parents can help their children make healthy food choices.

2. Materials and Methods

This is a secondary data analysis of data from a larger, mixed methods study designed to identify thoughts, expectations, and preferences of parents and children toward cooking and nutrition education programs promoting healthy eating. This paper was guided by the following research question: From the perspectives of both parents and children, how can parents help their children make healthy food choices?

2.1. Design

This study re-examined qualitative data from a larger mixed-methods study. The protocol was approved by the institutional review board at Baylor College of Medicine (H-44683).

2.2. Study Participants

Inclusionary criteria for the families included: child 8–13 years old; parent/guardian of a child 8–13 years old; both parent and child fluent in English or Spanish; child receives and/or is eligible for free or reduced price meals at school; healthy (i.e., no physical, health, or medical condition that would affect diet or participation in a telephone interview or focus group); parent and child living in the same household; the parent has primary responsibility for family food shopping/acquisition and/or meals; transportation to focus group (focus group participation only); families also needed to be willing to provide contact information, to participate in study activities, and have focus group/telephone interview audio recorded. Exclusionary criteria included unwillingness to have the telephone interview or focus group recorded and to take photos for the study.

2.3. Recruitment

Families living in under-resourced communities in the Greater Houston, TX metropolitan area were recruited for this study. A more detailed description of the recruitment procedures is reported elsewhere [24]. Briefly, recruitment started in early May 2019 and ended in mid-August 2019. Recruitment methods included contacting potential families from the volunteer database at the USDA/ARS Children's Nutrition Research Center (CNRC) and referrals from recruited families. All families provided written informed consent prior to participation. During the consent process, parents had the option for their family to participate in either separate telephone interviews or focus groups in their preferred language (English or Spanish). All families chose to participate in telephone interviews.

2.4. Data Collection

Data collection for the larger study began in June 2019 and ended in October 2019. In that study, parents and children completed online surveys, took photographs of situations that made it easy or hard to make healthy food choices, and completed telephone interviews. Surveys were available in English and Spanish, and telephone interviews were conducted in participants' preferred language (English or Spanish). Trained research coordinators conducted semi-structured telephone interviews [25]. Interviews were scripted and contained open-ended, non-leading questions; probes and prompts were used to clarify, expand, and understand responses. Separate scripts guided parent and child interviews. This paper reports demographic data, as well as parent and child responses to the following interview questions: "How can parents help their children to eat healthy?" (parents); "How could your parents help you make healthy food choices at home?" (child). To explore children's perspectives related to their personal eating habits, child responses to the following interview questions are also reported: (1) "On a scale of 1 (hard), 2 (not hard or easy), 3 (easy), how easy or hard is it to eat healthy?" (2) "What grade would you give your eating habits (i.e., A, B, C, D, F like in school grades)?" Each interview was digitally recorded, transcribed, and reviewed for accuracy prior to analysis.

2.5. Data Analysis

2.5.1. Surveys

A single dataset was created by combining the English and Spanish language surveys. Parent and child data were analyzed separately. Descriptive statistics (frequencies, percentages) were calculated for demographic and household characteristics.

2.5.2. Interviews

Two independent coders used hybrid thematic analysis to code and analyze verbatim transcripts [26]. Transcripts were reviewed for accuracy prior to analysis. To provide structure to the coding process, transcripts were initially coded using a priori codes guided by the research question. Emergent codes were generated as transcripts that were reviewed and coded to provide flexibility to the coding process and ensure that parent and child perspectives were fully captured. After coding was complete, the codes were reviewed for relevance to the research question. During this process, some codes were dropped, and others were grouped into categories based on their similarities. Then, categories were reviewed and grouped into higher-order categories as appropriate. Analysis was conducted on English language transcripts (i.e., English language transcripts and translated Spanish language transcripts). Separate parent and child codebooks were maintained and routinely updated to reflect new emergent codes, definitions, and key decisions. Frequencies were calculated for children's responses to rating scales and the grade they gave their eating habits. Their reasons for selecting a rating or grade were used to expand the findings and provide additional insight.

Verbatim quotes, used to support qualitative findings, were labeled as follows: P = Parent; C = child; A = Black/African American; H = Hispanic. To help differentiate the quotes, a number (from 1–18) was assigned to each parent/child dyad.

3. Results

3.1. Family Characteristics

Eighteen parent–child dyads enrolled in the study. All participating parents were mothers (100%), mostly 40–49 years old (61%), Black/African American (56%), Hispanic (44%), and married/living with significant other (61%). Over half of the children were female (56%) and Black/African American (56%). Half of the children's ethnicity (50%) was reported as Hispanic by the mothers. The ages of children participating included 8–10 years old (22%) and 11–13 years old (78%).

The highest level of household education varied, with 33% of families having less than a college education, 33% having some college coursework, 22% having a college degree, and 11% having a postgraduate degree. Annual household income for the majority of families (66%) was below $41,000. To add context, 39% of mothers reported two adults in the household, and 50% reported having two children under the age of 18 living in the household. Although the majority of mothers reported high/marginal food security (89%), more than half reported using one to three food assistance programs (67%). The majority of families (61%) spoke mostly English at home. All families recruited for the study met the inclusionary criteria.

3.2. Interview Findings

Interviews ranged from an average of 43 min (children) to 56 min (mothers). As previously stated, the a priori codes were generated from the research question prior to coding. Then, emergent codes were added throughout coding based on parents and children responses. After coding all transcripts, the emergent codes were reviewed, collapsed, and grouped into categories. Parents' responses were grouped into two categories: facilitators (what made it easy to help their child make healthy food choices) and barriers (what made it difficult to help their child make healthy food choices). Children's responses were also grouped into two categories: environmental support (how parents create healthy eating choices at home) and personal support (how parents actively influence the child to eat healthy). The categories are presented in Figure 1 (parent) and Figure 2 (child).

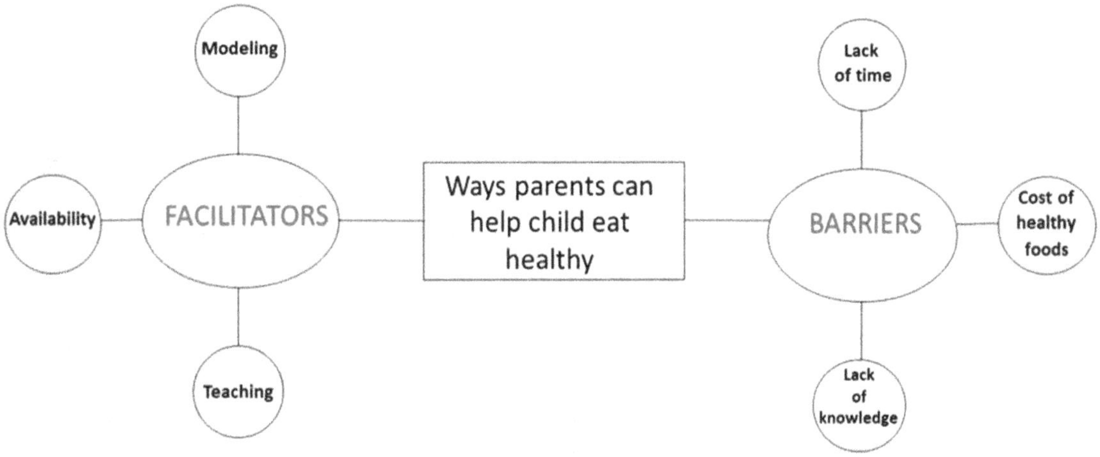

Figure 1. Visual representation of mothers' perspectives on ways parents can help their children eat healthy. (Note: Red font indicates the categories. Bold black font indicates the supporting categories that emerged.)

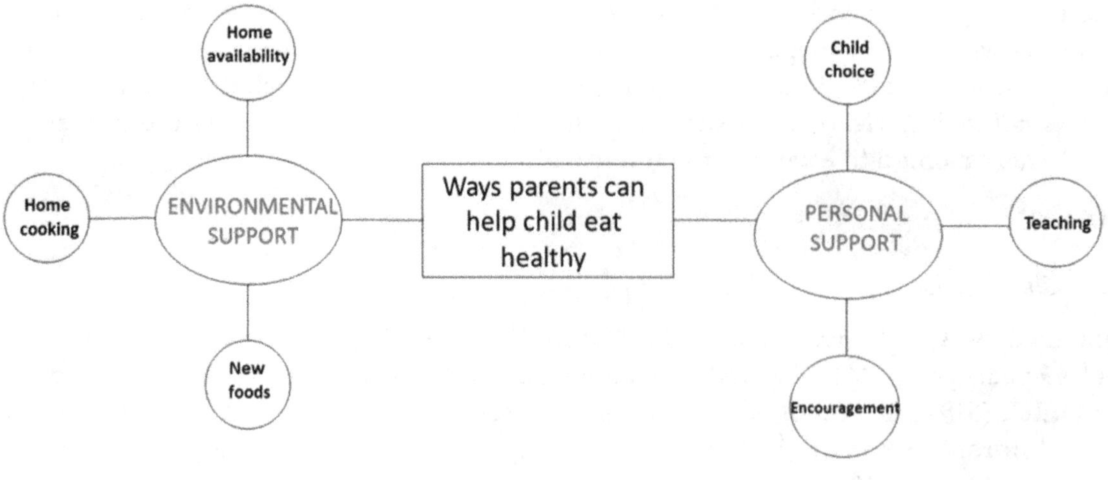

Figure 2. Visual representation of children's perspectives on ways parents can help their children eat healthy. (Note: Red font indicates the categories. Bold black font indicates the supporting categories that emerged.)

3.2.1. Parents

When parents were asked, "How can parents help their child eat healthy?" two main categories emerged: facilitators and barriers to helping their child eat healthy (Figure 1). Each is described in more detail below in order of prevalence and presented in Table 1.

Table 1. Categories and subcategories from qualitative data analysis of interviews with parents on ways parents can help their children eat healthy.

Categories	Subcategories	Definitions
Facilitators	• Modeling • Availability • Teaching	• Modeling healthy eating behaviors • Having healthy foods easily available • Teaching healthy eating behaviors
Barriers	• Lack of time • Cost of healthy foods • Lack of knowledge	• Lack of time to prepare or serve healthy foods • High cost of healthy foods • Lack of knowledge about healthy eating and cooking

Facilitators. Three ways parents could help their children make healthy food choices were mentioned: (1) modeling healthy eating behaviors, (2) having healthy foods easily available for the child (availability), and (3) teaching the child about healthy eating. Several mothers shared that modeling healthy eating is beneficial to a child: *"By eating healthy themselves. Kids follow what we do. And if they see a parent eating healthy, they are more likely to follow in their parent's footsteps"* (P.15A). Mothers shared examples of ways to make healthy foods easily available for their children. One mother mentioned, *"I think that ... the healthy way depends on what kind of food. Because I try to use those tricks in the soup so that they eat it. So that they can eat healthier. And with fruit, I try to keep as many containers full of fruit as possible, so that they don't have to wash them, so that they can see it [as] appetizing there, in the refrigerator"* (P.6H). A few mothers shared their perspective about teaching healthy eating habits to their children. For example, one mother taught her children about the benefits of healthy eating: *"By explaining to them that our food is our medicine, and our medicine has to be our food, because we are what we eat. By showing them the effects that diseases caused by unhealthy food have on different people"*(P.17H). Another mother shared teaching children about preparing healthy foods: *"I think that as a parent, we help them package up food portions, be it in Ziploc bags or in Tupperware, teaching them how to divide up food and have it prepared for when they come back from school, or some sport, grab it and eat"* (P.18H).

Barriers. Parents mentioned three types of barriers to helping children eat healthy: (1) lack of time, (2) cost of healthy foods, and (3) parent's lack of knowledge about healthy eating and cooking. Lack of time to prepare or serve healthy foods was noted as a barrier by several mothers. For example, one mother shared how time affects working mothers: *"Sometimes, you know, when the mother works or both parents work, especially the mother, there is no time to prepare, like, maybe healthy food. So, maybe, you know, 'cause you need to cook or to grill or whatever. So the things that are not healthy in a can or fast food that you buy, you know, it's easier, so the family ends up eating unhealthy because their mother would be tired and all that. But I think time really plays a role, especially if the mother is working"* (P.2A). However, stay-at-home mothers did not see lack of time as a barrier: *"Time? No, not right now because the children are on vacation. I'm here with them, I don't work. So, of course I can go to the store to buy the ingredients or whatever I need. No, time is no obstacle"* (P.12H).

The high cost of healthy foods was also seen as a barrier for some mothers: *"Economics. If a parent feels as though they don't have the money for the healthy food, they're likely to buy what's cheap"* (P.15A). One mother shared her personal experience with household finances impacting eating choices for her family: *"Yes, one of the first obstacles is that sometimes... The day you don't eat healthy at home is for lack of... it's because our budget is really low. But, we try to do the best we can"* (P.3H).

Knowledge also emerged as a barrier to helping children make healthy food choices. For example, one mother shared how lack of knowledge of " ... how to cook [or] prepare ... food" was a barrier to helping children eat healthy (P.11A). Another shared how some parents are not knowledgeable about healthy ingredient substitutions for meals they enjoy cooking: *"And they may not know that you can cook the foods you love but you don't have to use—you can use different ingredients to get the flavor and the taste you want"* (P.1A).

3.2.2. Children

When children were asked, "How could your parents help you make healthy food choices at home?" two main categories emerged: environmental and personal support by parents (Figure 2). Each is described in more detail below in order of prevalence and presented in Table 2.

Table 2. Categories and subcategories from coding of interviews with children on ways parents can help their children eat healthy.

Categories	Subcategories	Definitions
Environmental Support	• Home availability • Home cooking • New foods	• Healthy foods easily available at home • Cooking foods at home • Introduction to new or different foods
Personal Support	• Child choice • Teaching • Encouragement	• Giving child the opportunity to choose foods, preparation methods, and meals • Teaching healthy eating behaviors • Encouraging child to practice healthy eating behaviors

Environmental support. Three ways parents could encourage a child's healthy eating choices in the home environment were mentioned by children: (1) home availability (i.e., healthy foods easily available at home), (2) home cooking, and (3) introducing new foods. Several children suggested that their parents could make healthy foods more available. For example, one child shared, *"Maybe by like buying more healthier food like more fruits and vegetables"* (C.15A). Another child shared how their mother makes healthy foods available at home: *"Well, she would help me by like at home, we would find things in the house that would be healthy. Like, fruit in yogurt and stuff. Sometimes, we'll make, like, smoothies, like, but they would have, like, lots of vegetables. Well, like, vegetables and things inside. Plus, we have a lot of vegetable things we cook with"* (C.16A).

For home cooking, children also noted that preparing foods in a healthy way would be helpful: *"Or maybe when we cook not putting as much grease and butter and unhealthy foods like that"* (C.15A). Some children also suggested including more vegetables in meals. For example, one child shared, *" ... my mom and my dad could help me in the kitchen with different types of vegetables and different types of protein, things that I need"* (C.8A).

Introduction to new or different foods was also suggested by children: *"And—but I think to help us more she could, like, start influencing us by giving us more creative things and different foods that sometimes we've never tried. Because if you keep eating the same thing over and over, even though it's healthy, it might get boring and you don't want to eat it anymore"* (C.10H). Children shared examples of how their parents introduced new foods, including through sharing new recipes, watching their mothers cook, and cooking foods from different cultures. For example, one child shared her experience with cultural foods: *"Mainly, my mom influences me to try new food because since she's, like, from ... she's from Mexico, she, like, influenced me to try a lot of new foods from other places"* (C.10H). It is worth noting that a majority of children identified their mothers as an influence to try new foods.

Personal support. Children mentioned three types of personal support parents could use to help children eat healthy: (1) giving the child choice, (2) teaching, and (3) providing encouragement. Giving the child choice (i.e., opportunities to choose foods, preparation methods, and meals) was recommended by a few children. For example, one child shared how parents could ask questions about making healthy food choices: *"I think if they asked more about what type of food we want to eat that is healthy"* (C.2H). A few children expressed interest in making choices at the grocery store: *"Going with her to the grocery store to pick out the vegetables and fruits I want"* (C.7H).

For teaching, a child was interested in her mother teaching her to cook healthy: *"My mom could teach me how to cook healthier meals so that way when I [get] hungry I could just cook that and I would be able to eat healthy"* (C.13A). A few children shared that their mothers taught them about cooking through showing them: *"Mom teaches us how she does things. And then my mom does it"* (C.12H). For encouragement, one child shared how his mother encouraged him to make healthy snack choices: *"Well, sometimes ... because most of the time, I like to walk to the store and buy chips, but my mom told me that I shouldn't be walking to the store and getting chips because chips are unhealthy, so she just doesn't give me the money. She says if you go to the store you better come back with some fruit cups or something."* A child also shared how her mother encouraged her to make healthy choices at restaurants: *"So when we go places, like, for example Chick-fil-A and all that stuff that has a lot of grease, she encourages me to try, like, salads and stuff"* (C.16A). Simple words of encouragement with reasoning were also noted as helping a child with eating healthy: *"She says you won't know if you won't taste it"* (C.11A).

3.2.3. Children's Perspectives on Making Healthy Dietary Choices

Ease and Difficulty of Healthy Eating

When children were asked, "on a scale of 1 (hard), 2 (not hard or easy), 3 (easy), how easy or hard is it to eat healthy," the following ratings were reported: rating of 1 ($n = 3$), rating of 2 ($n = 5$), and rating of 3 ($n = 10$). Reasons for choosing the ratings varied. For example, one child who gave a rating of 1 noted eating habits as a reason healthy eating was difficult for the general population: *"Well, I think it's hard to eat healthy because some people might be so used to eating unhealthy that they'll just like they're are going to keep eating unhealthy. But they might eat something healthy not very often, but they'll probably eat it every once in a while"* (C.1A). Children shared a variety of reasons for choosing a rating of 2. A child mentioned how temptation can influence eating healthy: *"Because it's not hard to eat healthy, but it's not also easy to eat healthy. Because if it's easy to eat healthy but if you see stuff that's unhealthy and it looks good or smells good, you might want it"* (C.9A). Another shared how types of foods can influence eating choices: *"I chose two because it can be easy sometimes but not always is, but it's not hard either. It depends on the food I'm eating and the taste"* (C.14H).

Children also shared a variety of reasons for choosing a rating of 3. A few children noted parental and/or family influences on their eating choices. For example, one child shared how the entire family encourages healthy eating: *"Because in my household, my family, like my sisters, especially my older sister, my dad, my mom, they really, like, encourage us to eat foods that don't contain things that are bad for your body and healthy things"* (C.10H). Another child shared that her mother *"buys fruits and vegetables"* (C.4A). Some children also noted their eating habits as a reason for choosing a rating of 3: *"Because I like eating lots of apples and salads so it's much easier to do that"* (C.11A) and *"Because I normally eat healthy"* (C.13A). The benefits of healthy eating were also mentioned as a reason: *"Three cause it doesn't really matter really what you eat, you have to have a lot of—I mean, not a lot, less calories and you have to have a lot of vegetables and stuff like lettuce, carrots, tomatoes, a lot of things that will help your body"* (C.16A).

Personal Eating Habits Assessment

When children were asked, "What grade would you give your eating habits?" they reported the following grades: A (n = 3), B (n = 10), C (n = 2), and D (n = 2). Reasons varied for choosing the grades. For example, a child who reported an A for their eating habits mentioned his mother's cooking: *"'Cause most of the things I eat, my mom cooks and she cooks a lot with a lot of vegetables and stuff so to help be healthy"* (C.16A). Similarly, a child with an "A" grade mentioned eating healthy foods at home and school: *"At school, the food is very healthy. They give us balanced meals, but sometimes the taste just isn't so great. Sometimes it's a bit hard to eat. And at home it's an A, because most of the time, almost all the time it's very healthy and the taste is good so it's easier to eat"* (C.14H). Another described their favorite types of foods, while also noting fruit purchases made by his mother as the reason for reporting an A.

Several children who reported a "B" or "C" grade for their eating habits mentioned mixed eating habits (i.e., eating healthy and unhealthy foods) as a reason. One child shared the following: *"Because I don't, like, all the time it won't always be healthy food but sometimes it's healthy food. And then sometimes I do have sweets now and then"* (C.8A). One child noted differences in foods eaten in the home and school environment as a reason for a "B" grade: *"Because I eat great at home, but at school not that well"* (C.17H). Interestingly, one child compared their eating habits to their friends as the reason for a "B" grade: *"... because I'm not that healthy that I over overpass everything. But I do consider myself eating healthier than a lot of my friends"* (C.10H). Both children who reported a "D" grade shared a lack of vegetable consumption as the reason.

4. Discussion

The purpose of this research was to investigate the perspectives of minority parents and children on the ways in which parents could help their children make healthy eating choices. Although a few studies [27,28] have presented interview findings from parent–child dyads regarding healthy eating, this study is unique in that it highlights both parent and child perspectives of the ways parents could help their children eat healthy. This study is also distinctive as it presents interview findings from children about the ease and difficulty of eating healthy and an assessment of their personal eating habits.

For mothers in this sample, modeling, availability, and teaching served as the main facilitators for parents to help children practice healthy eating behaviors. Similar to our research, parental roles of modeling healthy eating behaviors [29,30], making healthy foods available [8,29], and teaching about healthy eating [29] have been reported by parents in other studies. Previous studies have also found that availability of healthy foods [8,31] in the home and modeling [31] have been associated with child's diet quality. Contrary to previous research, child's weight was not mentioned as a motivation to encourage healthy eating behaviors in children [27]. These findings suggest that interventions promoting healthy eating behaviors for minority children living in under-resourced communities should promote strategies such as modeling, making healthy foods available at home, and teaching children how to eat and cook healthy, while avoiding an emphasis on child's body weight.

For mothers in this sample, lack of time, cost of healthy foods, and lack of knowledge were highlighted as barriers to helping children practice healthy eating behaviors. Lack of time to prepare healthy meals [27,30,32–34] is consistently reported by parents as a barrier to healthy eating. This could be due to parents from under-resourced families working long hours and/or having multiple jobs [32]. However, a few mothers in our study did not report a lack of time as a barrier due to their role as stay-at-home mothers. Similar to mothers in our study, parents from previous studies, including those with limited income, also identified the cost of healthy foods as a barrier and also believed that healthy eating is expensive [21,27,30,32–34]. Lack of knowledge was also reported as a barrier by parents with limited income [32] and minority families [27]. These findings highlight the need for developing parent-focused interventions for minority and under-resourced communities with a focus on teaching time management strategies for preparing healthy meals, providing affordable options for purchasing healthy foods (e.g., purchasing fresh fruits and vegetables in season), and promoting nutrition and cooking skills knowledge.

Children reported that home availability, home cooking, and new foods were environmental support factors to be practiced by parents to help children eat healthy. Home availability [35], home cooking [36], and willingness to try new foods [37] were reported by children in other studies as ways in which parents helped them make healthy eating choices. In our study, both mothers and children reported that home availability of healthy foods can support the creation of a healthy home food environment. The availability of healthy foods is consistently supported in the literature as an agent for changing children's dietary behaviors [9,29]. In addition to availability, it is imperative that nutrition education/promotion interventions are inclusive of strategies on home cooking (e.g., healthful preparation methods, cooking with the child) and how to introduce new foods.

Children also reported that giving the child choice, teaching, and encouragement were personal support factors to helping children eat healthy. These factors were found to be similar to concepts in previous research, including instrumental and emotional social support for healthful eating from the parent's perspective [38] and positive parental parenting (i.e., feeding practices) [39]. Comparable to our study, middle school aged children in the northeastern United States noted that their food choices were influenced by their parent's guidance [40]. Interestingly, child choice was seen differently by children in Spain, as they did not have a choice in how the foods were prepared, but they were given an option for the amount and type of foods eaten [37]. Similar to our study, children noted that parents shared advice on fruit and vegetable consumption and encouraged them to eat foods prepared at home instead of foods prepared outside of the home [36].

Furthermore, similar to our study, teaching and encouragement were identified as active guidance in five research studies, and a positive relationship was found with vegetable consumption in one study [29]. In our study, the environmental and personal support factors were primarily influenced by mothers. The literature consistently supports mothers influencing the eating behaviors of their children [9]. It is important to note that both children and mothers mentioned teaching as a way parents can help their children eat healthy. Future research should explore the role of fathers in the environmental and personal support factors for children's dietary behaviors. Based on the above findings, intervention programs should include strategies for parents on ways to offer choices in healthy foods, teaching about them (e.g., types of healthy foods, benefits of healthy eating), and encouraging their child to eat them.

Our study highlighted another contribution to the literature: children's perspectives on the ease and difficulty of eating healthy. A variety of reasons (i.e., eating habits, benefits of healthy eating, and temptations) were mentioned in considering healthy eating choices. It is critical to note that a few of the children's responses reflected parental influences (i.e., maternal encouragement and purchasing of fruits and vegetables). Children's perspectives on their personal eating habits also contribute to the literature. A majority of the children rated their eating habits highly, while only a few rated their eating habits below a B. Similar to reasons for the ease and difficulty of eating healthy, children noted parental influences (i.e., home cooking, mother purchasing fruits) attributing to their eating choices. Comparable to our study, children in England shared parental influences on their eating choices [41]. Food choices at school, mixed eating habits, and a lack of vegetable consumption were also mentioned as reasons for the personal eating habits grade. Further investigation is needed into children's perspectives on their personal eating habits. Although parents believed that they needed to make ample effort to help their children eat healthy, children simply wanted environmental modifications (e.g., having healthy foods available, home cooked meals, introduction of new foods) and personal support from parents (e.g., the freedom to make their own food choices, lessons on healthy eating, healthy eating encouragement). This suggests that future interventions to encourage healthy eating among minority children and children living in under-resourced communities should focus on encouraging these types of changes.

The strengths of this study included semi-structured interviews and interviewers trained in qualitative methods. One limitation included the differences in mothers' responses to the interview question; there was a lack of clarity in whether mothers were speaking of their personal experiences or their beliefs about the experiences of other parents. A second limitation included children's responses to the interview questions on the ease and difficulty of healthy eating; the data did not lend itself to hybrid thematic analysis. Despite the limitations, the findings provide an opportunity to identify parent and child perspectives of the ways in which parents can help their children make healthy dietary choices.

5. Conclusions

Insights from minority parents and children are critical to the development of effective child obesity prevention and nutrition education programs for families living in under-resourced communities.

Strategies centered on environmental and personal support are needed for parents to help their children develop and practice healthy eating behaviors. It is important that child nutrition promotion strategies tailor to the perspectives of families with the priority of reducing diet-related disparities among racial/ethnic minorities and under-resourced communities.

Author Contributions: Conceptualization, C.C. and D.T.; methodology, D.T., J.M.D., N.O., and C.C.; validation, C.C. and D.T.; formal analysis, T.-A.C., C.C., and D.T.; investigation, C.C., D.V., and M.A.; data curation, C.C.; writing—original draft preparation, C.C.; writing—review and editing, C.C., D.T., M.A., D.V., J.M.D., N.O., T.-A.C., and S.A.; visualization, C.C.; supervision, D.T.; project administration, S.A.; funding acquisition, D.T. All authors have read and agreed to the published version of the manuscript.

Acknowledgments: We would like to thank the families who participated in this research.

References

1. Fryar, C.D.; Carroll, M.D.; Ogden, C.L. Prevalence of Overweight, Obesity, and Severe Obesity among Children and Adolescents Aged 2–19 Years: United States, 1963–1965 through 2015. Available online: https://www.cdc.gov/nchs/data/hestat/obesity_child_15_16/obesity_child_15_16.htm (accessed on 29 June 2020).
2. Mejia de Grubb, M.C.; Levine, R.S.; Zoorob, R.J. Diet and obesity issues in the underserved. *Prim. Care* **2017**, *44*, 127–140. [CrossRef] [PubMed]
3. Hales, C.M.; Carroll, M.D.; Fryar, C.D.; Ogden, C.L. Prevalence of obesity among adults and youth: United States 2011–2014. *NCHS Data Brief.* **2017**, *2017*, 1–8.
4. Ogden, C.L.; Carroll, M.D.; Fakhouri, T.H.; Hales, C.M.; Fryar, C.D.; Li, X.; Freedman, D.S. Prevalence of obesity among youths by household income and education level of head of household—United States 2011–2014. *MMWR Morb. Mortal. Wkly. Rep.* **2018**, *67*, 186–189. [CrossRef] [PubMed]
5. U.S. Department of Health and Human Services. Healthy People. Available online: https://www.healthypeople.gov/ (accessed on 29 June 2020).
6. Wilfley, D.E.; Saelens, B. Epidemiology and causes of obesity in children. In *Eating Disorders and Obesity: A Comprehensive Handbook*, 2nd ed.; Fairburn, C.G., Brownell, K.D., Eds.; The Guildford Press: New York, NY, USA, 2002; pp. 429–432.

7. Kumar, S.; Kaufman, T. Childhood obesity. *Panminerva Med.* **2018**, *60*, 200–212. [CrossRef] [PubMed]
8. Santiago-Torres, M.; Adams, A.K.; Carrel, A.L.; LaRowe, T.L.; Schoeller, D.A. Home food availability, parental dietary intake, and familial eating habits influence the diet quality of urban Hispanic children. *Child. Obes.* **2014**, *10*, 408–415. [CrossRef] [PubMed]
9. Scaglioni, S.; De Cosmi, V.; Ciappolino, V.; Parazzini, F.; Brambilla, P.; Agostoni, C. Factors influencing children's eating behaviours. *Nutrients* **2018**, *10*, 706. [CrossRef] [PubMed]
10. Beckerman, J.P.; Alike, Q.; Lovin, E.; Tamez, M.; Mattei, J. The development and public health implications of food preferences in children. *Front. Nutr.* **2017**, *4*, 66. [CrossRef]
11. French, S.A.; Tangney, C.C.; Crane, M.M.; Wang, Y.; Appelhans, B.M. Nutrition quality of food purchases varies by household income: The SHoPPER study. *BMC Public Health* **2019**, *19*, 231. [CrossRef]
12. Banfield, E.C.; Liu, Y.; Davis, J.S.; Chang, S.; Frazier-Wood, A.C. Poor adherence to US dietary guidelines for children and adolescents in the National Health and Nutrition Examination Survey population. *J. Acad Nutr. Diet.* **2016**, *116*, 21–27. [CrossRef]
13. Satia, J.A. Diet-related disparities: Understanding the problem and accelerating solutions. *J. Am. Diet. Assoc.* **2009**, *109*, 610–615. [CrossRef]
14. Block, J.P.; Subramanian, S.V. Moving beyond "food deserts": Reorienting United States policies to reduce disparities in diet quality. *PLoS Med.* **2015**, *12*, e1001914. [CrossRef] [PubMed]
15. Lucan, S.C.; Maroko, A.R.; Sanon, O.C.; Schechter, C.B. Unhealthful food-and-beverage advertising in subway stations: Targeted marketing, vulnerable groups, dietary intake, and poor health. *J. Urban. Health* **2017**, *94*, 220–232. [CrossRef] [PubMed]
16. Fleischhacker, S.E.; Evenson, K.R.; Rodriguez, D.A.; Ammerman, A.S. A systematic review of fast food access studies. *Obes. Rev.* **2011**, *12*, e460–e471. [CrossRef] [PubMed]
17. Hager, E.R.; Cockerham, A.; O'Reilly, N.; Harrington, D.; Harding, J.; Hurley, K.M.; Black, M.M. Food swamps and food deserts in Baltimore City, MD, USA: Associations with dietary behaviours among urban adolescent girls. *Public Health Nutr.* **2017**, *20*, 2598–2607. [CrossRef]
18. Gruber, K.J.; Haldeman, L.A. Using the family to combat childhood and adult obesity. *Prev. Chronic Dis.* **2009**, *6*, A106.
19. Laraia, B.A.; Leak, T.M.; Tester, J.M.; Leung, C.W. Biobehavioral factors that shape nutrition in low-income populations: A narrative review. *Am. J. Prev. Med.* **2017**, *52*, S118–S126. [CrossRef]
20. Evans, A.; Chow, S.; Jennings, R.; Dave, J.; Scoblick, K.; Sterba, K.R.; Loyo, J. Traditional foods and practices of Spanish-speaking Latina mothers influence the home food environment: Implications for future interventions. *J. Am. Diet. Assoc.* **2011**, *111*, 1031–1038. [CrossRef]
21. Nepper, M.J.; Chai, W. Parents' barriers and strategies to promote healthy eating among school-age children. *Appetite* **2016**, *103*, 15–64. [CrossRef]
22. Parks, E.P.; Kazak, A.; Kumanyika, S.; Lewis, L.; Barg, F.K. Perspectives on stress, parenting, and children's obesity-related behaviors in Black families. *Health Educ. Behav.* **2016**, *43*, 632–640. [CrossRef]
23. Taverno Ross, S.E.; Macia, L.; Documét, P.I.; Escribano, C.; Kazemi Naderi, T.; Smith-Tapia, I. Latino parents' perceptions of physical activity and healthy eating: At the intersection of culture, family, and health. *J. Nutr. Educ. Behav.* **2018**, *50*, 968–976. [CrossRef]
24. Thompson, D.; Callender, C.; Velazquez, D.; Gonzalez, A.; Adera, M.; Li, P.; Mackey, G.; Dave, J.M.; Olvera, N.; Chen, T.A.; et al. *Common Threads Grant—Final Report*; Baylor College of Medicine: Houston, TX, USA, 2020; unpublished work.
25. Jamshed, S. Qualitative research method-interviewing and observation. *J. Basic Clin. Pharm.* **2014**, *5*, 87–88. [CrossRef] [PubMed]
26. Fereday, J.; Muir-Cochrane, E. Demonstrating rigor using thematic analysis: A hybrid approach of inductive and deductive coding and theme development. *Int. J. Qual. Methods* **2006**, *5*, 80–92. [CrossRef]
27. Lilo, E.A.; Muñoz, M.; Cruz, T.H. Perceptions of healthy eating among Hispanic parent-child dyads. *Health Promot. Pract.* **2019**, *20*, 231–238. [CrossRef] [PubMed]
28. Danford, C.A.; Martyn, K.K. Exploring eating and activity behaviors with parent-child dyads using event history calendars. *J. Fam. Nurs.* **2013**, *19*, 375–398. [CrossRef] [PubMed]
29. Yee, A.Z.; Lwin, M.O.; Ho, S.S. The influence of parental practices on child promotive and preventive food consumption behaviors: A systematic review and meta-analysis. *Int. J. Behav. Nutr. Phys. Act.* **2017**, *14*, 47. [CrossRef] [PubMed]

30. van der Velde, L.A.; Schuilenburg, L.A.; Thrivikraman, J.K.; Numans, M.E.; Kiefte-de Jong, J.C. Needs and perceptions regarding healthy eating among people at risk of food insecurity: A qualitative analysis. *Int. J. Equity Health* **2019**, *18*, 184. [CrossRef]
31. Couch, S.C.; Glanz, K.; Zhou, C.; Sallis, J.F.; Saelens, B.E. Home food environment in relation to children's diet quality and weight status. *J. Acad. Nutr. Diet.* **2014**, *114*, 1569–1579.e1. [CrossRef]
32. Dave, J.M.; Thompson, D.I.; Svendsen-Sanchez, A.; Cullen, K.W. Perspectives on barriers to eating healthy among food pantry clients. *Health Equity* **2017**, *1*, 28–34. [CrossRef]
33. Oates, G.R.; Phillips, J.M.; Bateman, L.B.; Baskin, M.L.; Fouad, M.N.; Scarinci, I.C. Determinants of obesity in two urban communities: Perceptions and community-driven solutions. *Ethn. Dis.* **2018**, *28*, 33–42. [CrossRef]
34. Callender, C.; Thompson, D. Text messaging based obesity prevention program for parents of pre-adolescent African American girls. *Children* **2017**, *4*, 105. [CrossRef]
35. St. George, S.M.; Wilson, D.K. A qualitative study for understanding family and peer influences on obesity-related health behaviors in low-income African-American adolescents. *Child. Obes.* **2012**, *8*, 466–476. [CrossRef] [PubMed]
36. Banna, J.C.; Buchthal, O.V.; Delormier, T.; Creed-Kanashiro, H.M.; Penny, M.E. Influences on eating: A qualitative study of adolescents in a periurban area in Lima, Peru. *BMC Public Health* **2016**, *16*, 40. [CrossRef] [PubMed]
37. Lopez-Dicastillo, O.; Grande, G.; Callery, P. School children's own views, roles and contribution to choices regarding diet and activity in Spain. *Child. Care Health Dev.* **2013**, *39*, 109–117. [CrossRef] [PubMed]
38. Dave, J.M.; Evans, A.E.; Condrasky, M.D.; Williams, J.E. Parent-reported social support for child's fruit and vegetable intake: Validity of measures. *J. Nutr. Educ. Behav.* **2012**, *44*, 132–139. [CrossRef] [PubMed]
39. Haines, J.; Haycraft, E.; Lytle, L.M.; Nicklaus, S.; Kok, F.; Merdji, M.; Fisberg, M.; Moreno, L.A.; Goulet, O.J.; Hughes, S.O. Nurturing children's healthy eating: Position statement. *Appetite* **2019**, *137*, 124–133. [CrossRef] [PubMed]
40. Holsten, J.E.; Deatrick, J.A.; Kumanyika, S.; Pinto-Martin, J.; Compher, C.W. Children's food choice process in the home environment. A qualitative descriptive study. *Appetite* **2012**, *58*, 64–73. [CrossRef]
41. Pearce, A.; Kirk, C.; Cummins, S.; Collins, M.; Elliman, D.; Connolly, A.; Law, C. Gaining children's perspectives: A multiple method approach to explore environmental influences on healthy eating and physical activity. *Health Place* **2009**, *15*, 614–621. [CrossRef]

7

Machine Learning Models to Predict Childhood and Adolescent Obesity

Gonzalo Colmenarejo

Biostatistics and Bioinformatics Unit, IMDEA Food, CEI UAM+CSIC, E28049 Madrid, Spain; gonzalo.colmenarejo@imdea.org

Abstract: The prevalence of childhood and adolescence overweight an obesity is raising at an alarming rate in many countries. This poses a serious threat to the current and near-future health systems, given the association of these conditions with different comorbidities (cardiovascular diseases, type II diabetes, and metabolic syndrome) and even death. In order to design appropriate strategies for its prevention, as well as understand its origins, the development of predictive models for childhood/adolescent overweight/obesity and related outcomes is of extreme value. Obesity has a complex etiology, and in the case of childhood and adolescence obesity, this etiology includes also specific factors like (pre)-gestational ones; weaning; and the huge anthropometric, metabolic, and hormonal changes that during this period the body suffers. In this way, Machine Learning models are becoming extremely useful tools in this area, given their excellent predictive power; ability to model complex, nonlinear relationships between variables; and capacity to deal with high-dimensional data typical in this area. This is especially important given the recent appearance of large repositories of Electronic Health Records (EHR) that allow the development of models using datasets with many instances and predictor variables, from which Deep Learning variants can generate extremely accurate predictions. In the current work, the area of Machine Learning models to predict childhood and adolescent obesity and related outcomes is comprehensively and critically reviewed, including the latest ones using Deep Learning with EHR. These models are compared with the traditional statistical ones that used mainly logistic regression. The main features and applications appearing from these models are described, and the future opportunities are discussed.

Keywords: childhood obesity; obesity; overweight; machine learning; deep learning; statistical models; data science; BMI

---

1. Introduction

Obesity and overweight prevalence among children and adolescents has increased to a large extent during the last four decades [1,2]. For instance, the prevalence of overweight and obese children and adolescents between 5 and 19 years has soared from about 4% in 1975 to 18% in 2016 [3]. This increase is especially dramatic in developing countries [4], while in developed countries it seems to be slowing down and affects mainly the low-income sub-populations [5]. In absolute numbers, it is currently estimated that about 38 million children under the age of 5 are overweight or obese, while about 340 million children and adolescents aged 5–19 years are overweight or obese [3].

This large prevalence poses a threat to the current and future health systems. Childhood and adolescent obesity is related to different comorbidities during this age [6–10], as well as to a lower quality of life [11], but, in addition, it is also associated to *adult* comorbidities, like metabolic syndrome and diabetes [12], cardiovascular risk [13,14], and death [15,16]. This is probably due to the difficulty in its eradication once it is established, justifying the adoption of childhood preventive measures, rather than therapeutic ones [9].

Obesity, that is, excess adipose tissue in the body [17], has a complex, multifactorial etiology. Among the factors involved in its development, the most important ones are genetics, physical activity, sedentary lifestyle, diet, etc. [18] In addition, obesity has additional complications for its analysis during childhood and adolescence. This is largely due to the huge changes in height and weight during this period. If we measure the Body Mass Index (BMI) through it, we see a pattern of an initial increase until reaching a first peak at about 1 year, followed by a decrease up to the age of about 6 years, where it starts to rise again (the so-called *adipose rebound*) [18]. So big are these changes that there is no universal consensus in the definitions of "overweight" and "obese" based on BMI at these ages [17], and in most cases, they are defined using sex-, age- and population-specific percentiles, normally ≥ 85th percentile for overweight, and ≥ 95th percentile for obese, as will be discussed in Section 4 in detail. (It must be noted that in this Review we use the concept "obesity" in two ways: one is as excess adipose tissue in the body in general, and the other is a BMI-based category to classify individuals, normally for adults BMI ≥ 30 kg/m^2 and for children with multiple definitions as described in the text.)

Therefore, during this period, there happen large metabolic and hormonal changes that largely influence the adiposity at different ages. On top of that, there is still a large influence of specific pre-gestational and gestational factors, especially during early childhood, that have a large impact at these ages. The additional risk factors for obesity in childhood-adolescence have been reviewed recently [18,19]. Some of the most outstanding ones are parent's BMI, gestational weight gain of the mother, gestational diabetes, maternal smoking, birth weight, rapid infant growth, and high protein and/or free sugars consumption. There are also psychological factors, especially during the adolescence period.

In order to prevent childhood and adolescent obesity, the development of predictive models to identify potential individuals of high risk is of great utility. This allows the focusing of preventive measures towards the high-risk subpopulation, allowing a more cost-effective and personalized approach to weight reduction interventions. In addition, the use of predictive models allows, by their analysis, to rank the different risk factors in order of importance, so that we can identify those that would be more effective in order to design these interventions. Moreover, the models can be used as simulation tools where "what-if" analyses can be conducted, by varying one or more predictor variables and seeing what would be the effect in obesity for particular sub-populations (defined by, e.g., sex, age, diet, etc.).

Given the large complexity of obesity, especially during the childhood and adolescence period, with a large number of multidomain influencing factors interacting in convoluted ways, traditional statistical methods like (generalized) linear models show limitations and have focused mainly in analyses with a reduced number of predictor variables and with limited predictive power. As we will see in Section 3, these models in most cases use more or less the same set of predictor variables transformed in one way or another and aggregated a linear functional form. Another limitation of these methods is their inability to deal with high-dimensional data, where the number of predictor variables (columns) is close or even much higher than that the number of dataset instances (rows), as they typically require many more instances than predictor variables in order to provide reliable inferences and avoid overfitting. Such situation makes them to need huge samples for they to be used with large sets of predictor variables, resulting in difficult practical implementations.

In this way, Machine Learning (ML) techniques are especially gifted modelling tools for these datasets, typically of high-dimensional nature and with complex relationships between many multidomain variables. This is due to their capacity to deal with high-dimensional data so that they can be applied to model relatively small datasets having large numbers of predictor variables and with reduced overfit. In addition, ML methods are able to find complex, nonlinear relationships between the predictor variables and these and the response variable or variables in an automated way, not requiring to manually predefine and test a large set of potential relationships between these variables. Therefore, the predictive capacity, ease of application, and robustness of these models for complex data far outclasses those of the traditional statistical models. This is even more in the case of the recent Deep Learning (DL) branch of ML, which can tap from huge datasets both in instances and predictor variables to obtain models with extremely good predictive capacities. DL methods, in addition, are able to directly use complex data like images, text, social media, time series, etc., avoiding the need of lengthy *feature engineering* processes, as we will see in Section 2. This is increasing dramatically the scope of data sources that can be used in this field, allowing to identify novel risk factors.

Given the above described advantages of ML over statistical methods for this problem, it is no surprise that ML have started to be used in the area. Thus, this paper attempts to conduct a critical and comprehensive review of the work done in ML models applied so far to the area of childhood and adolescent obesity. This will include a brief unbiased summary of each of the works available in the area to predict childhood or adolescent BMI and/or obesity/overweight with ML, followed by a thorough discussion of the collective patterns found, results obtained and novel risks factors identified, advantages and limitations of the approach, and future perspectives. The discussion will include also a comparison with the statistical models of the same outcomes, which will have been briefly reviewed previously. In addition, models to predict related outcomes (e.g., success of weight decreasing therapies, social obesogenic environments, pediatric attention to obesity, etc.) will also be reviewed, as they are of increasing interest especially in the area of preventive interventions. We will see that this is a new field that has experienced a recent explosion, especially during the last five years, mainly through the use of massive databases of Electronic Health Records (EHR) and the application for the first time of DL techniques, which is starting to allow a more systematic analysis of large cohorts with many multidomain predictor variables and the introduction of complex data sources as predictors. As the reader will see, this is also a very heterogeneous field, both in terms of type of model (cross-sectional, longitudinal), label predicted by the model (obesity, overweight, success of obesity therapies, pediatric attention to obesity, etc.), aim of the predictions (explanatory, predictive, and simulation), and application of the model (prediction of risk subpopulation, optimization of obesity therapy, suggestion of novel therapeutic approaches, etc.), further extending those typical of statistical models. It is expected to provide an updated view of the field to researchers within multiple disciplines and interests: statisticians, engineers, data scientists, epidemiologists, pediatricians, nurses, and nutritionists.

The article will be organized as follows: after this Introduction, first, a summary of the ML field will be conducted in order to provide some basic knowledge for readers not experts in the field, trying to make the work as much self-contained as possible; second, the procedure to search and select the reviewed works will be described; third, the statistical models in the childhood/adolescence obesity area will be reviewed, in order to set a comparison point with the ML models; fourth, ML models targeted to the prediction of BMI or categorized versions of BMI will be reviewed; fifth, ML models targeted to the prediction of related outcomes will be reviewed; sixth, a final wrap-up discussion of the main patterns in the models summarized will close the paper.

2. Basic Concepts in Machine Learning

Machine Learning (ML) exploded in the 90s of last century as a new field of data analysis at the interface between Statistics and Artificial Intelligence. Although the initial concepts like Rosenblatt's perceptron [20] (a basic, 1-layer artificial neural network to perform binary classification), Naïve Bayes [21], Decision Trees [21], and k-Nearest Neighbors date back to the 50s–60s of the 20th century, it was during the last decade of it when the field started to enter into full maturity and be massively applied. This happened with the appearance of multi-layer neural networks, thanks to the invention of the *backpropagation* training algorithm [22], as well as other ML paradigms like Support Vector Machines [23] and, in the first decade of the 21st century, Random Forests [24] and Gradient Boosting Machines [25]. This emergence has been fostered by the confluence of CPU miniaturization and cheapening, massive accessibility of computational capacity, and the development of completely new ideas for statistical modeling.

This explosion has been followed, in the second decade of the 21st century, by the one of *Deep Learning* (DL). DL is an outgrowth from ML that comprises mainly artificial neural networks of very large numbers of layers (the term "deep" comes from here), together with specialized layers, like *convolutional* and *recurrent* ones, and additional adaptations to allow the training of these huge neural networks: non-saturable activation functions; new weight initialization schemes; faster optimizers; and the training of the network in small, random batches of the data (the so-called *mini-batch* training). The DL models contain typically millions of training parameters. The specialized layers find directly from complex data like images, sounds, texts, music, etc., patterns ("feature maps") that are fed into multi-layer fully-connected perceptrons, allowing the direct modeling of this complex data, without the need of manually generating compressed representations of these data, the so-called "feature engineering".

Again, DL has benefited from an additional increase of computational power easily accessible, mainly though both the use of GPUs instead of CPUs, and of cloud computing, as well as the availability of huge public datasets (e.g., YouTube, San Bruno, CA, USA; Wikipedia, Facebook, Menlo Park, CA, USA; etc.) and open competitions (Kaggle, San Francisco, CA, USA, etc.).

Generally speaking, ML has put more emphasis in *prediction* rather than *testing of a predefined hypothesis* like traditional statistical models, where the emphasis is more in inference. In the same way, the focus is more in a practical, engineering-oriented approach rather than on a rigorous theoretical background. ML can be defined as a set of algorithms that *automatically learn simplified representations of the data*. For example, we can present the ML algorithm with a set of data instances, like pictures of animals, together with a label for the species present in each picture. The algorithm would then be *trained* by automatically learning some abstract internal rules to associate each image to each label, by minimizing some kind of measure of the prediction error or *loss*. When presented with new pictures, the algorithm would then be able to assign a label (species name) to each of them.

ML models are able to cope with very complex datasets, even those with many more predictor variables than instances (*high-dimensional datasets*). For this reason, they tend to be more difficult to interpret ("black-box" type of models), although as we will see later, new techniques have been developed to facilitate understanding the inner working of the model.

From our purposes in this Review, we can talk about two main groups of ML models: *supervised* and *unsupervised*. Supervised models are those that use datasets comprising both a set of *predictor variables* and one or more *target variables* or *labels*. The model would then be trained to be able to predict the label(s) from new instances of the predictor variables: for instance, to predict if a child will be obese or not from his age, sex, parent's BMI, and food consumption. The other type of ML models, *unsupervised ones*, attempt to find, without the use of labels, transformations of the input data with easier visualization, less noise, etc., or try to identify groups in the data. These techniques include *Dimensionality Reduction* and *Clustering* techniques.

Within the area of supervised models, which are the ones we will see in the Review, there are two main groups: *classification* models, those where the predicted label is a categorical one (e.g., obese child yes or not), and *regression* models, those where the label is a numeric one (e.g., BMI).

The most important type of classification models is *binary classification*, where the label has only two categories, for instance "+" and "−". In this case, the model frequently outputs a probability p of one of the two classes (e.g., "+"; the probability of the alternate class "−" would be $1 - p$). Once we define a threshold t for this probability, if $p \geq t$ for a new instance, we would assign the category "+" to that instance; if, on the contrary, $p < t$, we would assign the category "−". At this point, several concepts are used to characterize the performance of the model (Figure 1), depending on whether the real category is "+" or "−", and whether the predicted category is "+" or "−".

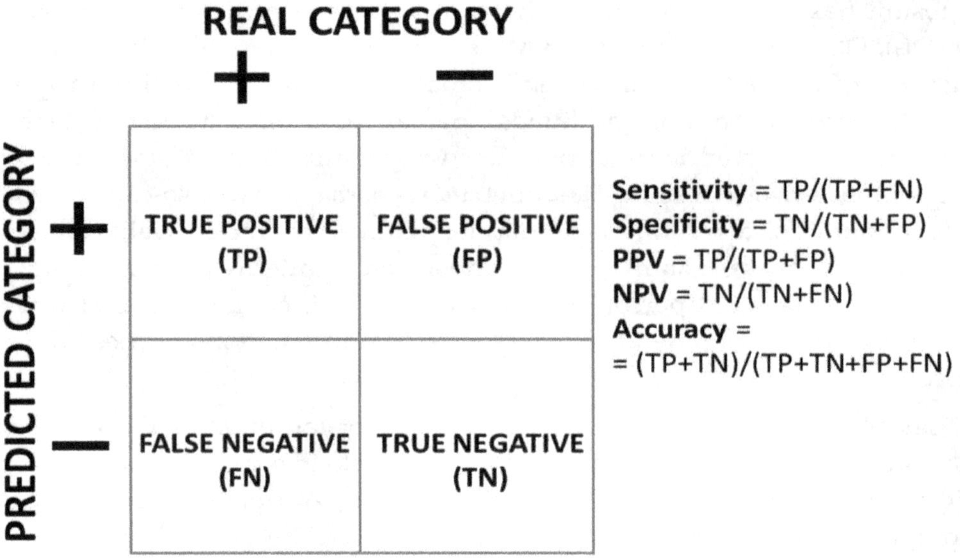

Figure 1. Measures of the performance of a binary classifier. Class labels are "+" and "−". Predicted category by the model is represented vs the real category, for all the possible situations.

Sensitivity (or *recall*) is the proportion of real positives that are predicted as positives. *Specificity* is the proportion of real negatives that are predicted as negatives. *Positive Predictive Value* (PPV), or *precision*, is the proportion of predicted positives that are real positives, and *Negative Predictive Value* (NPV) is the proportion of predicted negatives that are real negatives. *Accuracy* is the total proportion of correct predictions of all the predicted data.

A perfect model would have all these measures equal to 1. Obviously, this is almost never the case, and we have to cope with some proportion of errors. We can choose the threshold t so that it optimizes the purpose of our model. For example, if we are mainly interested in identifying as many real positives (e.g., future obese children) as possible, in order to apply to them some preventive weight-loss treatment, we would select a lower t and thus increase the sensitivity, even at the cost of increasing the false positives and, therefore, decreasing the specificity and the PPV. This approach would reach a point where we would identify so many false positives that would result in a prohibitive cost for treating many unnecessary cases or, if applying the treatment to a future normal-weight child has a negative effect, an unnecessary harm to too many members of our population. Alternatively, if we are more interested in finding a sample of children most of whom will be obese in the future, even if it is small (e.g., we can use it later for genotyping purposes), we would be more interested in optimizing the PPV; in this case, we would use a larger t, therefore increasing the false negatives. This would result in a decreased sensitivity and NPV. Again, we cannot increase t indefinitely, because there will be a point where the sample would be so small that would become useless. Therefore, there is always a balance between the cost and benefit, not just from the statistical point of view but also from the practical application of the model, which must be taken into consideration when optimizing the threshold of the model.

In order to characterize the discriminative capacity of the model, before selecting t, it is customary to use Receiver Operating Characteristic (ROC) curves. In this curve, the sensitivity is plotted against 1-specificity for all the values of the threshold (Figure 2).

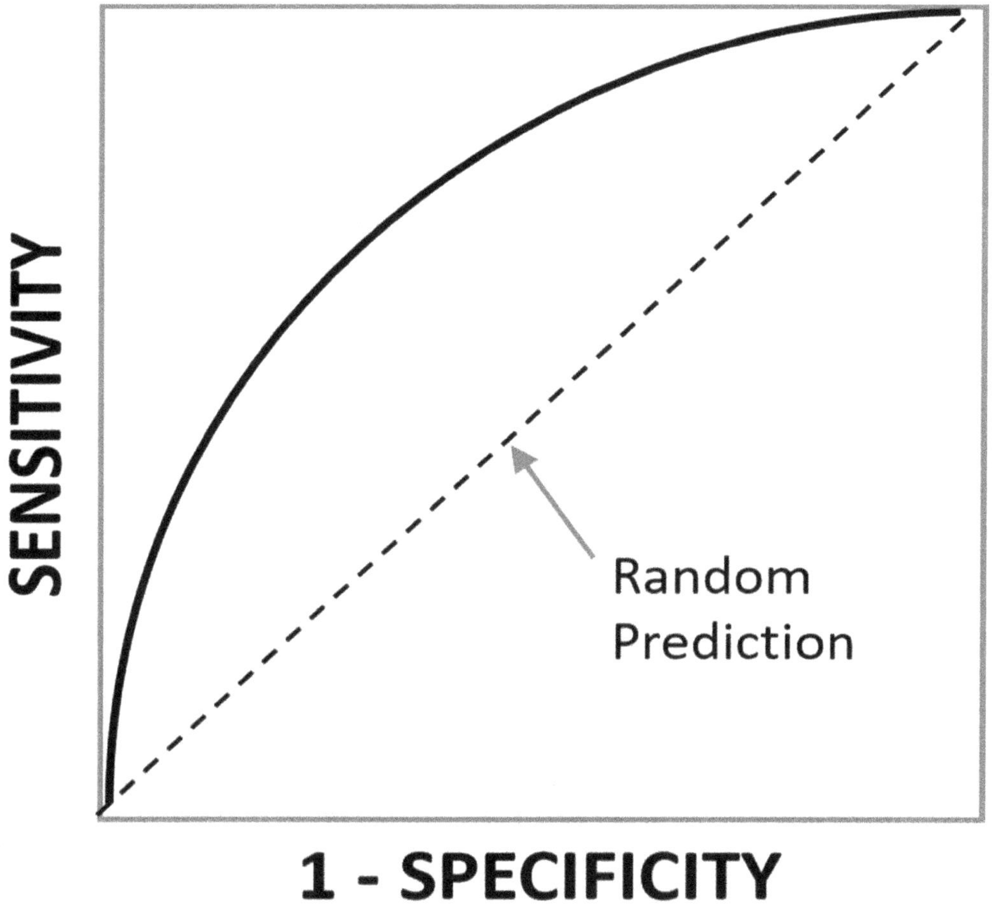

Figure 2. ROC curve of a binary classifier.

For a random classifier, the curve will be a diagonal going from (0, 0) to (1, 1). For a perfect classifier, the curve would go from (0, 0) to (0, 1) and then to (1, 1). Intermediate classifiers would have a curve in between these two extremes. A frequent measure of the discriminatory power of the classifier is the area under the curve of the ROC curve (AUCROC). A random classifier has an AUCROC of 0.5, and a perfect classifier has an AUCROC of 1. Real-life classifiers would have values in between, the better the closer to 1. The AUCROC equals the so-called *concordance index* or *c-index*.

When the classifier predicts a multi-class label, that is, with more than two classes, a measure of the prediction performance is the accuracy, defined above as the percentage of instances for which the label is predicted correctly. Another measure is the *categorical cross-entropy*. For a prediction instance i and an M-category label, it is defined as the Equation (1)

$$-\sum_{j=1}^{M} I_{ij} log P_{ij} \quad (1)$$

where I_{ij} is an indicator variable that is 0 if the predicted class j of instance i is not correct and 1 if it is. P_{ij} is the predicted probability for class j on the new instance i. For n predicted instances, the categorical cross-entropy would be the sum of each of the instances categorical cross-entropies. Therefore, it basically measures the match between the predicted probabilities for the different classes with the observed frequencies. The better the agreement between predicted and actual labels, the smaller the categorical cross-entropy, thus being an *error* or *loss* function that is minimized as the model is trained with the training data (in the case of accuracy, it would be maximized). For binary classifiers, the cross-entropy formula simplifies to $M = 2$, and we have the *binary cross-entropy*.

When we deal with regression, common measures of the error or loss are the *Mean Squared Error* (MSE, the Equation (2)):

$$MSE = \frac{1}{n}\sum_{i=1}^{n}(y_i - \hat{y}_i)^2 \tag{2}$$

where n is the number of predicted instances, y_i is the actual continuous label for instance i, and $\hat{y}_i$ is the predicted value of the label for that instance. Another is the *Mean Absolute Error* (MAE, the Equation (3)):

$$MAE = \frac{1}{n}\sum_{i=1}^{n}\left|y_i - \hat{y}_i\right| \tag{3}$$

where $|.|$ means absolute value.

When training a model with training data, there is a risk that the model learns too many details of the latter, which makes it perform worse when presented with new data. In this case, we say that the model is *overfit*. Normally, all the models we fit will fit better the training data than new datasets. Therefore, in order to assess the *practical* prediction performance of a model, we need to *validate* it with new data. We will see that there are different approaches for validation of models, which can be divided in two groups: *internal validation* methods and *external validation* methods.

The main feature of internal validation methods is that we resample several times from the whole dataset, fit a new model with the resample, and evaluate the model with the instances left out from the resample. From this repeated resampling, model fit, and evaluation, we get an estimation of the predictive performance of the modeling *process* with new data, although we do not really test a final model with new data. Internal validations are used normally when the data is scarce, so it is very difficult to obtain a new data set to externally validate the model.

There are two main general approaches for internal validation: *cross-validation* and *bootstrap*. In the former case, in its *k-fold* version, what we do is divide the total sample into k random subsets ("folds"; as for k, normally 5 or 10 is used). Then what we do is, for each fold, validate with this fold a model fitted with the $k - 1$ remaining folds. The estimated validation measure of the performance of the model (accuracy, cross-entropy, MSE, etc.) will be the average of the performances of the k models fitted with each k subsamples, each having with $k-1$ folds and evaluated in the corresponding hold-out fold.

Cross-validation schemes can also be used to estimate *hyperparameters* of our model (e.g., number of nearest neighbors in the k-Nearest Neighbors method, see below). What we do then is perform the cross-validation with a double loop of folds; in one loop, we vary the hyperparameter among several options, and in the other, we estimate the validation performance within each hyperparameter selection. We will select the hyperparameter value that optimizes the cross-validation performance estimate, and at the same time that performance will serve as estimate of the external performance of the model (fitted with that optimal hyperparameter value).

It must be taken into account that the models fitted with cross-validation use a smaller dataset than the whole dataset, so this can be a source of error of estimation of the performance. The other approach for internal validation, bootstrap, avoids this issue by generating repeatedly samples of the same size of the original one by sampling with replacement (allowing randomly repeated instances). The model is refitted for each of these random samples and then evaluated in both that sample and in the original sample or the left-out instances. By averaging the difference between the training performance in each sample and the performance in the original sample, we get an estimation of the so-called *optimism* in the training performance. Then, we would derive the model with the whole dataset, evaluate its performance, and correct it by the estimated optimism.

We see that in both cross-validation and bootstrap, we do not make a real evaluation of the external performance of the model but rather make an estimation of it from data that is used at the end in the derivation of the final model. The alternative is to use an *external validation sample*. This is data that is not used in the derivation of the model and is only used for validating the model. A simple approach here is to randomly split the original sample into a training dataset (e.g., 60–80% of the data) to fit the model with it and then a validation/testing dataset (40–20% of the data) to evaluate external performance. This has two drawbacks when compared with internal validation methods: on one hand, we miss some of the data in the model derivation; on the other hand, we make the estimation of the external performance with a normally small dataset, which would result in an estimate with high variance (depending on how "lucky" we are in the random split, we can have very different estimates). This is not an issue if we have a very large dataset, and the validation set is quite large. However, in case we have a small dataset, it is preferable to use internal validation measures, despite being a bit more optimistic than external validations.

In addition, the random split approach has an additional problem in that both the training and the validation datasets come from the same sample, and thus, it is likely that they are very similar, a situation that quite possibly does not to occur when using the model in real life. There are ways to avoid this issue, like clustering the original sample and then generating training and validation datasets from different clusters. Another approach is to train the model with one dataset and then validate it with a different dataset, e.g., a posterior in time dataset, a dataset from another country, etc. This is a more demanding comparison but is probably the closest to the real performance of the model in production. Obviously, this approach is very expensive in terms of datasets, so it is only available in a reduced number of situations.

We will finish this section by briefly describing the ML models we will see in the Review.

2.1. *Naïve Bayes (NB)*

This method uses Bayes rule together with the approximation of conditional independence of predictor variables given the response class. Bayes rule establishes the posterior probability of the target variable y (label) taking the value j, conditioned to the predictor variables $x_1, \ldots, x_n$ (the Equation (4)):

$$P(y = j|x_1, \ldots, x_n) = \frac{P(x_1, \ldots, x_n|y = j)P(y = j)}{P(x_1, \ldots, x_n)} \quad (4)$$

where $P(y = j)$ is the prior probability of y taking the value j, $P(x_1, \ldots, x_n|y = j)$ is the posterior probability of the predictor variables conditioned to y taking the value j, and $P(x_1, \ldots, x_n)$ are the prior probabilities of the predictor variables. These prior and conditional probabilities can be estimated from the respective empirical frequencies when the predictor variables are categorical. When they are continuous, they can be approximated by different kernel functions. When the independence approximation is applied in NB, this simplifies largely (the Equation (5)):

$$P(y = j|x_1, \ldots, x_n) = \frac{P(y = j) \prod_1^n P(x_i|y = j)}{P(x_1, \ldots, x_n)} \quad (5)$$

The predicted class for a set of $x_1, \ldots, x_n$ predictor values will be the one that maximizes the productory above, since the other factors are constant.

2.2. *k-Nearest Neighbors (kNN)*

The idea of this method is quite simple: For a new instance with predictor variables $x_1, \ldots, x_n$, assign the label most frequent between the k instances in the training data with predictor variables less distant (more similar, the k-*nearest neighbors*) to the new instance predictor variables. This is called the *majority voting* class assignment. When the label is a continuous one (regression), the predicted value is the (weighted) average of the labels of the k-nearest neighbors. In order to measure the distance between sets of predictor variables, different metrics can be used. Probably the most frequent is the Euclidean one. The value of k can be quite variable and depends heavily on the dataset. It can be obtained through cross-validation techniques.

2.3. Decision Trees (DT)

This method can be used for both regression and classification. The idea here is to generate rectangular partitions of the space of predictor variables, by successive splitting the data by (usually binary) splits in one variable that optimize some loss function (e.g., minimization of MSE for regression). At the end, the label we assign to each partition is one function of the labels of the data instances belonging to each partition, e.g., its mean, or the majority voting class. Then, for new instances, we will find the partition it belongs to and assign the label that corresponds to that partition. A simple schema with only two predictor variables is depicted in Figure 3.

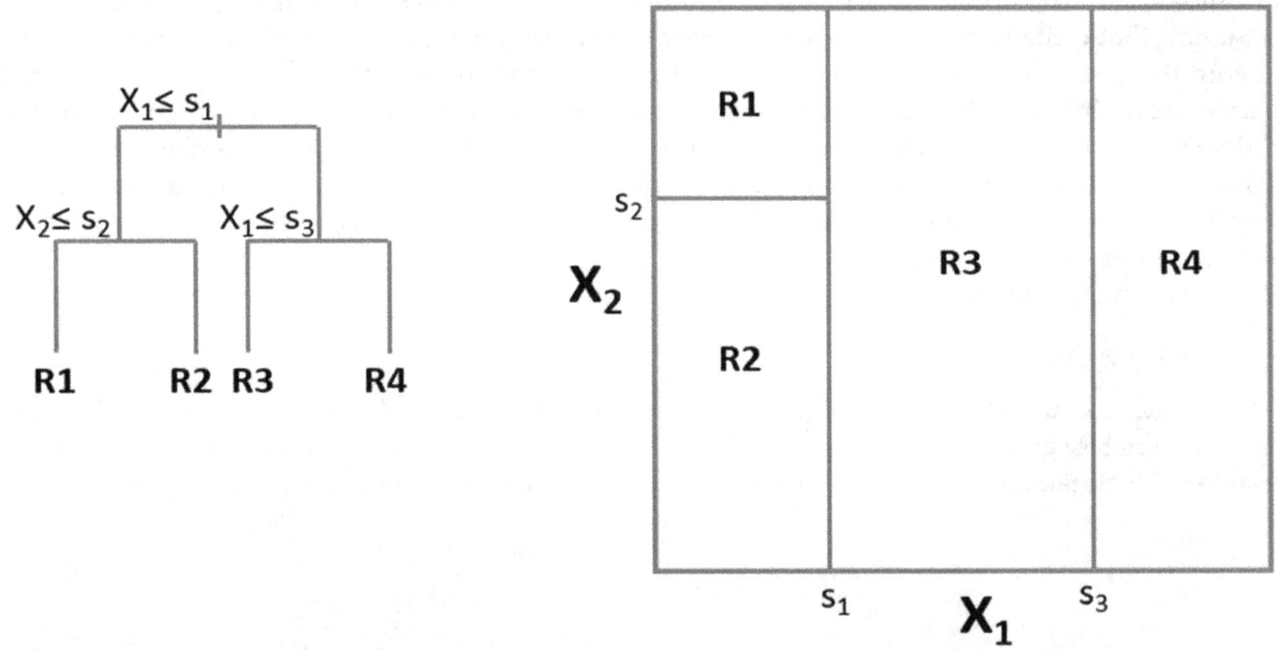

Figure 3. Depiction of Decision Tree for two variables, X_1 and X_2. R1, R2, R3, and R4 are partitions generated by the splits s_1, s_2, and s_3. The labels for the partitions would be a function of the labels of the instances in each partition in the training set.

Obviously, to grow a tree can become a very complicated task, given the combinatorial number of possible splits and variable sequences that can be created. Therefore, simplified algorithms for generating the tree have been devised. There are different ones, depending on the criteria for split, the selection of variables at each split, and the pruning of terminal nodes. These are CART [26], on one hand, and ID3 [27], which evolved to C4.5 (also called J48 in Weka's Java implementation) and later to C5.0. There is also the CHAID [28] algorithm, based on statistical tests and allowing non-binary splits.

The advantage of DT is the ease of interpretation, which can be aided by graphical displays; however, they are known for the high variance of their predictions, such that little variations of the dataset can result in very different trees and predictions.

2.4. Support Vector Machines (SVM)

This method was initially developed as a binary classifier. The approach is to build a hyperplane from the predictor variables with maximal margin, so that one half of the predictor space would result in a "+" label and the other in a "−" label. By maximal margin is meant a hyperplane that has the largest distance to the training instances of the infinite possible hyperplanes or, more correctly, the farthest minimum perpendicular distance to the training instances (since the "margin" is the minimum distance the training set points have to the hyperplane). Figure 4 displays a dataset of two predictor variables and the corresponding maximal margin hyperplane for the training instances.

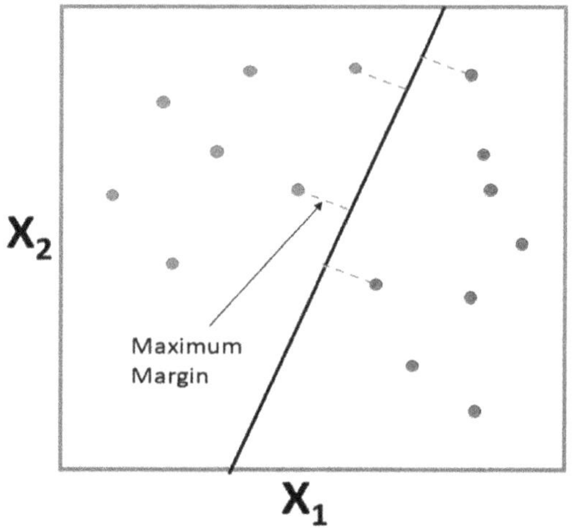

Figure 4. Maximum margin hyperplane for a predictor space of two variables. Two categories are perfectly classified by this hyperplane. The hashed lines indicate the maximum margin to the training set, obtained with this particular hyperplane. Training instances are presented as points in the plane, blue points corresponding to class "+" and red points to "−". The points located at a maximum margin to the hyperplane are the *support vectors*, since the plane only depends on these points of the training set.

For new testing instances, we just need to find which side of the hyperplane the new point lies in order to predict a label for it.

As a matter of fact, it is usually the case that the points are not perfectly separable. Therefore, instead of a maximum margin hyperplane, a "soft" margin one is obtained, by allowing some latitude for misclassified points with some specific criterion. This also makes the method more robust against small modifications of the dataset. In addition, in many situations, the boundary regions between the two classes are not linear. In this case, what we do is include as predictor variables additional specialized functions of these variables and instances, the so-called *kernels*, such that the dataset becomes linearly separable. There is a variety of kernels yielding different types of the SVM method: linear, polynomial, radial, etc. It turns out also that the computation of the hyperplane only requires the closest points to the boundary, which are called the *support vectors*, making the computation much faster. From this, the method takes its name.

Later developments of the method allowed it to deal with multiclass classification as well as regression.

2.5. Random Forest (RF)

RF are an example of ensemble methods, where a model of higher quality is built by aggregating multiple models of lower quality. The prediction for new instances will be obtained by averaging the prediction of all the simple models in the case of regression or, for classification problems, by the majority voting. In this way, we make predictions much more robust, with much less variance and with higher accuracy.

In the case of RF, we use an ensemble of hundreds or thousands of DTs. In addition, these DTs are built without pruning so that they will have little error, although large variance. However, since we are averaging many of them, the final variance will also be low. These DTs are built from bootstrap samples of the original training dataset (this is called *bagging* or bootstrap averaging). Moreover, to decorrelate the trees, at each split in the tree, only a random subset of predictor variables is used. In this way, the reduction of variance by averaging the trees is more efficient.

A very interesting property of the RFs is that they incorporate internally a direct estimation of the external validation error. Since the DT models are derived using bootstrap samples, for each instance in the training set, there will be a set of trees (approximately B/3, where B is the number of trees since they are fit using bootstrap samples) that will have been derived without that instance. By averaging the difference in label prediction for that instance in these trees and its actual label, we would have what is called an out-of-bag (OOB) estimate for that instance. Averaging over all the instances, results in an estimate of the external performance of the RF without the need to use cross-validation or bootstrap.

RFs are a very powerful predictive method, both for regression and classification, and very robust irrespective of the type of datasets. The issue with them is the difficulty of interpretation (this is general for all the ensemble methods), since they contain many different and decorrelated DTs using different predictor variables. An approach used to analyze them is the so-called *variable importance techniques*. The idea here is to analyze the effect that each predictor has (on average over all the DTs) on the error of the RF. One approach is to calculate, for each predictor, what error reduction it has had each time it has been used in the trees. This is summed for all the trees, and the largest sum will correspond to the most important predictor as on average it has produced the largest reduction of errors in all the trees. Another approach uses permutation of the variables. For each tree, we have its OOB prediction accuracy after applying it to its OOB samples. After that, the jth variable is permuted and the OOB prediction is recalculated and subtracted from the previous one. This is averaged over all the trees. This is also repeated for all the predictor variables. We would then obtain a ranking of the variables, with those with the largest reduction of OOB performance being the top ranked.

2.6. Gradient Boosting Machines (GBM)

This is another ensemble method, but one that uses *boosting* instead of bagging. By *boosting*, it is meant the iterative improvement of a weak model by adding sequentially new models that improve the previous fit. In the case of gradient boosting machines, normally the models are DTs, and the improvement is done by fitting the new model to the residuals of the model so far or, more generally, to the gradient of the loss function we are using. Newer versions, like XGboost, use the second derivatives instead of the first ones, in order to improve speed and performance.

GBM, especially XGBoost, are currently the most used ML algorithms for models using numeric tabular data or (when modeling more complex data) feature pre-engineered data. For problems using complex data directly (e.g., computer vision, speech recognition, natural language processing, etc.) Deep Learning methods are used instead (see below).

As it happens with RF, the interpretation of these ensemble models is complicated. However, in the same way, techniques like variable importance can be used to facilitate interpretation.

2.7. Regularized Linear Models (LASSO)

When fitting linear models, the residuals of the least squares fit decrease as we add more predictor variables. However, if the number of instances n is not so much larger than the number p of predictor variables, the estimates of the least squares increase their variance as p becomes closer to n so that the model becomes overfit, and the external or test performance of the model decreases. In the case of $n < p$, the variance become infinite, no unique fit exists, and the method becomes useless. However, this situation of high dimensionality is very typical in ML datasets. One way to fix this problem is to shrink or *regularize* the estimates, so they remain small and with low variance, and in some cases, they even become zero. One approach to regularization is *ridge regression*, where all predictor variables are maintained, but their betas are kept small by restraining the sum of squared betas to be less or equal than a small value. Although this approach improves external performance of the model, it keeps an interpretation issue as no irrelevant variables are removed. An alternative approach is the LASSO, where the sum of the absolute value of the betas is restrained to being less or equal than a small value. This has the advantage of making some betas equal to zero, thus performing an effective selection of important variables.

2.8. Bayesian Networks (BN)

A Bayesian Network is a directed acyclic graph of nodes that correspond predictor variables, plus one or more nodes that represent the label(s). The directed edges between the nodes represent causal relationships between the variables, through conditional dependence, and Bayes rule is used to determine the probability of the different possible values of the labels conditioned to particular values of the predictor variables. Nodes not connected would be conditionally independent. There is a large set of techniques to infer the structure and parameters of the network.

2.9. *Artificial Neural Networks (ANN)*

ANNs are ML methods that mimic the structure and mechanism of the nervous system. They are composed of layers of artificial neurons, with connections between neurons in consecutive layers. Each artificial neuron is an abstract unit that applies a weighted sum of its numeric inputs plus a bias parameter, and the resulting sum is passed to a so-called "activation function" to generate a numeric output. The first layer corresponds to the input variables; these variables are used as inputs of the next layer neurons, where each of its neurons generate an output, which is then used as input of the next layer neurons, and so on. The last layer contains typically one single neuron for one label or more for multilabel models. Figure 5 displays a typical fully connected, feedforward ANN (multilayer perceptron).

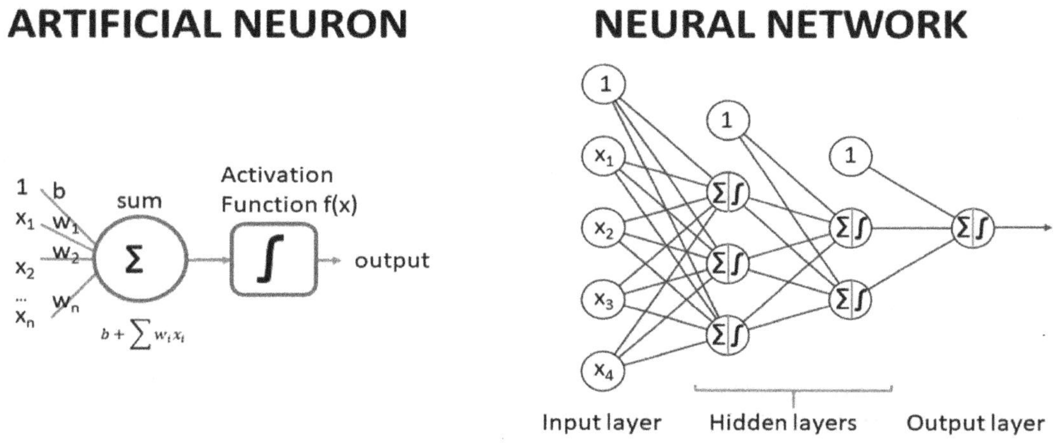

Figure 5. Typical structure of an artificial neuron and a fully connected feedforward neural network. The x_i are the predictor variables, the w_i are the weights and b is the biass.

The input layer contains the input variables (no transformation), while the last layer generates the output of the model and is called the output layer. In between, there are one or more layers, which are called "hidden" layers. Each neuron has a weight per input plus a bias parameter; all these weights and biases of all the neurons are the parameters of the network, which are optimized to minimize a loss function.

The first model or ANN was the perceptron by Rosenblat [20], which was designed as a one-neuron simple binary classifier after the mathematical neuron devised previously by McCulloh–Pitts [29]. The development of ANN to solve problems not linearly separable was allowed by the invention of the backpropagation algorithm [22], which allowed the training of multilayer perceptrons.

ANN became very popular in the 90s of last century, when they were amply used in many areas. At that time, they required feature engineering for many problems, and they were more or less abandoned in the first decade of the 21st century after the appearance of RF and GBM, since ANNs were slow to train, expensive computationally, and prone to overfitting. However, they have become very popular in the second decade of this century with the advent of the field of Deep Learning.

2.10. *Deep Learning (DL)*

The ML models we have seen so far have two main issues. On one hand, their performance in many cases shows *saturation*: This means that they reach a point when, irrespective of how big we grow the training set, the performance does not increase significantly. On the other hand, they work with numeric, tabular data, so they are unable to handle complex data like images, speech, text, etc. In order to model this type of data, it is required to convert it to numerical predictor variables in a very ad hoc and manual fashion. This is the so-called "feature engineering" problem. They are "shallow" methods, that is, unable to learn hierarchical representations of complex data.

These two problems are solved to a large extent with DL. DL consists mainly in ANNs with very large numbers of layers (that is the reason for the "Deep" in the name) and, therefore, huge numbers of training parameters. In this way, they are able to tap from huge datasets and increase steadily their performance without saturation.

On the other hand, some specialized layers have been developed that are able to automatically generate numerical representations (*feature maps*) of complex data. That is the case of *convolutional layers*, that are able to reformat tensor data of different dimensions. For example, in the case of 1D convolutional layers, they are able to find representations for serial data like text for language translation models; 2D convolutional layers are appropriate to model images like in computer vision models; while 3D layers can handle volumetric data like medical 3D images or video data.

Another specialized layers are the *recurrent layers*, where the output of the layer goes both to the next layer and to itself, allowing to find long-term and long-distance patterns by the use of ad hoc developed layers: Long Short-Term Memory (LSTM) [30] and Gated Recurrent Units (GRU) [31]. This type of layers is very appropriate also for serial data and is mostly used in natural language processing (NLP) applications.

Many of these specialized layers can be stacked sequentially and thus generate automatically hierarchies of representations with increasing levels of abstraction. This allows the model to learn very convoluted aspects of the data, which is not possible with the traditional ML methods. In addition, this hierarchical representation of the data can be applied to generate new specialized models with small datasets by reusing more general models fitted with much larger datasets. For example, we can develop one very efficient model to classify cats from a dataset of relatively few pictures of them by reusing some of the more abstract pre-fit layers of a more general model developed to classify animals from a huge dataset of pictures and adding to them some new layers that would be fit with the new small dataset of cat pictures. The previous layers would have learnt to identify the general shape of an animal, while the new layers would fit the specific features of cats. This is the process called *transfer learning*.

At the end of these layers, normally a multilayer perceptron is added to generate the output, whether numerical (regression) or categorical (classification).

DL is revolutionizing the ML area and is being applied in completely new fields, like drug discovery, music generation, self-driving cars, etc. They are also applied to biomedicine, [32,33] and as we will see, they have started to be used in the childhood obesity area.

After this summary of the main types of ML models, we proceed to describe the selection process of works reviewed in this paper.

3. Bibliographic Search and Selection of Works for Reviewing

An attempt was made for comprehensiveness in the bibliographic search, both in terms of time and publication media. Since the field of ML/DL applications is a very hot one, growing in an extremely fast way, it is not infrequent to find material published in congress proceedings, arXiv, etc. In addition, since this field shows a large interdisciplinarity, being at the interface between statistics, artificial intelligence, and biomedicine and including statisticians, engineers, pediatricians, nutritionists, and nurses in its research body, typical search engines used in biomedicine like Scopus, PubMed, etc., were not used in the search, as they missed many of the available references. Instead, Google Scholar was used for the bibliographic search. The search was performed by iteratively querying the engine with appropriate keywords in order to find papers that applied ML to predict childhood/adolescent obesity/overweight (e.g., childhood OR child OR adolescent AND machine learning OR data mining, etc.), extracting the matches and matching references in the corresponding bibliographies, and updating the queries after the titles of the matching references if necessary. This procedure was repeated until no new matches were obtained. Concept papers not applied to a particular dataset were not included.

On next section, the most outstanding statistical models in the literature to predict childhood and adolescent obesity will be briefly reviewed. These will be used as comparison point to the ML models, that will be reviewed afterwards.

4. Statistical Models to Predict Childhood/Adolescent Obesity

There has been a lot of work performed to derive statistical models to predict childhood/adolescent obesity [34–47]. Although in principle it is advisable not to categorize variables when deriving models, whether predictor or target ones, given that the process results in a loss of information, most of the work in this area has focused on classification models for overweight, obesity, or combinations of them. The reason is obviously that most of the clinical interest is in detecting the conditions that can lead to pathological complications, and these are overweight and obesity, not BMI or similar endpoints in general. Another pathological nutritional status is undernutrition, but it is outside the scope of this Review. In the case of children and adolescents, given the large variability of both height and weight during this period of life, there is no general consensus in the definitions of overweight and obese [17], and the single-cutoff definitions used with adults, namely BMI ≥ 25 kg/m^2 for overweight and BMI ≥ 30 kg/m^2 for obesity, following the WHO definition, [3] are not valid. Instead, the common practice in the case of children/adolescents is to refer the BMI to an age- and sex-based (in some cases ethnicity too) distribution of BMI of the population at hand. The most common criterion is to define as overweight a child whose BMI is equal or above the 85th percentile for that sex and age and as obese a child whose BMI is equal or above the 95th percentile. As we will see, in most of the cases, these percentiles are obtained from the Centers of Disease Control (CDC) data if the sample is from the US [48] or alternatively from WHO growth charts [3], charts from the International Obesity Task Force (IOTF) [49], or growth charts from samples in other countries (e.g., UK90 for UK [50]).

Previous recent reviews in the area are those of Butler et al. [51], Ziauddeen et al. [52], and Butler et al. [53], all of them from 2018. Here, we will briefly review all the works found there and additional ones, in order to provide some sort of baseline predictive models to compare with the ML ones. A total of 14 papers have been found. Table 1 summarizes the main features of these models.

The most used tool to develop the statistical models is logistic regression, which is applied to predict binary outcomes. Here, a linear equation is used to predict the log-odds of a binary variable displaying one of its two alternative categories vs. the other, like being obese or being overweight vs. normal weight. This is the case of all the works but two exceptions. One is the work by Cortés-Martín et al. [47], where proportional-odds ordinal logistic regression is used, which is an statistical model appropriate to predict ordinal variables. In this case, the predicted outcome was the three ordered categories of BMI, namely normal weight vs. overweight vs. obese for children and adolescents (5–17 years). The other case is the work by Mayr et al. [38] where the authors use quantile regression with boosting to derive prediction intervals (which are at the end quantiles of the BMI for future observations) for BMI at different ages in childhood.

In addition, in the paper by Pei et al. [40], the standardized BMI at 5 years was also predicted by means of linear regression, together with obesity at 10 years with logistic regression. Moreover, in the paper by Druet et al. [35], a metanalysis is performed from the odds-ratios obtained from several logistic regressions for 10 different cohorts of variable nationality to estimate an odds-ratio for childhood obesity as a function of the 0–1 year weight gain standard deviation score (SDS).

Table 1. Summary of statistical models.

Article (year)	Training Set Size	Number of Predictors	Country	Outcome Predicted *	Statistical Method	Validation	Type of Prediction **
Steur et al. [34] (2011)	1687	6	The Netherlands	OW 8 years	Stepwise Logistic Regression	Bootstrap	L
Druet et al. [35] (2012)	47,661; 8236	4	UK, France, Finland, Sweden, US, Seychelles	Childhood OB OR; Childhood OB	Metanalysis; Stepwise Logistic Regression	External	L
Levine et al. [36] (2012)	Not specified	5	UK	OB 5 years	Logistic regression	None	L
Morandi et al. [37] (2012)	4032	6	Finland	OB 7 years; OW 7 years; OB 16 years; OW 16 years; OB 7 and 16 years; OW 7 and 16 years	Stepwise Logistic Regression	External	L
Mayr et al. [38] (2012)	Not specified	10	Germany	Childhood OB prediction intervals	Quantile regression with boosting	Simulation and Internal	L
Manios et al. [39] (2013)	2294	5	Greece	OB 9–13 years	Logistic regression	None	L
Pei et al. [40] (2013)	1515	5	Germany	zBMI 10 years; OW 10 years	Linear regression; Logistic regression	Cross-validation	L
Weng et al. [41] (2013)	10,810	7	UK	OW 3 years	Stepwise Logistic Regression	External	L
Santorelli et al. [42] (2013)	1735	4	UK	OB 2 years	Stepwise Logistic Regression	External	L
Graversen et al. [43] (2015)	4111	3	Finland	OW adolescence	Logistic Regression	Bootstrap, External	L
Manios et al. [44] (2016)	5946	5	Greece	OB 6–15 years	Logistic Regression	None	L
Robson et al. [45] (2016)	166	5	US	OB 5 years	Stepwise Logistic Regression	Bootstrap	L
Redsell et al. [46] (2016)	980	7	UK	OW 5 years	Logistic regression	External validation of Weng et al. [41]	L
Cortés-Martín et al. [47] (2020)	415	7	Spain	NW/OW/OB 5–17 years	Ordinal Logistic Regression	Bootstrap	CS

* NW = normal weight; OW = overweight; OB = obese; ** L = longitudinal model; CS = cross-sectional model.

The rest of the papers aim at the prediction of overweight or obesity at one or several ages or a range of ages exclusively by means of logistic regression. Papers focused on the prediction of overweight are those of Steur et al. [34] (at 8 years), Weng et al. [41] (3 years), Graversen et al. [43] (at adolescence), and Redsell et al. [46] (5 years). Papers focused on the prediction of obesity are those of Druet et al. [35] (7–14 years), Levine et al. [36] (5 years, stratified by sex), Manios et al. [39,44] (9–13 years), Pei et al. [40] (10 years, as said before), Santorelli et al. [42] (2 years) and Robson et al. [45] (5 years). In the paper by Morandi et al. [37] both endpoints are predicted: overweight and obesity at both 7 and 16 years; in addition, predictions are made for *persistent* overweight and obesity, that is, overweight and obesity at *both* 7 and 16 years. By considering the definition of overweight and/or obesity in these works, some [34,35,37,39,41,46] used the IOTF criteria, others [40,44,47] used the WHO one, and other [45] used the CDC criteria.

When using logistic regression, in most of the cases, [34,35,37,41,42,45,46] a stepwise variable selection is performed from a pull of predictor variables to select the final ones to use in the definitive model or models. In one case [39,44], a score is derived "by hand" by combining odds-ratios obtained from simple logistic regressions of different variables and then used in a simple [39] or multiple [44] logistic regression to estimate its odds-ratio. In two other cases [36,43], the predictor variables are predefined, and in one case [40] several predefined predictor variables are used at the beginning, but then, the model is rederived with only the significant ones.

As regarding the predictor variables, the most popular ones, in decreasing order, are parental BMI (8 times), sex and birth weight (7 times), smoking mother during gestation (6 times), weight gain at some previous period (5 times), parental education (4 times), exclusive breastfeeding during some initial period (3 times), etc. Sometimes, versions of these variables are used, like categorized ones (e.g., obesity instead of BMI) or standardized ones. Some other times, mother's version (instead of parental ones) are used, e.g., mother's BMI, or mother's education. There are two cases where a set of genetic polymorphisms are used; in one case [37], incorporated as a score obtained as sum of risk alleles, they appeared to add no significant predictive capacity, but in the other, [47] in the form of components of a Multiple Component Analysis (MCA), they did.

The cohorts used in the derivation of the models are of variable origin: Netherlands [34], UK [36,41,42], Finland [37,43], Germany [38,40], Greece [39,44], USA (Latino community) [45], and Spain. [47] In the case of the metanalysis previously mentioned [35], the 10 different cohorts are also from multiple countries: UK, France, Finland, Sweden, USA, and Seychelles. We can see that most of the work has been performed in developed countries with mostly Caucasian samples, which limits their applicability. The sizes of the cohorts are also variable: They range from 166 [45] to around 13,000. [41] The metanalysis [35] includes more than 47,000 cases in the 10 cohorts.

In terms of model validation, some of the models [35,37,41,43,44,46] were externally validated (as a matter of fact, the works by Manios et al. [44] and Redsell et al. [46] are external validations of the previous models described in Manios et al. [39] and Weng et al. [41]), while other models were internally validated through bootstrap [34,45,47] or cross-validation [38,40]. In two cases, [42,43] both internal and external validation was used, while in one case [36] no validation was performed at all.

If we focus in the comparison of performances of the different logistic regression models, we can use the AUCROC (that equals the so-called c-index or concordance index) as a criterion for discrimination. Depending on where the linear predictor threshold of the model is set to assign one category or its alternative to the predictions, we can have very different sensitivities and specificities, as well as PPV (precision) and NPVs; to select the threshold we must take into account the purpose of the model, as well as the possible costs of false positives and/or false negatives. However, as a *global* measure of the discriminative capacity of the model, before its practical application by selecting a threshold, the AUCROC is a well-established criterion. Obviously, for two models with the same AUROC, one internally validated and the other externally validated, we will prefer the one externally validated, especially if it is with a large, unrelated cohort, because it will approximate more closely a real-life prediction than the internal validation that is based on data reutilization.

In this way, the models of the different works using external validation would be ranked in the following order of decreasing AUROC: Santorelli et al. [42] (0.89), Morandi et al. [37] (0.79), Druet et al. [35] (0.77), Weng et al. [41] (0.75), Redsell et al. [46] (0.67), and Manios et al. [44] (0.64). In the case of the paper by Graversen et al. [43], the AUROC is provided only for the internal validation. These values should be taken with caution, given that they do not compare the same "difficulty" in prediction, e.g., if the testing cohort is very similar to the training one, a very large AUROC could be obtained very easily; for example, an external validation with a different cohort to the training one is a more demanding task that an external validation with a random split of the same cohort, even if the latter is not used for training. Moreover, the difficulty depends on the relatedness between the predictor and target variables, e.g., the prediction of obesity at age 9 is more difficult if the predictor variable is weight gain between 0 and 1 years than if the predictor variable is weight gain between 7 and 8 years.

On the other hand, the ranking of models for internal validation by decreasing AUROC is Robson et al. [45] (0.78) and Steur et al. [34] (0.75). Mayr et al. [38] and Pei et al. [40] do not provide AUROC values. In principle, the evidence of predictive capacity of these models is weaker given that they have not been externally validated.

Finally, we should mention that, in terms of the type of prediction, all the models have a longitudinal setting, that is, they aim at predicting the endpoint *in the future* from *predictor variables taken in a previous point in time*, at least partially, e.g., predict overweight at 8 years using birth weight and mother smoking at gestation. These are designated in Table 1 as "L" type of prediction. The only exception is the work by Cortés-Marín et al., which has no predictive but explanatory purpose and therefore uses a cross-sectional setting, where the predictor variables are taken at the same time than the endpoint. This is designated in Table 1 as "CS" type of prediction. Here, the aim is to obtain the relative strengths of associations of variables of different domains with putative explanatory character (diet, age, sex, genetic polymorphisms, microbiota), although given the cross-sectional setting of the model, no demonstration of causality can be obtained from it but rather of putative variables to consider for a further test with a longitudinal setting.

5. Machine Learning Models to Predict Childhood/Adolescent Obesity Based on BMI

In this section, we will review the ML models derived to predict BMI (regression) and/or categorized versions of it (classification), e.g., normal-weight, overweight, obesity, etc.

To our knowledge, there are only two previous reviews of ML models to predict childhood/adolescent obesity. One early paper in 2010 by Adnan et al. [54] described the scarce work performed before it; another very recent paper [55] reviews the work up to 2020, together with the area of computerized decision support for the prevention and treatment of childhood obesity. However, the latter paper, being arranged as a systematic review, lacks many of the publications in the area of ML, and some of the ones described there could be more appropriately defined as statistical models (e.g., generalized linear mixed models and linear and logistic regression) or are targeted to the prediction of physical activity in children.

In what follows, we will use more or less a chronological order in the description of the works conducted in the area. As we will see, the field has experienced an explosion very recently, especially through the use of electronic health records (EHR) as sources of very large datasets. ML methods will be abbreviated as in Section 2. Table 2 summarizes the main features of the models that will be described.

The first attempts to use ML to predict childhood obesity are those of Novak and Bigec, back in 1995 [56] and 1996 [57]. In these papers, they describe the use of ANN to predict childhood obesity. However, the work is of preliminary nature and is more a description of the ANN theory and method, without providing a description of the results of a particular model derived from a particular sample.

This work was followed by that of Zhang et al. in 2009 [58]. Here, the aim is to compare the performance of ML models with the traditional logistic regression model. By using an UK cohort (the so-called Wirral database of >16,000 children), they developed several models to predict overweight at 3 years from previous data, using predictor variables available at 8 months or at 2 years. These variables were all child features like sex, BMI at 8 months, adjusted SDS of height at different visits, weight gain between pairs of visits, etc. Different ML methods were used: DT, Association Rules, ANN, Linear SVM, RFB (Radial Basis Function) SVM, BN, and NB. In the case of the prediction at 8 months, the ANN showed the largest accuracy, although the RBF (Radial Basis Function) SVM displayed the largest sensitivity (probably more useful for clinical purposes). For the prediction at 2 years, the largest accuracy was obtained with the Bayesian methods, although the largest sensitivity was observed in the case of RBF SVM again. Logistic regression had the largest specificity, but the sensitivity and accuracy were much worse than the ML models. They also derived models to predict obesity, but the quality of them was very low. No validation was performed in any of the models developed.

Table 2. Machine Learning (ML) models to predict BMI or its categories.

Article (year)	Training Set Size	Number of Predictors *	Country	Outcome Predicted **	ML Method	Validation	Type of Prediction ***
Novak and Bigec [56] (1995)	ND ****	ND	Slovenia	Childhood OB	ANN	Not described	ND
Novak and Bigec [57] (1996)	ND	ND	Slovenia	Childhood OB	ANN	Not described	ND
Zhang et al. [58] (2009)	16,523	10	UK	OW 3 years	DT, ANN, NB, BN, SVM, association rules, logistic regression	None	L
Rehkopf et al. [59] (2011)	2150	41	US	Girls Change in BMI percentile (9 to 19 years); onset of OW or OB	RF	None	L
Adnan et al. [60] (2012)	140	20	Malaysia	Children OB 9–11 years	NB	None	CS
Adnan et al. [61] (2012)	320	8	Malaysia	Children OW/OB	NB	None	CS
Adnan et al. [62] (2012)	180	19	Malaysia	Children OW/OB	NB	None	CS
Lazarou et al. [63] (2012)	600	5	Cyprus	OW 10–12 years	DT	Bootstrap	CS
Pochini et al. [64] (2014)	15,425	9	US	OW 14–18 years; OB 14–18 years	DT; Logistic Regression	External	CS
Dugan et al. [65] (2015)	7519	167	US	OB 2 years	DT; RF; NB; BN	Cross-validation	L
Lingren et al. [66] (2016)	5857	9	US	Severe OB 1–6 years	Rule based; SVM; NB	External	CS
Abdullah et al. [67] (2017)	4245	29	Malaysia	OB 12 years	BN; DT; NB; ANN; SVM	None	L
Rios-Julian et al. [68] (2017)	221	16	Mexico	OW 6–13 years	DT; Logistic Model Trees; ANN; RF; Logistic Regression	None	CS
Wiechmann et al. [69] (2017)	238	ND	US	OW 2–5 years	DT	None	CS
Zheng and Rugggiero [70] (2017)	5127	9	US	OB 14–18 years	Logistic Regression; DT; kNN; ANN	Cross-validation	CS
Gupta et al. [71] (2019)	40,817	1737	US	BMI and OB 3–20 years	DL(RNN)	External	L
Hammond et al. [72] (2019)	2759	19,290		OB 5 years	Logistic penalized Regression; RF; GBM; LASSO	Bootstrap cross-validation; External	L
Lee et al. [73] (2019)	~ 600,000	21	South Korea	OB 24–80 months	DT	External	L
Park et al. [74] (2019)	76	379	US	BMI progression in childhood	LASSO	Cross-validation; External	L
Singh and Tawfit et al. [75] (2019)	ND	ND	UK	BMI 14 years	Linear Regression; ANN	External	L
Kim et al. [76] (2019)	11,206	19	South Korea	BMI categories	BN	None	CS
Pang et al. [77] (2019)	10,881	102	US	OB 2–7 years	GBM	External	L

* When several models are derived, the largest number of predictors is reported; ** NW = normal weight; OW = overweight; OB = obese; *** L = longitudinal model; CS = cross-sectional model; **** ND = Not described. ML Method abbreviation as in Section 2.

A work in 2011 by Rehkopf et al. [59] used and American cohort (the NHLBI Growth and Health Study) of ca. 2000 white or black girls 8 or 9 years old that were followed for 10 years to predict the change from 9 to 19 years in the CDC BMI percentile and the transition from normal-weight to overweight or obese by means of RF models. They took 41 predictor variables from different domains: diet, physical activity, psychological, and social and parent health in order. They applied variable importance techniques by permutation to estimate the relative importance of these variables. For the first outcome, body dissatisfaction, drive for thinness, physical appearance (psychological), income and parental education (social), and other psychological variables were the most important variables. In the case of the transition to overweight or obesity, the most important predictor was income, followed by psychological variables. Again, no internal/external validation of the model was performed.

Following their review in 2010 [54], Adnan et al. published in 2012 three papers in this area [60–62] to predict the nutritional status (normal-weight, overweight and obese) by means of NB and a cohort of 140 Malaysian children 9–11 years old. They applied 19 predictor variables of different domains obtained from literature review: children features, lifestyle (including physical activity and diet), and family/environment. In the first work [60], they observed that the use of these variables improved the accuracy of obesity prediction by NB as compared to the work by Zhang et al. [58]. This approach was improved in the second paper [61] by using a genetic algorithm to select predictor variables in order to avoid the problem in NB with many variables where the predicted posterior probabilities turn to zero each time at least one of the predictor variables prior probability is zero. The third paper [62] adopted two additional methods for variable selection for NB models: variable importance with CART and Euclidean distances. The models were not validated in any of the papers.

Another work from 2012 is that of Lazarou et al., [63] where diet variables were used to predict overweight + obesity vs. normal-weight. A Cypriot cohort of ca. 600 children 10–12 years old was used with a cross-sectional setting. They used questionnaires of eating frequencies of food groups as predictor variables (fried food, fish and seafood, delicatessen meat, soft drinks, and sweets and junk food). By developing many DTs, for both boys and girls, they were able to derive rules of overweight + obesity risk as a function of diet patterns and sex. The approach was validated by bootstrap, but the results were not shown. Finally, they developed logistic regression models using as predictor variables PCA components of the diet variables; only one of the PC of the girls model was significant.

One paper in 2014 by Pochini et al. [64] predicted overweight and obesity in high-school students (14–18 years old) from 9 lifestyle predictor variables, using both logistic regression and DT, again, in a cross-sectional setting. The sample modeled was a cohort of ca. 15,000 high-school students in Columbia, USA (from the 2011 CDC Youth Behavior Risk Survey). For obesity, logistic regression significant factors were consumption of fruit/vegetables, smoking, being physically active, having regular breakfast, drinking fruit juice, and drinking soda; the remaining variables in the DT after pruning were physically active and tobacco. For the overweight prediction, the logistic significant variables were having regular breakfast and being physically active. For the DT, no variable remained after pruning; before pruning, the variables were breakfast, fruit juice, and sleep. In the case of the DT, the models were externally validated with a 30% of the original sample.

Dugan et al. [65], in 2015, used multiple ML methods to predict obesity at 2 years using predictor variables obtained before that age. The data came from a clinical decision support system, CHICA, that contained information from a multiethnic cohort in USA of >7000 children. Random Tree, RF, J48, ID3, NB, and BN were tried out. The best performing algorithm was ID3, with an accuracy of 85%, sensitivity of 89%, PPV of 84%, and NPV of 88%. Using some sort of variable importance by removing variable by variable, they found that the strongest predictors were overweight before 24 months, followed by being very tall before 6 months. All the models were internally validated through 10-fold cross-validation.

In 2016, a paper by Lingren et al. [66] was published aimed at the identification of putative cases of severe early childhood obesity from children 1–6 years old above the 99th BMI percentile, to separate them from those due to medications, pathologies, etc. The objective was to develop a cohort for further genotyping studies, in order to understand the genetic basis for severe early childhood obesity. Therefore, they attempted to optimize the PPV, in order to be most effective in the detection of these children. The dataset used corresponded to a cohort of >5000 of EHR from two children hospitals, one in Boston and another in Cincinnati. The predictor variables used were structured data (demographics, anthropometrics, ICD-9 diagnosis codes, and medications) as well as unstructured data (narrative) by NLP. They used both rule-based methods and ML methods (SVM and NB) that were tested in an external split of the original data. In general, the rule-based method worked better, but the ML one had more flexibility to leverage PPV and sensibility and to select variable sets.

Abdullah et al. published a paper [67] in 2017, where they used ML to predict obesity at 12 years from a Malaysian cohort of >4000 children 12 years old. The predictor variables were obtained from questionnaires and included three domains: socio-demographic, physical activity, and diet. Multiple methods for variable selection were tested, as well as multiple ML methods: BN, DT (J48), NB, ANN, and SVM. The best results were obtained with J48, together with consistency + linear forward variable selection. In this case, the models were not validated.

A later paper in the same year by Rios-Julián et al. [68] attempted to predict obesity + overweight (following the CDC criteria) vs. normal-weight by using BMI and other anthropometric variables in a community of Me'Phaa ethnicity in Mexico. They modeled a cohort of 221 children 6–13 years old by using different ML models: J48, logistic model trees, ANN, RF, and logistic regression. Three groups of variables were tried on: all; all but skinfold thickness; and sex, age, height, weight, BMI, and skinfold thickness. They obtained not very different results for the different variable groups and models, and in general, all the models yielded excellent predictions. All the models were internally validated by 10-fold cross-validation.

Moreover, in 2017 Wiechman et al. published a paper [69] that used DTs (C4.5 type) to gain insight on the factors influencing child obesity in Hispanic preschoolers in the USA. The sample analyzed was a cohort of children of 238 families, 2–5 years old, of Hispanic ethnicity. They develop shallow C4.5 decision trees to predict overweight by using variables from different domains: demographics, caregiver feeding style, feeding practices, home environment, dietary information, beverage consumption, social support, family life, integrated behavior model, and spousal support. They found some clues for obesity development: If the mother cares for the child or if she works but the father has high-level education, the child has less probability of being overweight. If the child is fed to avoid tantrums, the child tends to be more obese. The models were not validated.

The last paper in 2017 is that of Zheng and Ruggiero [70]. They used a dataset comprising a cohort of >5000 high-school (14–18 years) students in the USA. They predicted obesity between 14 and 18 years from 9 variables within three different domains: energy update, physical activity, and sedentary behavior. They used logistic regression, DT, kNN, and ANN. The best models were ANN and kNN, and all the ML models performed much better than logistic regression. All were internally validated by 10-fold cross-validation.

The year 2019 saw an explosion of ML and DL models to predict childhood obesity. We have identified up to 7 papers in this area, together with other aimed at related endpoints that will be described in the next section. Several of them make use of EHR as sources of data. We finish this section by describing these works.

An example of DL models is that of Gupta et al. [71] They used a cohort of EHR from ca. 68,000 children/adolescents with visits to medical centers for at least 5 years, in order to predict BMI and obesity from 3 to 20 years in groups of 3 consecutive years using data from the 3 previous years, resulting in multiple models. Recurrent NN of the LSTM type were used, with predictor variables from the EHR including medical conditions observed, drugs prescribed, procedures requested, and measurements taken, together with static demographic data. Data was split into three subsets: 60% for training, 20% for hyperparameter validation, and 20% for external validation. The whole training dataset was used to train a global model, and then, by transfer learning, specialized models for each sub-cohort were obtained by retraining the global model with the corresponding subset of data. In order to identify important variables, they used embedding, while to identify important time intervals, they used attention techniques. The RNN was compared with RF and linear regression, which do not take into account the longitudinal information, and the RNN gave a much better performance. The performance of the models decays with the temporal distance between the acquisition of the predictor variables and the time of BMI prediction in the future, as expected.

Another work that used EHR data is that of Hammond et al. [72], who used a multiethnic cohort obtained from multiple providers in a safety net in New York city that included >3000 children. The authors predict obesity at year 5 by using logistic penalized regression, RF, and GB. In addition, obesity was predicted by deriving regression models for z-BMI using LASSO, RF, and GB and applying an obesity cutoff for the z-BMI predicted. They used feature engineering to generate predictor variables from the EHR: demographic information, home address, vital signs, and medications from the children when they were < 2 years old and from the mother vital signs, diagnosis codes; procedures; and laboratory results before, during, and post-pregnancy. They developed different models for boys and girls. The most important predictors were weight-for-length z-score, BMI between 19 and 24 months, and the last BMI measure before age 2. The best models have an AUCROC of 81.7% for girls and 76.1% for boys. Internal validation was conducted by bootstrap CV and external validation with a previously selected test split.

One case of work aiming at understanding risk factors for childhood obesity is that of Lee et al. [73]. They used a South Korean longitudinal cohort of ca. 1 million children and used DT models to predict obesity vs. normal-weight between 24 and 80 months (overweight children are removed). They used a set of 21 predictor variables of different domains: socioeconomic status (SES (modelled after attending medical aid or not), maternal factors (e.g., pregestational obesity, abdominal obesity, hypertension, smoking, etc.), paternal factors (obesity, abdominal obesity, and hypertension), and child factors (preterm, exclusive breastfeeding, high consumption of sugar sweetened beverages, etc.)) The model was externally validated with a 40% test split, resulting in an accuracy of 93%. By using a CHAID-type of variable selection, the most important predictor variable was mother obesity, followed by parental obesity and SES; other important factors were old pregnancy and gestational diabetes and hypertension. Child factors were exclusive breastfeeding, consumption of sugar-sweetened beverages, and irregular breakfasting. Interestingly, they observed that child's z-score for weight at birth and z-score for weight-for-height were not selected.

A South-Korean dataset was also used in order to understand factors affecting obesity is that of Kim et al. [76], although in this case it deals with *adolescent* obesity. They used a cohort of >11,000 students from South Korea and 19 predictor variables from questionnaires of different domains: sociological, anthropometric, smartphone use, obesity, other. They predict the three categories of BMI: underweight, normal, and overweight, by means of a General Bayesian Network (GBN), and compare it with many different ML methods resulting in GBN displaying the best fit: the best accuracy is 53.7%, and the AUCROC is 0.758. No validation is performed. The variable most related to BMI class is pocket money. More interestingly, they use the GBN to perform a "what-if" analysis by modifying the values of different variables or combination of variables in order to get an understanding of putative mechanisms for risk of obesity. For instance, the combination of high pocket money and low wealth increases a lot the probability of obesity, etc.

An adolescent cohort was also used by Singh et al. [75] but in this case from the UK. The Millenium cohort of UK of children born between 2000 and 2001, particularly the subsets MC2 to MC5, was modeled in order to predict the BMI at 14 years (MC6). The data was externally validated with a test split of 25%. Linear SVM, linear regression, and ANN were tried, and the best performance was obtained by the ANN, followed by the SVM.

A work that uses XGBoost is that of Pang et al. [77]. The authors predict obesity in the period 2–7 years from data in windows in the 0–2 years period with a cohort of ca. 27,000 children from Philadelphia in the Pediatric Big Data repository. Variables included vital signs, laboratory values, and provider information, resulting in a total of 102 predictors. Data was divided into train 1 (40%), train 2 (40%), and hold-out (20%) to determine hyperparameters iteratively and train/test the model. Different ML models were tried, and the best was XGBoost, giving an AUCROC of 0.81, and for the threshold that gives a recall of 0.8, the precision, F1, accuracy, and specificity were 30.9%, 44.6%, 66.14%, and 63.27%, respectively. They analyzed the models with variable importance techniques, resulting in weight-for-height at month 24, weight at month 24, weight for height at month 18, and race being the most important ones. Different races, ethnicities, and caregivers had different importance distributions. Using sensitivity analysis, it was observed that the prediction of obesity at later times degrades, as expected.

An interesting alternative set of predictive variables to the ones described so far is the use of neuroimaging biomarkers. This is the case of the work by Park et al., [74] who used resting-state functional magnetic resonance imaging (rs-fMRI) to derive predictive models for BMI progression (and indirectly future BMI) of adolescents. A cohort of 76 individuals from the Enhanced Nathan Kline Institute Rockland Sample (NKI-RS) database of white and African American preadolescents (average age of 11.94 years) was used. Their BMI was measured in a first visit, followed by a second visit about 1.5 years later. From the fMRI of their brain in the first visit, both considering subcortical volume and cortical surface, 379 Degree-Centrality (DC) values of different parts of the brain were extracted. These were used with LASSO to predict the BMI progression (DeltaBMI/Deltat) and indirectly BMI in the second visit. Only six DC remained after the variable selection in the LASSO. These variables were entered in a linear regression model. The model was internally validated with leave-one CV, giving and Intra Class Correlation (ICC) for DeltaBMI of 0.70, and ICC for BMI of 0.98, and (when predicting the binary variable increase/decrease of BMI) an AUCROC of 0.82. Brain regions of the selected DCs were correlated with the eating disorder, anxiety, and depression. The approach was applied to a local South Korean dataset of 22 young adults (average age of 21.4), and the results were similar, suggesting robustness of the first model.

6. Machine Learning Models to Predict Related Outcomes

Some other works in the literature make use of ML to derive predictive models not of BMI or BMI categories, but of related endpoints. Table 3 summarizes these models.

Table 3. Summary of ML models to predict BMI-related outcomes.

Article (Year)	Training Set Size	Country	Outcome Predicted	ML Method	Validation
Nau et al. [78] (2015)	99 (communities)	US	Obesogenic environment	RF	None
Hasan et al. [79] (2018)	40191 (utterances)	US	Success of communication strategies to promote weight reduction behavior	DL	External
Öksüz et al. [80] (2018)	20	Switzerland	Success of weight decrease therapy	SVM, kNN, DT, GBM	Cross-validation
Turer et al. [81] (2018)	7192	US	Doctors attention to childhood obesity	Ad hoc algorithm	External
Duran et al. [82] (2019)	1333	US	Body fat% (excess)	ANN	External

ML Method abbreviation as in Section 2.

For instance, a work by Duran et al. [82] describes the use of ANN models to predict body fat percentage (BF%) and its excess (BF% above 85th percentile), which is an alternative measure of obesity to those based on BMI. A cohort ca. 2000 non-Hispanic white children less than 20 years old were used here. Different models were derived for boys and girls. The predictors used were age, height, weight, and waist circumference. The ANN were compared with the prediction using z-BMI and z-WC. In the case of boys, ANN has better accuracy, sensibility, and specificity than the simple models, especially the z-WC one; in the case of girls, the ANN performs similarly to the z-BMI one and better than the z-WC one. The models were internally validated and externally validated with a test split.

On the other hand, there are models aimed at the prediction of the success of therapies or treatments to decrease childhood obesity. One case is described in a work by Hasan et al. [79], where they used RNN (both LSTM and GRU types) and probabilistic models to try to predict the positive or negative reception by obese adolescents of communication sequences by a counselor in interviews to promote weight reduction behavior. The authors used a dataset of 129 motivational interviews between a counselor and an adolescent (accompanied by a caregiver) for promoting weight reduction behavior. These interviews included 50,239 encoded sequences of utterances ending or not in a positive change talk or positive commitment language by the adolescent or caregiver. Given the high imbalance of the sequences of utterances (most of them are successful ones), they evaluated the models through either synthetic oversampling of the negative sequences or under-sampling of the positive ones. The models were trained with 80% of the data and externally evaluated with 20% of the data. In the case of under sampling, the LSTM models with target replication (LSTM-TR) resulted in the best models in terms of F1, precision, and recall. The probabilistic models were much worse. When using oversampling, the LSTM-TR was again the best model. These models can therefore be used to design communication strategies that achieve the best success.

Another example of prediction of therapy success is the work by Öksüz et al. [80] They used a cohort of 20 overweight or obese children 11–16 years old in Switzerland to predict the success of a weight-decrease 6-months therapy (defined as BMI after therapy < 0.4 BMI units than before). As predictors, they measured the heart rate at several intervals during a run test and a cooldown period, plus weight, age, BMI, and height. They tried different ML methods: several SVM, kNN, DT, and GB. Nested cross validation was used to train and internally validate the models given the small sample size. The best model used linear SVM, giving an accuracy of 85%. They used permutation tests to estimate the relative importance of the predictors, and several heart rate ones are the most important. These ML models performed better than the prediction of two domain experts.

A related task is the detection from EHR of attention by pediatricians to childhood obesity and associated medical risks. This is the case of the paper by Turer et al. [81]. They used a dataset of doctor visits of >7000 overweight/obese children 6–12 years old in several centers in Texas. They developed a rule-based classification algorithm to detect from EHR doctor's behaviors that indicate therapeutic "attention towards excess BMI", "attention towards excess BMI + comorbidities (medical risk)", and "no attention". They used different types of evidence, in addition to pathology codes, from EHR indices: diagnosis codes, orders for laboratories, medications, and referrals. The algorithm was externally validated by manual review of EHR data of 309 additional visits. Sensitivity to BMI alone was 96%, while to BMI/Medical risk was 96.1%.

We end this section with an interesting paper by Nau et al. [78] describing a predictive model for obesogenic vs. obesoprotective community environments. Here, the aim is predicting not the obesity for a particular child or adolescent, but rather if the features of a community are those that foster childhood obesity within it, or on the contrary, they protect against it. These authors analyzed 99 communities in Pennsylvania, 50 of them in the high quartile of child obesity prevalence and 49 others other in the lowest quartile. Therefore, it uses community-aggregated data to try to predict obesogenic vs. obesoprotective communities. They used 44 variables as potential predictors in different domains: food services, social, physical activity establishments, and land use. They used variable importance measures with RF to identify the most important variables. A total of 13 were deemed important above noise; unemployment was the most important, followed by population density, social disorganization, proportion of people with less than high school education, population change, no car ownership, etc. These are physical activity and social variables. The most important food services variables are counts of snacks stores and counts of fast food chains score. Models were also obtained without social variables that are considered causal of the others; the results gave similar ranking of the other variables. It seems that well-off communities are more protected against obesity. It was also observed that classification accuracies were different for high and low obesity communities, indicating different structures/hierarchy of variables for these two groups. The models, however, were not internally or externally validated.

7. Discussion

In the present Review, we have seen a large amount of models to predict childhood/adolescent obesity. We have grouped them into two types: statistical ones and ML ones. The former models use traditional statistical techniques, mainly logistic regression, [34–37,39–46] although there are cases using linear regression [40], quantile regression [38], and ordinal logistic regression. [47] The ML models use a wide variety of ML methods: ANN [56–58,67,68,70,75], SVM [58,66,67], DT [58,64,65,67–70,73], NB [58,60–62,66,67], BN [58,65,67,76], LASSO [72,74], kNN [70], RF [59,65,68,72], GBM [72,77], and DL (RNN [71]).

In general, when in the same work logistic/linear regression is compared with ML models when fitting the same dataset [58,64,68,70,72,75], the latter give better results than the former in terms of prediction performance. This confirms that ML techniques are able to yield better predictions, not just by fitting better the training set but also through giving better results in internal and/or external validations.

On the other hand, if we analyze the models in terms of predictor variables, we see that the statistical models make use in most of the cases of a reduced set of well-established risk factors for childhood obesity: parental BMI, sex and birth weight, smoking mother during gestation, weight gain at some previous period, parental education, exclusive breastfeeding during some initial period, etc. Only the work by Cortés-Martín et al. [47] uses a wider set of predictor variables, including a Mediterranean diet score, multiple SNPs, and a marker of microbiota (urolithin metabotype), in addition to sex, age, and ethnicity. On the contrary, in multiple ML models, we observe other types of variables, alone or in combination with the "traditional" predictor variables. For example, the work of Rehkopf et al. [59] uses psychological predictor variables, that of Lazarou et al. [63] focuses mainly on diet, while that of Park et al. [74] utilizes rs-fMRI predictor variables. There are also several papers that use lifestyle variables (including both diet- and physical activity-related variables) [59–62,64,69,70]. Works that stand out for their use of specially wide sets of multidomain predictor variables are those of Rehkopf et al. [59] (diet; physical activity; and psychological, social, and parental health); Wiechman et al. [69] (demographics, caregiver feeding style, feeding practices, home environment, diet, social support, spousal support, family life, etc.); and Kim et al. [76] (wealth, smartphone use, pocket money, academic performance, sleeping quality, etc.) The latter work is interesting also because it makes a "what-if" analysis where some variables are modified, and their concerted effect on the predicted obesity is evaluated; this is an interesting approach to use ML models as simulation tools to suggest possible therapeutic or preventive interventions.

Therefore, we could say that the statistical models are probably more oriented towards earlier ages, where the number of factors affecting is less variable, or to predicting shorter times in the future. We would be mainly doing a short extrapolation of the BMI curve: Obese children would be those who were obese some short time before, and in the case of babies or early age children, gestational factors like smoking mother or gestational diabetes would also be of importance. These are simpler models with immediate implementation in the clinics, as they contain a small number of easily retrieved predictor variables. On the contrary, once the multidomain factors of obesity, like diet, physical activity, psychological variables, genetic, family environment, sociological, etc., enter the scene, which takes place in late childhood or adolescence, ML models are more appropriate. This is also for predictions spanning large periods of time, like the model by Gupta et al. that was developed to predict BMI and obesity from 3 to 20 years, or when we require higher accuracy in the prediction. In addition to prediction purposes, these ML models are useful in that they can be used to rank these wide sets of variables by importance, thus allowing to better identify the strongest risk factors and generate new ideas for future preventive interventions [59,71,73,74,77,83]. In the case of longitudinal models, the strongest influence times can also be derived through attention techniques [71].

A specially interesting situation from the point of view of predictor variables are the ML models that use EHR [65,66,71,72,77], since they appear as very powerful approaches to predict childhood/adolescent obesity by tapping from the large databases of medical records with many patients and extended sets of predictor variables, including measurements, drug prescriptions, conditions observed, and procedures requested. These are especially amenable of DL techniques of the RNN type, which are specialized in dealing with time serial data like this. As described above, one case in the models presented here is that of Gupta et al. [71], where they were able to deliver excellent predictions of BMI and obesity along the whole childhood and adolescence growth curve. Another interesting use of RNN in this framework would be the extraction of information from narrative data in the medical records by means of NLP; an example of predictor variables extracted through NLP is the work by Lingren et al. [66].

These ML/DL models using EHR could be implemented in hospitals and primary health care centers to provide predictions and alerts through *dynamic, online* training. By this, we mean a model that is fed continuously with new data and is retrained periodically to enhance its predictions with the new data. This is opposed to *static, offline* training where the model is fit with a definite dataset and only once and forever. All the models we have reviewed are in the last category.

EHR offer also very interesting opportunities as Big Data sources for remining through ML/DL models. For example, we have seen the case of the work by Lingren et al. [66] where the EHR was exploited to identify a cohort of severe early childhood obesity for further genotyping efforts. Many other applications are possible, like analyzing and predicting comorbidities through statistical network analysis [84–86], phenotyping, diagnosing, pharmacoepidemiology and pharmacovigilance, etc. [87].

In addition, we should mention the fruitful application of ML/DL models to the field of childhood obesity prevention, not just through the identification of risk subpopulations but through the analysis of different aspects of the preventive intervention. We have seen that these models can be useful to optimize obesity prevention strategies [79], predict its success [80], and identify doctor's behaviors attentive or not of childhood obesity and related risks in the clinics [81] and, from a community point of view, social environments with obesogenic properties that should be targeted with preventive governmental policies [78].

To summarize, ML/DL approaches offer extraordinary advantages and new insights for childhood and adolescent obesity prediction and prevention over statistical methods. The following points summarize them:

- They have increased the prediction accuracy over the statistical models, given their ability to model complex, nonlinear relationships between variables, as well as the very large number of parameters that they contain, especially in the case of DL, avoiding the saturation in prediction performance. This is always beneficial irrespective of the application, as the more accurate is a model the more practical it is in real life.
- They allow to model directly and automatically high-dimensional data, which is not possible in the case of traditional statistical models. For the latter, one has to make use of questionable variable selection techniques, and at the cost of making biased inferences.
- They have expanded the predictor variable set from the "traditional" one in statistical models (well-established risk factors) to a much wider, multidomain one: psychological, diet, social, lifestyle, smartphone use, academic performance, sleeping quality, drug prescriptions, spousal support, rs-fMRI, and other domains of variables. In this way, they have been able to find new insights about novel "risk" factors of a completely new nature.
- They are able to use new complex data sources other than numeric ones: text, images, RMN, social media, etc.; this is especially the case with DL, which can use that data directly, without previous "feature engineering". This is another way to expand the number and domain of predictor variables.

- They (especially DL) are appropriate tools for the modeling of EHR, as described in the examples reviewed. In particular, the EHR offer an incredible opportunity for remining efforts, in order to find new insights from these data sources that can suggest opportunities for further research and therapeutic approaches.
- They have provided new applications, besides the prediction of risk subpopulations, e.g., identification of samples for genotyping from EHR, optimization of utterances in counseling interventions to decrease adolescent obesity, analysis of pediatrician attention to obesity and related risks from EHR, etc.
- They have been used not just as prediction or explanatory tools but also as simulation tools, so that they can be used to get new insights about possible therapeutic approaches.

To be fully fair, we should as well mention the *disadvantages* of ML methods over statistical ones. The first one is that making statistical inferences (parameter estimation and hypothesis test) in these models is more complicated than in statistical models. However, it is not impossible, and resampling and simulation techniques could be used if required. Another drawback of ML models is that they are more difficult to interpret, and they are typically called "black-box" type of models. This is an area of intense research, and we have seen above several examples of techniques to solve this problem, namely, the techniques of variable importance, embedding, and attention.

Seeing the advantages and disadvantages of both types of methods, we can ask: when is ML more appropriate, and when are statistical models? The following patterns have emerged:

- If the interest is mainly in interpretability, inference, and simple models of reduced numbers of predictor variables, instead of predictive performance, statistical models should be more appropriate. Again, this is more the case with early childhood and for clinical applications not requiring high accuracy.
- The opposite is applicable: If we want to have very good predictive performance and are less worried about interpretability and inference, ML should be used.
- If we have a high-dimensional sample, ML should be used, for example, if we want to analyze a wide, multidomain set of predictor variables. This is more the case with exploratory studies from which we want to gain new insights about new risk factors: psychological, social, genetics or genomics, microbiome and metagenomics, neuroimaging, diet, lifestyle, etc. As said above, these models are more likely to be relevant as the child grows and especially during adolescence.
- If we want to use complex data as predictors (images, text, time series, social media, etc.) DL is the one to go for.
- If we want to use EHR, ML (DL) should be applied.
- It is likely that new applications will go mainly through the use of ML or DL, as these are more powerful to tap from Big Data sources: Internet, social media, mobile and wireless devices, sensors, etc. These applications would include computerized decision support systems, simulation applications, novel preventive interventions, analysis of social obesogenic environments, etc.

Hopefully this Review will help the wide set of researchers in the field, including pediatricians, nurses, nutritionists, statisticians, data scientists, engineers, and epidemiologists, to get an updated view of these novel approaches and the opportunities they open, in order to approach in a more effective and creative way the prevention of childhood and adolescent obesity. We are at the beginning of a qualitatively new phase that can revolutionize this field in the near future.

Author Contributions: Conceptualization and writing, G.C. The author has read and agreed to the published version of the manuscript.

Acknowledgments: The author acknowledges the Community of Madrid Government for providing the funds for Open Access publication of this article.

References

1. Abarca-Gómez, L.; Abdeen, Z.A.; Hamid, Z.A.; Abu-Rmeileh, N.M.; Acosta-Cazares, B.; Acuin, C.; Adams, R.J.; Aekplakorn, W.; Afsana, K.; Aguilar-Salinas, C.A.; et al. Worldwide trends in body-mass index, underweight, overweight, and obesity from 1975 to 2016: A pooled analysis of 2416 population-based measurement studies in 128·9 million children, adolescents, and Adults. *Lancet* **2017**, *390*, 2627–2642. [CrossRef]
2. Ng, M.; Fleming, T.; Robinson, M.; Thomson, B.; Graetz, N.; Margono, C.; Mullany, E.C.; Biryukov, S.; Abbafati, C.; Abera, S.F.; et al. Global, regional, and national prevalence of overweight and obesity in children and adults during 1980–2013: A systematic analysis for the global burden of disease study 2013. *Lancet* **2014**, *384*, 766–781. [CrossRef]
3. WHO. Obesity and Overweight. Available online: https://www.who.int/news-room/fact-sheets/detail/obesity-and-overweight (accessed on 15 June 2020).
4. De Onis, M.; Blössner, M.; Borghi, E. Global prevalence and trends of overweight and obesity among preschool children. *Am. J. Clin. Nutr.* **2010**, *92*, 1257–1264. [CrossRef]
5. Chung, A.; Backholer, K.; Wong, E.; Palermo, C.; Keating, C.; Peeters, A. Trends in child and adolescent obesity prevalence in economically advanced countries according to socioeconomic position: A systematic review. *Obes. Rev.* **2016**, *17*, 276–295. [CrossRef]
6. Kumar, S.; Kelly, A.S. Review of childhood obesity: From epidemiology, etiology, and comorbidities to clinical assessment and treatment. *Mayo Clin. Proc.* **2017**, *92*, 251–265. [CrossRef]
7. Gibson, L.Y.; Allen, K.L.; Davis, E.; Blair, E.; Zubrick, S.R.; Byrne, S.M. The psychosocial burden of childhood overweight and obesity: Evidence for persisting difficulties in boys and girls. *Eur. J. Pediatr.* **2017**, *176*, 925–933. [CrossRef] [PubMed]
8. Rankin, J.; Matthews, L.; Cobley, S.; Han, A.; Sanders, R.; Wiltshire, H.D.; Baker, J.S. Psychological Consequences of Childhood Obesity: Psychiatric Comorbidity and Prevention. Available online: https://www.dovepress.com/psychological--consequences-of-childhood-obesity-psychiatric-comorbidi-peer-reviewed-article-AHMT (accessed on 29 June 2020).
9. Pandita, A.; Sharma, D.; Pandita, D.; Pawar, S.; Tariq, M.; Kaul, A. Childhood Obesity: Prevention is Better Than Cure. Available online: https://www.dovepress.com/childhood-obesity-prevention-is-better-than-cure-peer-reviewed-article-DMSO (accessed on 29 June 2020).
10. Fox, C.K.; Ryder, J.R.; Gross, A.C.; Kelly, A.S. Obesity in children and adolescents. In *Obesity*; Sbraccia, P., Finer, N., Eds.; Endocrinology; Springer International Publishing: Cham, Switzerland, 2019; pp. 295–322. [CrossRef]
11. Anderson, Y.C.; Wynter, L.E.; Treves, K.F.; Grant, C.C.; Stewart, J.M.; Cave, T.L.; Wouldes, T.A.; Derraik, J.G.B.; Cutfield, W.S.; Hofman, P.L. Assessment of health-related quality of life and psychological well-being of children and adolescents with obesity enrolled in a New Zealand community-based intervention programme: An observational study. *BMJ Open* **2017**, *7*, e015776. [CrossRef] [PubMed]
12. Liang, Y.; Hou, D.; Zhao, X.; Wang, L.; Hu, Y.; Liu, J.; Cheng, H.; Yang, P.; Shan, X.; Yan, Y.; et al. Childhood obesity affects adult metabolic syndrome and diabetes. *Endocrine* **2015**, *50*, 87–92. [CrossRef] [PubMed]
13. Juonala, M.; Magnussen, C.G.; Berenson, G.S.; Venn, A.; Burns, T.L.; Sabin, M.A.; Srinivasan, S.R.; Daniels, S.R.; Davis, P.H.; Chen, W.; et al. Childhood adiposity, adult adiposity, and cardiovascular risk factors. *N. Engl. J. Med.* **2011**, *365*, 1876–1885. [CrossRef]
14. Twig, G.; Yaniv, G.; Levine, H.; Leiba, A.; Goldberger, N.; Derazne, E.; Ben-Ami Shor, D.; Tzur, D.; Afek, A.; Shamiss, A.; et al. Body-Mass index in 2.3 million adolescents and cardiovascular death in adulthood. *N. Engl. J. Med.* **2016**, *374*, 2430–2440. [CrossRef]
15. Abdullah, A.; Wolfe, R.; Stoelwinder, J.U.; de Courten, M.; Stevenson, C.; Walls, H.L.; Peeters, A. The number of years lived with obesity and the risk of all-cause and cause-specific mortality. *Int. J. Epidemiol.* **2011**, *40*, 985–996. [CrossRef] [PubMed]
16. Reilly, J.J.; Kelly, J. Long-term impact of overweight and obesity in childhood and adolescence on morbidity and premature mortality in adulthood: Systematic review. *Int. J. Obes.* **2011**, *35*, 891–898. [CrossRef]
17. Sweeting, H.N. Measurement and definitions of obesity in childhood and adolescence: A field guide for the uninitiated. *Nutr. J.* **2007**, *6*, 32. [CrossRef] [PubMed]

18. González-Muniesa, P.; Mártinez-González, M.-A.; Hu, F.B.; Després, J.-P.; Matsuzawa, Y.; Loos, R.J.F.; Moreno, L.A.; Bray, G.A.; Martinez, J.A. Obesity. *Nat. Rev. Dis. Primers* **2017**, *3*, 1–18. [CrossRef]
19. Larqué, E.; Labayen, I.; Flodmark, C.-E.; Lissau, I.; Czernin, S.; Moreno, L.A.; Pietrobelli, A.; Widhalm, K. From conception to infancy—Early risk factors for childhood obesity. *Nat. Rev. Endocrinol.* **2019**, *15*, 456–478. [CrossRef]
20. Rosenblatt, F. *The Perceptron—A Perceiving and Recognizing Automaton*; Cornell Aeronautical Laboratory: Buffalo, NY, USA, 1957.
21. Maron, M.E. Automatic indexing: An experimental inquiry. *J. ACM* **1961**, *8*, 404–417. [CrossRef]
22. Rumelhart, D.E.; Hinton, G.E.; Williams, R.J. Learning representations by back-propagating errors. *Nature* **1986**, *323*, 533–536. [CrossRef]
23. Cortes, C.; Vapnik, V. Support-vector networks. *Mach. Learn.* **1995**, *20*, 273–297. [CrossRef]
24. Breiman, L. Random forest. *Mach. Learn.* **2001**, *45*, 5–32. [CrossRef]
25. Friedman, J.H. Greedy Function Approximation: A Gradient Boosting Machine. *Ann. Stati.* **2001**, *29*, 1189–1232. [CrossRef]
26. Breiman, L.; Friedman, J.; Stone, C.J.; Olshen, R.A. *Classification and Regression Trees*; Taylor & Francis: New York, NY, USA, 1984.
27. Quinlan, J.R. Induction of decision trees. *Mach. Learn.* **1986**, *1*, 81–106. [CrossRef]
28. Kass, G.V. An exploratory technique for investigating large quantities of categorical data. *Appl. Stat.* **1980**, *29*, 119. [CrossRef]
29. McCulloh, W.S.; Pitts, W.H. A logical calculus of the ideas immanent in nervous activity. *Bull. Math. Biophys.* **1943**, *5*, 115–133. [CrossRef]
30. Hochreiter, S.; Schmidhuber, J. Long short-term memory. *Neural Comput.* **1997**, *9*, 1735–1780. [CrossRef] [PubMed]
31. Cho, K.; van Merrienboer, B.; Gulcehre, C.; Bahdanau, D.; Bougares, F.; Schwenk, H.; Bengio, Y. Learning Phrase Representations Using RNN Encoder-Decoder for Statistical Machine Translation. Available online: https://arxiv.org/abs/1406.1078 (accessed on 25 March 2019).
32. Wainberg, M.; Merico, D.; Delong, A.; Frey, B.J. Deep learning in biomedicine. *Nat. Biotechnol.* **2018**, *36*, 829–838. [CrossRef] [PubMed]
33. Mamoshina, P.; Vieira, A.; Putin, E.; Zhavoronkov, A. Applications of deep learning in biomedicine. *Mol. Pharm.* **2016**, *13*, 1445–1454. [CrossRef] [PubMed]
34. Steur, M.; Smit, H.A.; Schipper, C.M.A.; Scholtens, S.; Kerkhof, M.; de Jongste, J.C.; Haveman-Nies, A.; Brunekreef, B.; Wijga, A.H. Predicting the risk of newborn children to become overweight later in childhood: The PIAMA birth cohort study. *Int. J. Pediatr. Obes.* **2011**, *6*, e170–e178. [CrossRef]
35. Druet, C.; Stettler, N.; Sharp, S.; Simmons, R.K.; Cooper, C.; Davey Smith, G.; Ekelund, U.; Lévy-Marchal, C.; Jarvelin, M.-R.; Kuh, D.; et al. Prediction of childhood obesity by infancy weight gain: An individual-level meta-analysis: Infancy weight gain and childhood obesity. *Paediatr. Perinat. Epidemiol.* **2012**, *26*, 19–26. [CrossRef]
36. Levine, R.S.; Dahly, D.L.; Rudolf, M.C.J. Identifying infants at risk of becoming obese: Can we and should we? *Public Health* **2012**, *126*, 123–128. [CrossRef]
37. Morandi, A.; Meyre, D.; Lobbens, S.; Kleinman, K.; Kaakinen, M.; Rifas-Shiman, S.L.; Vatin, V.; Gaget, S.; Pouta, A.; Hartikainen, A.-L.; et al. Estimation of newborn risk for child or adolescent obesity: Lessons from longitudinal birth cohorts. *PLoS ONE* **2012**, *7*, e49919. [CrossRef]
38. Mayr, A.; Hothorn, T.; Fenske, N. Prediction intervals for future BMI values of individual children—a Non-parametric approach by quantile boosting. *BMC Med. Res. Methodol.* **2012**, *12*, 6. [CrossRef] [PubMed]
39. On behalf of the "Healthy Growth Study" Group; Manios, Y.; Birbilis, M.; Moschonis, G.; Birbilis, G.; Mougios, V.; Lionis, C.; Chrousos, G.P. Childhood obesity risk evaluation based on perinatal factors and family sociodemographic characteristics: Core index. *Eur. J. Pediatr.* **2013**, *172*, 551–555. [CrossRef] [PubMed]
40. For the GINIplus and LISAplus Study Group; Pei, Z.; Flexeder, C.; Fuertes, E.; Thiering, E.; Koletzko, B.; Cramer, C.; Berdel, D.; Lehmann, I.; Bauer, C.-P.; et al. Early life risk factors of being overweight at 10 years of age: Results of the German birth cohorts GINIplus and LISAplus. *Eur. J. Clin. Nutr.* **2013**, *67*, 855–862. [CrossRef] [PubMed]
41. Weng, S.F.; Redsell, S.A.; Nathan, D.; Swift, J.A.; Yang, M.; Glazebrook, C. Estimating overweight risk in childhood from predictors during infancy. *Pediatrics* **2013**, *132*, e414–e421. [CrossRef]

42. Santorelli, G.; Petherick, E.S.; Wright, J.; Wilson, B.; Samiei, H.; Cameron, N.; Johnson, W. Developing prediction equations and a mobile phone application to identify infants at risk of obesity. *PLoS ONE* **2013**, *8*, e71183. [CrossRef]
43. Graversen, L.; Sørensen, T.I.A.; Gerds, T.A.; Petersen, L.; Sovio, U.; Kaakinen, M.; Sandbaek, A.; Laitinen, J.; Taanila, A.; Pouta, A.; et al. Prediction of adolescent and adult adiposity outcomes from early life anthropometrics: Prediction of adolescent and adult adiposity. *Obesity* **2015**, *23*, 162–169. [CrossRef]
44. Manios, Y.; Vlachopapadopoulou, E.; Moschonis, G.; Karachaliou, F.; Psaltopoulou, T.; Koutsouki, D.; Bogdanis, G.; Carayanni, V.; Hatzakis, A.; Michalacos, S. Utility and applicability of the "Childhood Obesity Risk Evaluation" (CORE)-Index in predicting obesity in childhood and adolescence in Greece from early life: The "National Action Plan for Public Health". *Eur. J. Pediatr.* **2016**, *175*, 1989–1996. [CrossRef]
45. Robson, J.O.; Verstraete, S.G.; Shiboski, S.; Heyman, M.B.; Wojcicki, J.M. A risk score for childhood obesity in an urban Latino cohort. *J. Pediatr.* **2016**, *172*, 29–34.e1. [CrossRef]
46. Redsell, S.A.; Weng, S.; Swift, J.A.; Nathan, D.; Glazebrook, C. Validation, optimal threshold determination, and clinical utility of the infant risk of overweight checklist for early prevention of child overweight. *Child. Obes.* **2016**, *12*, 202–209. [CrossRef]
47. Cortés-Martín, A.; Colmenarejo, G.; Selma, M.V.; Espín, J.C. Genetic polymorphisms, mediterranean diet and microbiota-associated urolithin metabotypes can predict obesity in childhood-adolescence. *Sci. Rep.* **2020**, *10*, 7850. [CrossRef]
48. Ogden, C.L.; Flegal, K.M. Changes in Terminology for Childhood Overweight and Obesity. *Natl. Health Stat. Rep.* **2010**, *25*, 1–5.
49. Cole, T.J. Establishing a standard definition for child overweight and obesity worldwide: International survey. *BMJ* **2000**, *320*, 1240. [CrossRef]
50. Freeman, J.V.; Cole, T.J.; Chinn, S.; Jones, P.R.; White, E.M.; Preece, M.A. Cross sectional stature and weight reference curves for the UK, 1990. *Arch. Dis. Child.* **1995**, *73*, 17–24. [CrossRef] [PubMed]
51. Butler, É.M.; Derraik, J.G.B.; Taylor, R.W.; Cutfield, W.S. Prediction models for early childhood obesity: Applicability and existing issues. *Horm. Res. Paediatr.* **2018**, *90*, 358–367. [CrossRef]
52. Ziauddeen, N.; Roderick, P.J.; Macklon, N.S.; Alwan, N.A. Predicting childhood overweight and obesity using maternal and early life risk factors: A systematic review: Predicting childhood overweight. *Obes. Rev.* **2018**, *19*, 302–312. [CrossRef] [PubMed]
53. Butler, É.M.; Derraik, J.G.B.; Taylor, R.W.; Cutfield, W.S. Childhood obesity: How long should we wait to predict weight? *J. Pediatr. Endocrinol. Metab.* **2018**, *31*, 497–501. [CrossRef]
54. Adnan, M.H.B.M.; Husain, W.; Damanhoori, F. *A Survey on Utilization of Data Mining for Childhood Obesity Prediction*; IEEE: Kuching, Malaysia, 2010; pp. 1–6.
55. Triantafyllidis, A.; Polychronidou, E.; Alexiadis, A.; Rocha, C.L.; Oliveira, D.N.; da Silva, A.S.; Freire, A.L.; Macedo, C.; Sousa, I.F.; Werbet, E.; et al. Computerized decision support and machine learning applications for the prevention and treatment of childhood obesity: A systematic review of the literature. *Artif. Intell. Med.* **2020**, *104*, 101844. [CrossRef]
56. Novak, B.; Bigec, M. Application of artificial neural networks for childhood obesity prediction. In *Proceedings of the 1995 Second New Zealand International Two-Stream Conference on Artificial Neural Networks and Expert Systems*; IEEE Computer Society Press: Dunedin, New Zealand, 1995; pp. 377–380. [CrossRef]
57. Novak, B.; Bigec, M. Childhood obesity prediction with artificial neural networks. In Proceedings of the Ninth IEEE Symposium on Computer-Based Medical Systems; IEEE Computer Society Press: Ann Arbor, MI, USA, 1996; pp. 77–82. [CrossRef]
58. Zhang, S.; Tjortjis, C.; Zeng, X.; Qiao, H.; Buchan, I.; Keane, J. Comparing data mining methods with logistic regression in childhood obesity prediction. *Inf. Syst. Front.* **2009**, *11*, 449–460. [CrossRef]
59. Rehkopf, D.H.; Laraia, B.A.; Segal, M.; Braithwaite, D.; Epel, E. The relative importance of predictors of body mass index change, overweight and obesity in adolescent girls. *Int. J. Pediatr. Obes.* **2011**, *6*, e233–e242. [CrossRef]
60. Adnan, M.H.B.M.; Husain, W.; Rashid, N.A. *Parameter Identification and Selection for Childhood Obesity Prediction Using Data Mining*; IACSIT Press: Singapore, 2012; Volume 35, pp. 75–79.
61. Adnan, M.H.M.; Husain, W.; Rashid, N.A. Hybrid approaches using decision tree, naïve bayes, means and euclidean distances for childhood obesity prediction. *Int. J. Softw. Eng. Appl.* **2012**, *6*, 8.

62. Muhamad Adnan, M.H.B.; Husain, W.; Abdul Rashid, N. A hybrid approach using naïve bayes and genetic algorithm for childhood obesity prediction. In *2012 International Conference on Computer & Information Science (ICCIS)*; IEEE: Kuala Lumpur, Malaysia, 2012; pp. 281–285. [CrossRef]
63. Lazarou, C.; Karaolis, M.; Matalas, A.-L.; Panagiotakos, D.B. Dietary patterns analysis using data mining method. An application to data from the CYKIDS study. *Comput. Methods Programs Biomed.* **2012**, *108*, 706–714. [CrossRef]
64. Pochini, A.; Wu, Y.; Hu, G. Data mining for lifestyle risk factors associated with overweight and obesity among adolescents. In *2014 IIAI 3rd International Conference on Advanced Applied Informatics*; IEEE: Kokura Kita-ku, Japan, 2014; pp. 883–888. [CrossRef]
65. Dugan, T.M.; Mukhopadhyay, S.; Carroll, A.; Downs, S. Machine learning techniques for prediction of early childhood obesity. *Appl. Clin. Inform.* **2015**, *6*, 506–520. [CrossRef]
66. Lingren, T.; Thaker, V.; Brady, C.; Namjou, B.; Kennebeck, S.; Bickel, J.; Patibandla, N.; Ni, Y.; Van Driest, S.; Chen, L.; et al. Developing an algorithm to detect early childhood obesity in two tertiary pediatric medical centers. *Appl. Clin. Inform.* **2016**, *7*, 693–706. [CrossRef]
67. Abdullah, F.S.; Manan, N.S.A.; Ahmad, A.; Wafa, S.W.; Shahril, M.R.; Zulaily, N.; Amin, R.M.; Ahmed, A. Data mining techniques for classification of childhood obesity among year 6 school children. In *Recent Advances on Soft Computing and Data Mining*; Herawan, T., Ghazali, R., Nawi, N.M., Deris, M.M., Eds.; Springer International Publishing: Cham, Switzerland, 2017; Volume 549, pp. 465–474.
68. Rios-Julian, N.; Alarcon-Paredes, A.; Alonso, G.A.; Hernandez-Rosales, D.; Guzman-Guzman, I.P. Feasibility of a screening tool for obesity diagnosis in mexican children from a vulnerable community of me'phaa ethnicity in the state of Guerrero, Mexico. In *2017 Global Medical Engineering Physics Exchanges/Pan American Health Care Exchanges (GMEPE/PAHCE)*; IEEE: Tuxtla-Gutierrez, Mexico, 2017; pp. 1–6. [CrossRef]
69. Wiechmann, P.; Lora, K.; Branscum, P.; Fu, J. Identifying discriminative attributes to gain insights regarding child obesity in hispanic preschoolers using machine learning Techniques. In *2017 IEEE 29th International Conference on Tools with Artificial Intelligence (ICTAI)*; IEEE: Boston, MA, USA, 2017; pp. 11–15. [CrossRef]
70. Zheng, Z.; Ruggiero, K. Using machine learning to predict obesity in high school students. In *2017 IEEE International Conference on Bioinformatics and Biomedicine (BIBM)*; IEEE: Kansas City, MO, USA, 2017; pp. 2132–2138. [CrossRef]
71. Gupta, M.; Phan, T.-L.T.; Bunnell, H.T.; Beheshti, R. Obesity Prediction with EHR Data: A Deep Learning Approach with Interpretable Elements. Available online: https://arxiv.org/abs/1912.02655 (accessed on 25 March 2019).
72. Hammond, R.; Athanasiadou, R.; Curado, S.; Aphinyanaphongs, Y.; Abrams, C.; Messito, M.J.; Gross, R.; Katzow, M.; Jay, M.; Razavian, N.; et al. Predicting childhood obesity using electronic health records and publicly available data. *PLoS ONE* **2019**, *14*, e0215571. [CrossRef]
73. Lee, I.; Bang, K.-S.; Moon, H.; Kim, J. Risk factors for obesity among children aged 24 to 80 months in korea: A decision tree analysis. *J. Pediatr. Nurs.* **2019**, *46*, e15–e23. [CrossRef]
74. Park, B.; Chung, C.-S.; Lee, M.J.; Park, H. Accurate neuroimaging biomarkers to predict body mass index in adolescents: A longitudinal study. *Brain Imaging Behav.* **2019**. [CrossRef]
75. Singh, B.; Tawfik, H. A machine learning approach for predicting weight gain risks in young adults. In *2019 10th International Conference on Dependable Systems, Services and Technologies (DESSERT)*; IEEE: Leeds, UK, 2019; pp. 231–234. [CrossRef]
76. Kim, C.; Costello, F.J.; Lee, K.C.; Li, Y.; Li, C. Predicting factors affecting adolescent obesity using general bayesian network and what-if analysis. *Int. J. Environ. Res. Public Health* **2019**, *16*, 4684. [CrossRef]
77. Pang, X.; Forrest, C.B.; Le-Scherban, F.; Masino, A.J. Understanding early childhood obesity via interpretation of machine learning model predictions. In *2019 18th IEEE International Conference on Machine Learning and Applications (ICMLA)*; IEEE: Boca Raton, FL, USA, 2019; pp. 1438–1443. [CrossRef]
78. Nau, C.; Ellis, H.; Huang, H.; Schwartz, B.S.; Hirsch, A.; Bailey-Davis, L.; Kress, A.M.; Pollak, J.; Glass, T.A. Exploring the forest instead of the trees: An innovative method for defining obesogenic and obesoprotective environments. *Health Place* **2015**, *35*, 136–146. [CrossRef]
79. Hasan, M.; Kotov, A.; Carcone, A.I.; Dong, M.; Naar, S. Predicting the outcome of patient-provider communication sequences using recurrent neural networks and probabilistic models. *AMIA Jt. Summits Transl. Sci. Proc.* **2018**, *2018*, 64–73.

80. Öksüz, N.; Shcherbatyi, I.; Kowatsch, T.; Maass, W. A data-analytical system to predict therapy success for obese children. In Proceedings of the Thirty Ninth International Conference on Information Systems, San Francisco, CA, USA, 13–16 December 2018; pp. 1–16.
81. Turer, C.B.; Skinner, C.S.; Barlow, S.E. Algorithm to detect pediatric provider attention to high BMI and associated medical risk. *J. Am. Med. Inform. Assoc.* **2018**. [CrossRef]
82. Duran, I.; Martakis, K.; Rehberg, M.; Semler, O.; Schoenau, E. Diagnostic performance of an artificial neural network to predict excess body fat in children. *Pediatr. Obes.* **2019**, *14*, e12494. [CrossRef]
83. Marcos-Pasero, H.; Colmenarejo, G.; Aguilar-Aguilar, E.; Ramírez de Molina, A.; Reglero, G.; Loria-Kohen, V. Ranking of a wide multidomain set of predictors of children obesity by machine learning variable importance techniques. **2020**, submitted.
84. Capobianco, E.; Liò, P. Comorbidity networks: Beyond disease correlations. *J. Complex. Netw.* **2015**, *3*, 319–332. [CrossRef]
85. Brunson, J.C.; Agresta, T.P.; Laubenbacher, R.C. sensitivity of comorbidity network analysis. *JAMIA Open* **2020**, *3*, 94–103. [CrossRef]
86. Emmert-Streib, F.; Tripathi, S.; de Matos Simoes, R.; Hawwa, A.F.; Dehmer, M. The human disease network. *Syst. Biomed.* **2013**, *1*, 20–28. [CrossRef]
87. Bennett, T.D.; Callahan, T.J.; Feinstein, J.A.; Ghosh, D.; Lakhani, S.A.; Spaeder, M.C.; Szefler, S.J.; Kahn, M.G. Data science for child health. *J. Pediatr.* **2019**, *208*, 12–22. [CrossRef]

8

A Snapshot of European Children's Eating Habits: Results from the Fourth Round of the WHO European Childhood Obesity Surveillance Initiative (COSI)

Julianne Williams [1,*], Marta Buoncristiano [1], Paola Nardone [2], Ana Isabel Rito [3], Angela Spinelli [2], Tatjana Hejgaard [4], Lene Kierkegaard [5], Eha Nurk [6], Marie Kunešová [7], Sanja Musić Milanović [8], Marta García-Solano [9], Enrique Gutiérrez-González [9], Lacramioara Aurelia Brinduse [10], Alexandra Cucu [10], Anna Fijałkowska [11], Victoria Farrugia Sant'Angelo [12], Shynar Abdrakhmanova [13], Iveta Pudule [14], Vesselka Duleva [15], Nazan Yardim [16], Andrea Gualtieri [17], Mirjam Heinen [18], Silvia Bel-Serrat [18], Zhamyla Usupova [19], Valentina Peterkova [20], Lela Shengelia [21], Jolanda Hyska [22], Maya Tanrygulyyeva [23], Ausra Petrauskiene [24], Sanavbar Rakhmatullaeva [25], Enisa Kujundzic [26], Sergej M. Ostojic [27], Daniel Weghuber [28], Marina Melkumova [29], Igor Spiroski [30], Gregor Starc [31], Harry Rutter [32], Giulia Rathmes [1], Anne Charlotte Bunge [1], Ivo Rakovac [1], Khadichamo Boymatova [33], Martin Weber [34] and João Breda [1]

1 WHO European Office for the Prevention and Control of Noncommunicable Diseases, 125009 Moscow, Russian Federation; buoncristianom@who.int (M.B.); giuliarathmes@icloud.com (G.R.); anne-charlotte.bunge@charite.de (A.C.B.); rakovaci@who.int (I.R.); rodriguesdasilvabred@who.int (J.B.)

2 Italian National Institute of Health (Istituto Superiore Di Sanità), 00161 Rome, Italy; paola.nardone@iss.it (P.N.); angela.spinelli@iss.it (A.S.)

3 National Institute of Health Dr. Ricardo Jorge, 1600 560 Lisbon, Portugal; ana.rito@insa.min-saude.pt

4 Danish Health Authority, 2300 Copenhagen S, Denmark; thv@sst.dk

5 National Institute of Public Health, University of Southern Denmark, 1455 Copenhagen K, Denmark; leki@sdu.dk

6 Department of Nutrition Research, National Institute for Health Development, 11619 Tallinn, Estonia; eha.nurk@tai.ee

7 Institute of Endocrinology, Obesity Unit, 116 94 Prague, Czechia; mkunesova@endo.cz

8 Croatian Institute of Public Health, University of Zagreb, School of Medicine, 10000 Zagreb, Croatia; sanja.music@hzjz.hr

9 Spanish Agency for Food Safety and Nutrition, 28014 Madrid, Spain; mgarcias@mscbs.es (M.G.-S.); egutierrez@mscbs.es (E.G.-G.)

10 Department of Public Health and Management, University of Medicine and Pharmacy Carol Davila, 030167 Bucharest, Romania; lbrinduse@gmail.com (L.A.B.); alexandra.cucu@insp.gov.ro (A.C.)

11 Department of Cardiology, Institute of Mother and Child, 01-211 Warsaw, Poland; anna.fijalkowska@imid.med.pl

12 Primary Health Care, Ministry for Health, 1940 Floriana, Malta; victoria.farrugia-santangelo@gov.mt

13 National Center of Public health, Ministry of Health of the Republic of Kazakhstan, 010000 Nur-Sultan City, Kazakhstan; shynar_a@mail.ru

14 Centre for Disease Prevention and Control, LV-1005 Latvia, Riga; iveta.pudule@spkc.gov.lv

15 National Center of Public Health and Analyses, 1431 Sofia, Bulgaria; v.duleva@ncpha.government.bg

16 Turkish Ministry of Health, Public Health General Directorate, 34400 Istanbul, Turkey; nazan.yardim@saglik.gov.tr

17 Health Authority, Department of Health and Social Security, 47893 San Marino, San Marino; andrea.gualtieri.authority@pa.sm

18 National Nutrition Surveillance Centre, University College Dublin, Dublin, Ireland; mirjam.heinen@ucd.ie (M.H.); silvia.belserrat@ucd.ie (S.B.-S.)

19 Republican Center for Health Promotion and Mass Communication, 720040 Bishkek, Kyrgyzstan; jama.usupova@mail.ru

20 Institute of Paediatric Endocrinology, National Medical Research Centre for Endocrinology of the Ministry of Health of the Russian Federation, 117036 Moscow, Russian Federation; peterkovava@hotmail.com

[21] National Center for Disease Control and Public Health of Georgia, 0198 Tbilisi, Georgia; l.shengelia@ncdc.ge
[22] Institute of Public Health, 1007 Tirana, Albania; lhyska2002@yahoo.it
[23] Internal Diseases Department of the Scientific Clinical Centre of Mother and Child Health, 744036 Ashgabat, Turkmenistan; ovezmyradovag@who.int
[24] Department of Preventive Medicine, Lithuanian University of Health Sciences, 44307 Kaunas, Lithuania; ausra.petrauskiene@lsmuni.lt
[25] Department for Organization of Health Services to Children, Mothers, Adolescents and Family Planning, Ministry of Health and Social Protection of Population, 734025 Dushanbe, Tajikistan; sanavbar2010@list.ru
[26] Institute of Public Health of Montenegro, Podgorica, Montenegro; enisa.kujundzic@ijzcg.me
[27] Applied Bioenergetics Lab, University of Novi Sad, 21000 Novi Sad, Serbia; sergej.ostojic@chess.edu.rs
[28] Department of Pediatrics, Paracelsus Medical University, 5020 Salzburg, Austria; d.weghuber@salk.at
[29] Arabkir Medical Centre-Institute of Child and Adolescent Health, 0014 Yerevan, Armenia; mmelkumova@mail.ru
[30] Institute of Public Health, Faculty of Medicine, Ss. Cyril and Methodius University, 1000 Skopje, North Macedonia; i.spiroski@iph.mk
[31] Faculty of Sport, University of Ljubljana, 1000 Ljubljana, Slovenia; gregor.starc@fsp.uni-lj.si
[32] Department of Social and Policy Sciences, University of Bath, Bath BA2 7AY, UK; hr526@bath.ac.uk
[33] WHO Country Office for Tajikistan, 734019 Dushanbe, Tajikistan; boymatovak@who.int
[34] WHO Child and Adolescent Health and Development, WHO Regional Office for Europe, 2100 Copenhagen, Denmark; weberm@who.int
* Correspondence: williamsj@who.int

Abstract: Consuming a healthy diet in childhood helps to protect against malnutrition and noncommunicable diseases (NCDs). This cross-sectional study described the diets of 132,489 children aged six to nine years from 23 countries participating in round four (2015–2017) of the WHO European Childhood Obesity Surveillance Initiative (COSI). Children's parents or caregivers were asked to complete a questionnaire that contained indicators of energy-balance-related behaviors (including diet). For each country, we calculated the percentage of children who consumed breakfast, fruit, vegetables, sweet snacks or soft drinks "every day", "most days (four to six days per week)", "some days (one to three days per week)", or "never or less than once a week". We reported these results stratified by country, sex, and region. On a daily basis, most children (78.5%) consumed breakfast, fewer than half (42.5%) consumed fruit, fewer than a quarter (22.6%) consumed fresh vegetables, and around one in ten consumed sweet snacks or soft drinks (10.3% and 9.4%, respectively); however, there were large between-country differences. This paper highlights an urgent need to create healthier food and drink environments, reinforce health systems to promote healthy diets, and continue to support child nutrition and obesity surveillance.

Keywords: nutrition; child; obesity; surveillance; health; noncommunicable diseases; children; fruit; vegetables; soft drinks

1. Introduction

It is important for a child to eat a healthy diet in order to prevent malnutrition (stunting, wasting, micronutrient deficiencies, obesity) and noncommunicable diseases (NCDs) [1,2]. Low-quality diets are now believed to be the single biggest risk factor for the global burden of disease [3]. In recent decades, changes in dietary patterns and physical activity behaviors have been identified as likely contributors to a rise in childhood obesity [4,5]. Research from the latest round of the WHO European Childhood Obesity Surveillance Initiative (COSI) carried out in 2015–2017 indicates that 29% of boys and 27% of girls aged seven to nine years had overweight and there was a prevalence of obesity of 12% in boys and 9% in girls [6]. At the same time, in certain parts of the WHO European Region, there is a double burden of malnutrition, characterized by the coexistence of undernutrition (being underweight for one's age, too short for one's age (stunted), too thin for one's height (wasted), or deficient in vitamins and minerals (micronutrient malnutrition)), along with overweight, obesity, or noncommunicable diseases, within individuals, households, and populations, and across the life course [7,8].

The prevalence of overweight and obesity is increasing worldwide [9]. According to the WHO Global Monitoring Framework for NCDs, which is a set of 25 indicators and 9 voluntary targets are used to track progress toward reaching global targets in 2015–2020, not a single country in the WHO European Region is likely to meet Global Monitoring Target 7, which aims to "halt the rise in diabetes and obesity" [10].

Ensuring that children consume healthy diets is important for achieving the UN Sustainable Development Goals (SDGs) related to no hunger (SDG Goal 2), good health and well-being (SDG Goal 3), quality education (SDG Goal 4), no poverty (SDG Goal 1), economic growth (SDG Goal 8), and more [11,12]. Food preferences and eating habits established in childhood and adolescence tend to be maintained into adulthood [13], making nutrition in childhood an important public health issue.

A healthy diet includes adequate quantities and appropriate proportions of fruit, vegetables, legumes (e.g., lentils and beans), nuts, and whole grains [14], and limits the intake of free sugars [15,16], salt [17], saturated fats, and highly processed foods. A healthy diet eliminates trans fats of all kinds. Consumption of sugar-sweetened beverages should be limited, as it has been associated with increased body weight [18] and dental caries [19].

The WHO European Childhood Obesity Surveillance Initiative provides data on the eating behaviors of children across the WHO European Region. Established in 2007, COSI collects high-quality data on the childhood obesity prevalence and energy-balance-related behaviors [20]. These data enable countries to set national targets, monitor trends over time, make comparisons between countries, and over time, to evaluate the effectiveness of obesity prevention efforts. In addition to collecting high-quality anthropometric measurements from primary-school-aged children, COSI also collects information on children's dietary and physical activity patterns, screen time, sleep, and more.

Given the importance of nutrition in childhood, alongside the rising trend in childhood obesity, this study used the most recent results from the COSI study to describe the eating behaviors of children aged 6–9 years from across the WHO European Region.

2. Materials and Methods

Data were collected between 2015 and 2017, as part of COSI round four. Among the thirty-six countries participating in round four, 23 of them collected information on children's dietary behaviors using parental reports on a "family form". These countries were: Albania, Bulgaria, Croatia, Czechia, Denmark, Georgia, Ireland, Italy, Kazakhstan, Kyrgyzstan, Lithuania, Latvia, Malta, Montenegro, Poland, Portugal, Romania, Russian Federation (Moscow only), San Marino, Spain, Tajikistan, Turkey, and Turkmenistan. Children's parents or caregivers were asked to complete a questionnaire that contained indicators of energy-balance-related behaviors (including diet) and family socioeconomic status. Completion of the form was voluntary and participants could opt out or choose not to participate at any time.

The COSI study follows the International Ethical Guidelines for Biomedical Research Involving Human Subjects [21]. Local ethics approval was also granted. Details for this approval are found in Supplementary Box S1. More details on the data collection procedures are provided elsewhere [20,22,23].

Parents were asked: "over a typical or usual week, how often does your child eat or drink the following kinds of foods or beverages"? This was followed by a tick box, where parents answered "never", "less than once a week", "some days (1–3 days)", "most days (4–6 days)", or "every day". Parents were asked to report on a number of food items, shown in Supplementary Figure S1. For this paper, we reported on the consumption of fresh fruits, vegetables (excluding potatoes), savory snacks (e.g., potato crisps, corn chips, popcorn, peanuts), sweet treats (e.g., candy bars or chocolates), and sugar-containing soft drinks. These questions were selected because they provided a summary that was related to common sources of nutrients of interest [24]. Countries chose country-specific examples for the food examples for "savory snacks (like potato crisps, corn chips, popcorn, peanuts)", or "sweets (like candy bars or chocolate)". These examples were identified by leading nutrition experts within the country and approved by the government-appointed principal investigator of the study. All questionnaires were translated from English into the local language, and then back-translated into English to check for discrepancies with the original English form.

For each country, we calculated the percentage of children who consumed these foods "every day", "most days (four to six days per week)", "some days (one to three days per week)", or "never or less than once a week". We reported these results stratified by country, sex, and region. Geographic regions were based on the United Nations Standard Geographical regions, which are based on continental regions and are further subdivided into sub-regions and intermediary regions that are drawn to obtain greater homogeneity in the sizes of the population, demographic circumstances, and accuracy of demographic statistics [25]. We did not include sub-regional pooled estimates because these subregions include countries that are not participating in COSI, and therefore a sub-regional estimate would not provide an accurate assessment of the situation in that geographical area.

For each variable, we calculated the frequency of consumption according to country and sex. We tested for differences between sex in the distribution of the responses using the Rao–Scott chi-square test, a design-adjusted version of the Pearson's χ^2 test. We applied post-stratification weights to adjust for the sampling design, oversampling, and nonresponse proportions in order to infer results from the sample of the population. These were available and applied for all countries, with the one exception of Lithuania, where an unweighted analysis was carried out. All analyses took account of the complex survey nature of the data (i.e., multiple stages, clustering, and stratification). Pooled estimates were calculated, including only one target age group per country in order to balance the contribution of each country to the pooled estimates and to limit the differences in children's age as much as possible. An adjusting factor was applied to the post-stratification weights to take account of differences in the population sizes of the countries involved. The adjusting factor was based on the number of children belonging to the targeted age group according to Eurostat figures or national official statistics for 2016.

A *p*-value of 0.05 was used to define statistical significance. All statistical analyses were performed in the statistical software package Stata version 15·1 (StataCorp LLC, College Station, TX, USA).

3. Results

A total of 132,489 children from 23 countries were included in the analysis. The number of participants per country varied widely, from 306 children in San Marino to 43,696 in Italy (Table 1). Most of the children (75.2%) were seven years of age and 51.3% were boys.

The pooled estimates indicated that most children (78.8%) consumed breakfast every day, but around 2.3% consumed breakfast "never or less than once a week" and 8.6% consumed breakfast only on "some days" (one to three days a week). The pooled estimates indicated that 42.5% of children consumed fresh fruit "every day" and 7.5% "never consumed it or consumed it less than once a week". Around a quarter (22.6%) of all children consumed vegetables "every day", and 14.0% consumed it "never or less than once a week." The pooled estimates indicated that 5.2% of children consumed savory snacks "every day", but 57.9% consumed savory snacks "never or less than once a week". Around one in ten children (10.3%) consumed sweets "every day" and a third (32.8%) consumed sweets "never or less than once a week". Around one in ten (9.4%) children consumed soft drinks every day.

Table 1. Number of children invited to participate in COSI/WHO Europe Round 4 (2015–2017), the number of children included in the analysis, and the percentage of children participating by sex, age, and country.

Country [a]	Children Invited to Participate [b]		Children Included in the Analysis [c]			Percentage of Children Participating by Sex and Age (%) [d]				
	Total Number	Proportion Whose Family Form Was Filled in (%)	Boys (n)	Girls (n)	Total (n)	Boys (%)	6-Year-Olds	7-Year-Olds	8-Year-Olds	9-Year-Olds
Albania	7113	36.2	1315	1212	2527	52.5	0.1	24.2	52.0	23.7
Bulgaria	4090	83.1	1702	1698	3400	51.5	0	100.0	0	0
Croatia [e]	7220	76.0	1318	1333	2651	51.1	0	0	100.0	0
Czechia	n.a.	n.a.	670	736	1406	50.7	49.5	50.5	0	0
Denmark	3202	29.9	511	446	957	52.7	27.4	70.2	2.4	0
Georgia	4143	78.4	1667	1579	3246	51.2	1.6	85.1	13.0	0.3
Ireland	2704	32.4	438	436	874	52.6	38.2	60.2	1.6	0
Italy	50,902	95.2	22,425	21,271	43,696	51.5	0	0.5	66.3	33.1
Kazakhstan	6026	82.3	2149	2162	4311	50.6	0	0.4	51.0	48.6
Kyrgyzstan	8773	86.6	3798	3769	7567	50.7	10.5	43.5	39.5	6.5
Lithuania	5527	69.8	1930	1882	3812	50.6	0.4	66.4	33.0	0.2
Latvia	8143	71.5	2752	2955	5707	48.2	7.9	43.8	9.1	39.3
Malta	4329	73.4	1589	1590	3179	50.0	0.1	69.7	30.1	0.1
Montenegro	4094	66.8	1441	1295	2736	52.8	31.2	48.4	20.1	0.2
Poland	3828	76.9	1451	1494	2945	50.2	0	0	100.0	0
Portugal	7475	85.6	3167	3224	6391	50.7	25.2	49.0	24.0	1.7
Romania	9094	73.6	3312	3298	6610	49.1	0.4	28.4	47.5	23.8
Russian Federation	3900	52.6	1006	1046	2052	50.2	18.8	72.8	8.3	0.1
San Marino	329	93.6	138	168	306	45.1	0	0	64.7	35.3
Spain	14,908	70.1	5290	5163	10,453	50.9	25.4	25.2	24.9	24.6
Tajikistan	3502	93.5	1623	1647	3270	51.6	7.7	90.8	1.4	0.2
Turkmenistan	4085	95.3	1944	1947	3891	49.9	0	79.9	20.1	0
Turkey	14,164	81.7	5335	5167	10,502	50.9	11.4	82.3	6.0	0.3
Total	198,683	79.5	66,971	65,518	132,489	51.3	0	75.2	18.2	6.6

n.a.—not available. [a] Figures refer to primary school children from Albania (ALB), Bulgaria (BUL), Croatia (CRO), Czechia (CZH), Denmark (DEN), Georgia (GEO), Ireland (IRL), Italy (ITA), Kazakhstan (KAZ), Kyrgyzstan (KGZ), Lithuania (LTU), Latvia (LVA), Malta (MAT), Montenegro (MNE), Poland (POL), Portugal (POR), Romania (ROM), Moscow city (RUS), San Marino (SMR), Spain (SPA), Tajikistan (TJK), Turkmenistan (TKM), and Turkey (TUR). [b] Total figures were calculated including only countries with available information about the number of children invited to participate in the surveillance. [c] All children with complete information on sex, whose age was between six and nine years old and with information on eating habits from the family form. [d] Pooled values were estimated, including the following age groups/countries: 7-year-olds from Bulgaria, Czechia, Denmark, Kyrgyzstan, Georgia, Ireland, Latvia, Lithuania, Malta, Montenegro, Portugal, Spain, Tajikistan, Turkey, and Turkmenistan; 8-year-olds from Albania, Croatia, Poland, and Romania; and 9-year-olds from Kazakhstan. The figures were estimated by applying post-stratification weights. [e] For Croatia, only data on 8-year-olds were available for comparison at the European level. The proportion of children whose parents or caregivers filled in the family form was calculated in the whole sample (not only for 8-year-olds).

3.1. *Consumption of Breakfast*

The percentage of children who consumed breakfast every day ranged from 48.9% in Kazakhstan to 96.4% in Portugal (Figure 1). Between-country and between-region differences in breakfast consumption were not tested for significance, although there were visible between countries and no clear patterns according to region. There were no significant differences in breakfast consumption between boys and girls (Supplementary Table S1).

3.2. *Consumption of Fresh Fruit*

The frequency of consuming fresh fruit everyday ranged widely between the regions. The consumption of fresh fruit every day was highest in the Southern European countries, with 80.8% in San Marino, 72.6% in Italy, and 63.1% in Portugal (Figure 1, Supplementary Table S2). Meanwhile, the daily fresh fruit consumption was low in the Central Asian countries—Kyrgyzstan 18.1%, Kazakhstan 33.3%, and Tajikistan 33.5%—with an exception of Turkmenistan with 70.1%. The same trend was visible for differences in the proportion of children who consumed fresh fruit "never or less than once a week", ranging from 3.0% in San Marino, 3.3% in Portugal, and 2.2% in Montenegro to 21.4% in Tajikistan and 22.6% in Kyrgyzstan.

There were significant differences in fresh fruit consumption between sexes, with girls more likely to eat fruit on a daily basis compared to boys (Supplementary Table S2).

3.3. *Consumption of Vegetables*

Daily vegetable consumption ranged from 9.1% in Spain to 68.1% in Turkmenistan and 74.3% in San Marino (Figure 2). The percentage of children who consumed vegetables "never or less than once a week" was higher in Western Asian countries, with 20.4% in Turkey and 17.1% in Georgia compared with 1.3% in Czechia and 1.4% in Turkmenistan. There were significant between-sex differences, with boys tending to eat vegetables less frequently than girls (Supplementary Table S3).

3.4. *Consumption of Savory Snacks (Like Potato Crisps, Corn Chips, Popcorn, or Peanuts)*

We observed large differences between countries and regions of Europe in the frequency of consuming savory snacks like potato crisps, corn chips, popcorn, or peanuts. Low values for the daily consumption of savory snacks were observed in the Northern European countries, where Denmark reported 0%, Lithuania and Latvia 0.6%, and Ireland 1.5% (Figure 2). In contrast, in the Southern European and Asian countries, daily consumption of savory snacks was more frequently reported. Albania reported a percentage of 21.5% of children who consumed savory snacks every day, as well as Tajikistan with 11.3% and Montenegro and Turkmenistan with 9.0% (Table S4). In Malta, only 7.7% of the children never or less than once week, while in the Russian Federation, 90.8% of children consumed these foods "never or less than once a week". Similar results were seen in Lithuania (83.1% consumed savory snacks "never or less than once a week") and in Latvia (80.2% never or less than once a week). There were no significant differences in the consumption of savory snacks between boys and girls (Supplementary Table S4).

3.5. *Consumption of Sweets (Like Candy Bars or Chocolate)*

Daily consumption of sweet snacks like candy bars or chocolate ranged from 0.4% in Denmark to 21.1% in Turkmenistan and 22.8% in Bulgaria (Figure 2). The percentage of children who never or less than once a week consumed sweet snacks ranged from 3.9% in Malta to 56.7% in Spain and 67.8% in Portugal. There were no clear regional trends in the distribution of daily sweet snack consumption and there were no significant sex differences (Supplementary Table S5).

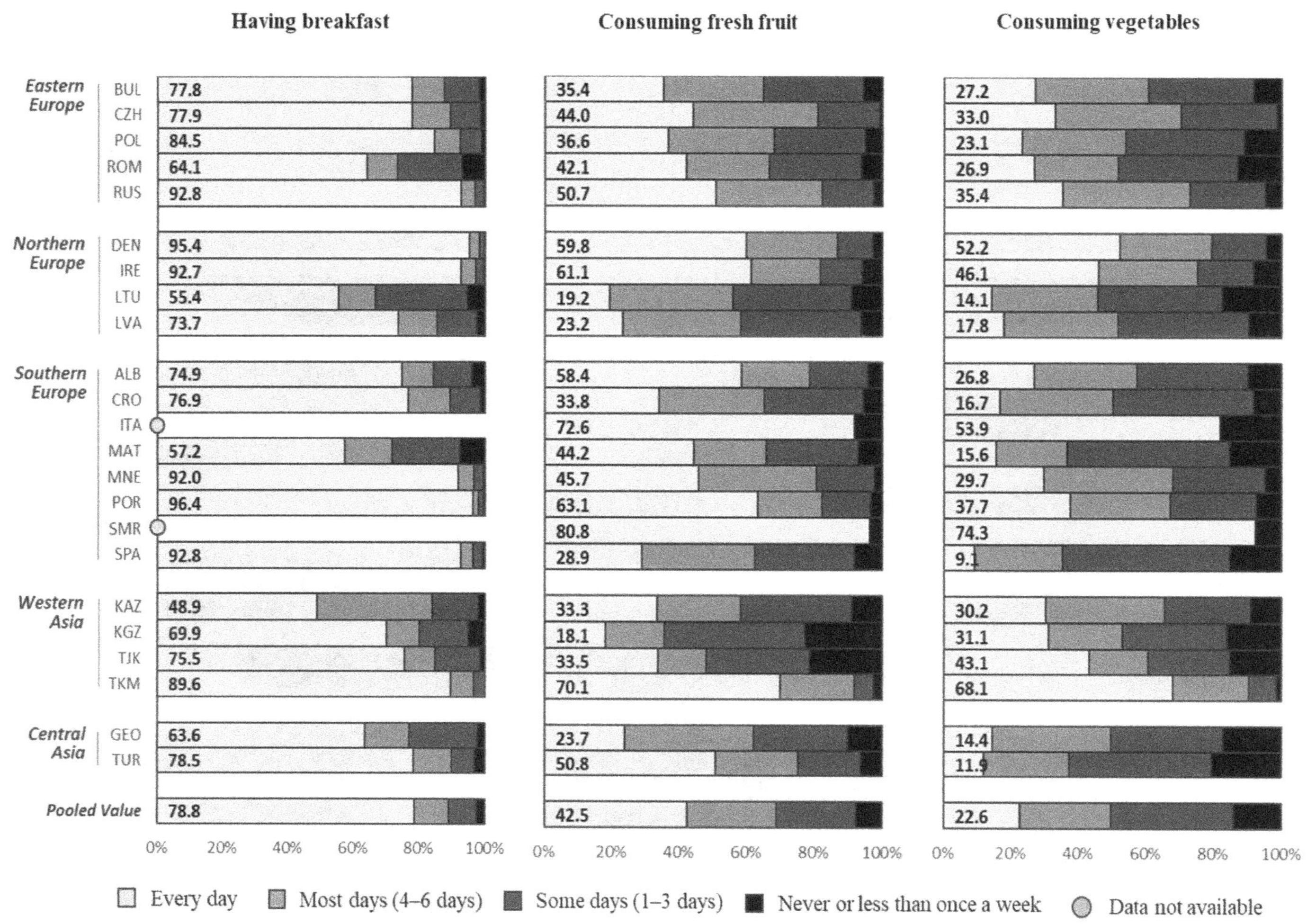

Figure 1. Frequency of consuming breakfast, fresh fruit, and vegetables among boys and girls by country [a]. COSI/WHO Europe round 4 (2015–2017). [a] Pooled values were estimated, including the following age groups/countries: 7-year-olds from Bulgaria, Czechia, Denmark, Kyrgyzstan, Georgia, Ireland, Latvia, Lithuania, Malta, Montenegro, Portugal, Spain, Tajikistan, Turkey, and Turkmenistan; 8-year-olds from Albania, Croatia, Poland, and Romania; and 9-year-olds from Kazakhstan.

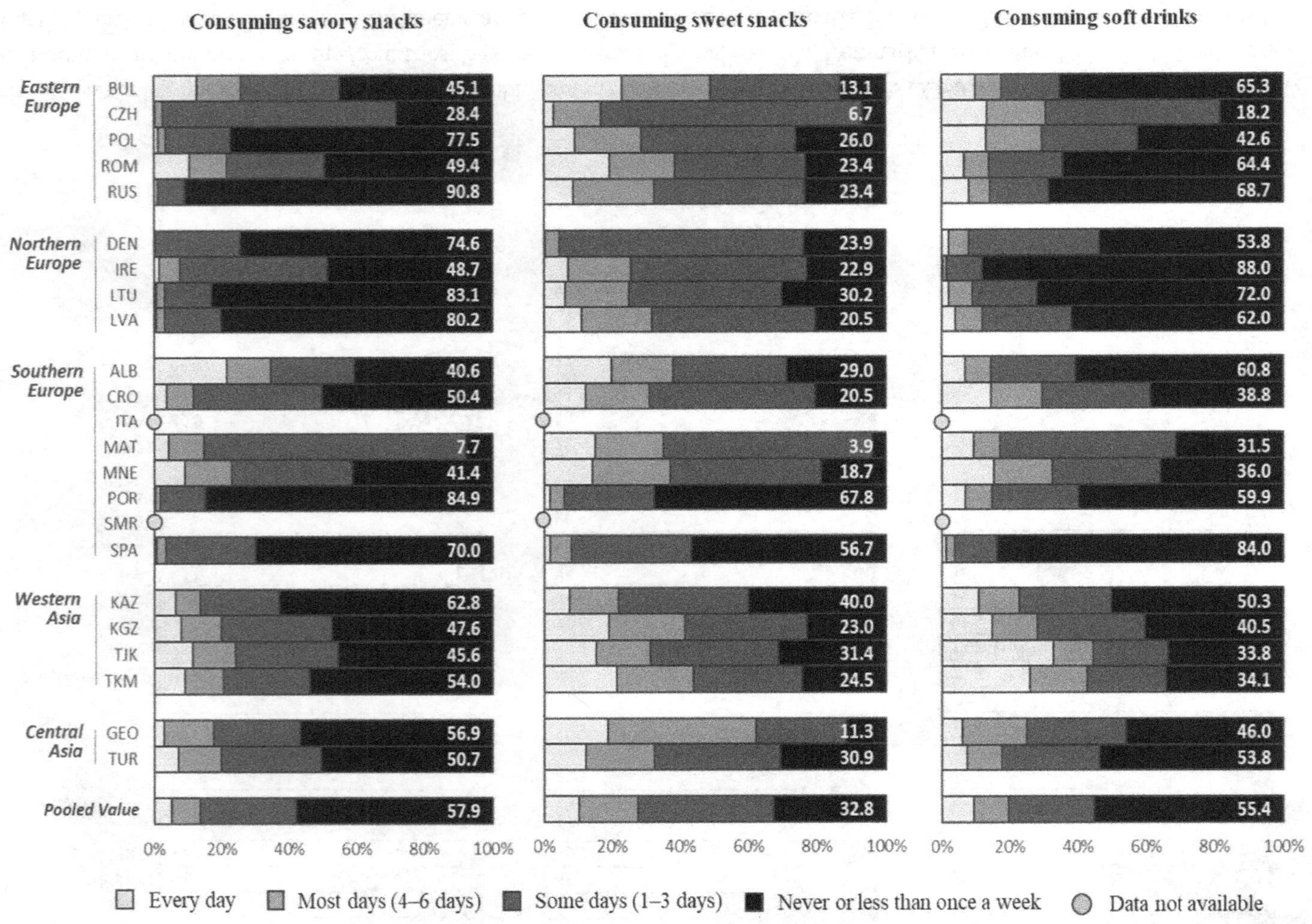

Figure 2. Frequency of consuming savory snacks, sweet snacks, and soft drinks among boys and girls by country [a]. COSI/WHO Europe round 4 (2015–2017). [a] Pooled values were estimated, including the following age groups/countries: 7-year-olds from Bulgaria, Czechia, Denmark, Kyrgyzstan, Georgia, Ireland, Latvia, Lithuania, Malta, Montenegro, Portugal, Spain, Tajikistan, Turkey, and Turkmenistan; 8-year-olds from Albania, Croatia, Poland, and Romania; and 9-year-olds from Kazakhstan.

The frequency of consuming soft drinks every day was lowest in Northern European countries, with a value of 0.4% in Ireland, 2.0% in Lithuania, and 2.1% in Denmark (Figure 2). In comparison, in the Central Asian countries of Tajikistan (32.8%) and Turkmenistan (25.8%), daily soft drink consumption was relatively high among some children. There was a lower percentage of children who never or less than once a week consumed soft drinks in the Central Asian countries (33.8% in Tajikistan, 34.1% in Turkmenistan, 40.5% in Kyrgysztan, 50.3% in Kazakhstan) compared to the Northern European countries (88.0% in Ireland, 72.0% in Lithuania, 62.0% in Latvia, 53.8% in Denmark). We observed no significant differences between boys and girls (Supplementary Table S6).

4. Discussion

The purpose of this study was to provide a snapshot that updates the general picture of the dietary habits of European children. Our data present a largely confirmatory picture of the current understanding, with some bright spots in terms of dietary habits but also many areas of opportunity.

The bright spots include high levels of breakfast consumption, with around 80% of children consuming breakfast every day. Daily breakfast consumption was the lowest in Kazakhstan, with fewer than half of the children consuming it every day, whilst almost all the children consumed it every day in Portugal and Denmark. The pooled results align with findings from another systematic review of 286,804 children and adolescents (2 to 18 years) living in 33 countries, which found that the prevalence of skipping breakfast ranged from 10–30%, with an increasing trend in adolescents, especially girls [26]. However, there is also evidence to suggest that breakfast consumption may decrease as children get older. A recent report from the Health Behaviour in School-Aged Children (HBSC) survey of findings from 227,441 young people aged 11, 13, and 15 years living in 45 countries/regions found that more than four out of 10 adolescents do not eat breakfast every school day, and that girls across all ages tend to skip breakfast and eat fewer meals with their family than boys [27].

The areas of opportunity for improving children's diets are related to increasing the consumption of fruits and vegetables. We found that only 42.5% of children consumed fruit and 22.6% consumed vegetables on a daily basis, but there were wide between-country differences. Daily fruit consumption ranged from 80.8% in San Marino to only 18.1% in Kyrgyzstan and 19.2% in Lithuania. Three-quarters (74.3%) of the children in San Marino consumed fresh vegetables every day compared to 9.1% of children in Spain, 11.9% in Turkey, 14.1% in Lithuania, and 14.4% in Georgia. Data on fruit and vegetable consumption trends from 33 countries participating in the HBSC surveys from 2002, 2006, and 2010 indicate that many adolescents do not consume fruit and vegetables on a daily basis, but there was an increase in daily fruit and vegetable consumption between 2002 and 2010 in the majority of countries [28]. Even so, findings from the latest HBSC report (2017/2018) found that almost two in three adolescents do not eat enough nutrient-rich foods, such as fruits and vegetables [27]. A recent review on dietary patterns found that among adolescents, the average fruit and vegetable consumption is below recommended levels in almost all populations [29].

This study also highlights the need for continued efforts to discourage the consumption of foods that are high in salt, sugar, and fat, and low in nutritional value. The pooled estimates related to the frequency of consuming savory snacks, sweets, and soft drinks suggest that 5.2%, 10.3%, and 9.4% of children consume these foods daily, respectively, but there was a wide between-country variation. The percentage of children consuming savory snacks every day ranged from 0% in Denmark and 0.1% in the Russian Federation to 21.5% in Albania. Daily consumption of sweet snacks ranged from 0.4% in Denmark to 21.1% in Turkmenistan and 22.8% in Bulgaria. Consumption of daily soft drinks ranged from 0.4% in Ireland to 32.8% in Tajikistan. This aligns with similar findings from the latest results from the HBSC, which also indicates that one in four adolescents eat sweets and one in six consume sugary drinks at least once a day [27]. Few available data have been found on savory snack consumption or sodium intake among children, but for the majority of the included populations, levels were far above the recommended five grams per day [29].

Based on the data from 23 countries, this study found wide between-country differences in children's healthy and unhealthy eating habits, but few clear patterns according to region. These differences were likely due to a complex range of factors. Eating patterns and food preferences in childhood are shaped by individual, interpersonal, and environmental factors, including a child's family, cultural background, social environment, socioeconomic status, and school environment [30]. Children today are increasingly exposed to environments where energy-dense and nutrient-poor foods are promoted [31] and readily available, which can make eating a healthy diet challenging. Other factors to consider include cultural differences, differences in school food environments, differences in home food environments, differences in family traditions and mealtimes, differences in the level of adherence to national dietary guidelines, price differences (which may affect the affordability and accessibility of healthy or unhealthy foods and differences in the availability of fruit or vegetables), and more.

These data lend further support to existing calls for urgent action to improve child nutrition. Schools may improve nutrition by following quality standards for school meals and providing students with access to healthy foods and beverages (such as fresh fruits, vegetables, and fresh water), and nutrition education [32]. Examples of successful initiatives include the European Union's School Fruit and Vegetable Scheme [33] and the WHO's Nutrition-Friendly Schools Initiative [34].

Another possible action to improve nutrition is through fiscal incentives or subsidies to promote better nutrition, both for encouraging the consumption of healthy foods (such as fruit or vegetables, or discouraging the consumption of unhealthy foods, such as sugary drinks). The United States Department of Agriculture provides reimbursement to states that operate nonprofit breakfast programs in schools [35]. Taxation on sugar-sweetened beverages has been shown to be effective in the reduction of sugar consumption [36,37]. Another potential intervention is the reformulation of processed foods [38], which has shown promise for the reduction of both sugar [39] and salt [40,41].

Current food and beverage marketing practices predominantly promote low-nutrition foods and beverages, and have a direct effect on children's nutrition knowledge, preferences, purchase behavior, consumption patterns, and diet-related health [42]. Governments should restrict the marketing of unhealthy foods to children, particularly in the digital world, where advertising may be especially persuasive [43]. Implementation of the WHO recommendations on the marketing of foods and non-alcoholic beverages to children is one indicator in the Global Monitoring Framework [44].

A comprehensive approach involving action at many levels is required to improve children's diets [45]. In addition to improving food environments (within schools, at home, and in other places where children gather), action is needed to engage parents and other adults who care for children [46]. Parents or caretakers often play a key role in ensuring the availability of nutritious foods, not only at home but also at school (in instances when children bring a packed lunch to school). Parents or caregivers can also help to ensure that children consume appropriate portion sizes, and there may be opportunities for governments to provide better guidance and support for parents and caregivers [47]. Front-of-pack labeling can help provide parents with information to support healthier eating choices and food purchases [48], although a recent Cochrane review suggests that more research may be needed regarding the effects that food labeling may have on consumer choices [49]. Nutritious diets may be more expensive, and this may contribute to socioeconomic disparities in health [50]; therefore, efforts must be made to ensure access to healthy and affordable foods, especially for vulnerable groups. Results from COSI indicate that the prevalence of obesity and severe obesity among children in Europe was common among children whose mothers had a lower level of education [51].

This study had several limitations. First, this study used a dietary questionnaire that has not been validated and which did not collect information on the portion sizes of foods. Future work is needed to validate this questionnaire and identify possible methods of assessing portion sizes of various foods that are consumed per day in order to identify the prevalence of children meeting certain nutrition recommendations (such as consuming five portions of fruits and vegetables per day). Further work is needed to validate questions about "sweets" and "savory snacks" where there may be cultural variation in the ways that these categories are understood. Another limitation is that the dietary indicators used in this paper are not comprehensive. For example, we reported here on "sweet treats, such as candy bars or chocolate" but there are other sweet foods, such as "biscuits, cakes, or doughnuts" (Supplementary Figure S1) that were assessed in a separate question but not reported in this paper.

This study was limited by a cross-sectional study design and a reliance on parental reports of children's diet behaviors, which may have limited accuracy [52,53]. Other limitations include possible social desirability bias or non-response bias. We do not know how the responders in this study varied from non-responders, but previous research indicates that healthier individuals with a higher socioeconomic status are more likely to respond to health surveys [54] or dietary surveys [55], and this may result in an overestimation of the prevalence of healthy behaviors. Another limitation is that this study did not account for seasonal differences in the availability of fruit and vegetables; responses to this questionnaire were collected during the autumn, winter, or spring months when fruit and vegetable availability may have been lower than during the summer months, particularly in Central Asia.

One of the main strengths of this study was that it collected data from a large sample of children across a diverse range of countries using nationally-representative sampling methods and following a common protocol.

This project is an ongoing one and will be updated in future years. It is a valuable dataset that represents the collaboration of many committed experts and provides important visibility into the habits of European children. Accurate data on children's weight status, eating habits, and other energy-balance-related behaviors provide a vital underpinning for government actions to implement and evaluate effective and appropriate strategies to combat under-nutrition and obesity. Investment in high-quality surveillance is essential to ensure more children can benefit from good nutrition and improved health during childhood and onward through the life course.

Supplementary Materials: The following are available online at Box S1: Description of national ethics approval for countries featured in this paper who were participating in the WHO European Childhood Obesity Surveillance Initiative (COSI) Round 4 (2015-2017), Table S1: Frequency of breakfast consumption among boys and girls, by country. COSI/WHO Europe Round 4 (2015-17), Table S2: Frequency of fresh fruit consumption among boys and girls, by country. COSI/WHO Europe Round 4 (2015-17), Table S3: Frequency of vegetable consumption among boys and girls, by country. COSI/WHO Europe Round 4 (2015-17), Table S4: Frequency of savory snack consumption among boys and girls, by country. COSI/WHO Europe Round 4 (2015-17), Table S5: Frequency of sweet snacks consumption among boys and girls, by country. COSI/WHO Europe Round 4 (2015-17), Table S6: Frequency of soft drinks consumption among boys and girls, by country. COSI/WHO Europe Round 4 (2015-17), Figure S1: Description of the WHO European Childhood Obesity Surveillance Initiative question related to child dietary habits, COSI Round 4 (2015-17).

Author Contributions: Conceptualization, J.B., M.B., and J.W.; formal analysis: M.B. and J.W.; data curation, M.B. and J.W.; writing—original draft preparation, J.W., G.R., P.N., M.B., and A.C.B.; writing—review and editing, J.W., M.B., P.N., G.R., A.C.B., A.I.R., A.S., T.H., L.K., E.N., M.K., S.M.M., M.G.-S., E.G.-G., L.A.B., A.C., S.M.O., D.W., M.M., H.R., G.R., A.C.B., I.R., S.A., M.H., S.B.-S., J.H., S.R., I.S., G.S., K.B., M.W. and J.B.; supervision, J.B., I.R., A.S., T.H., M.K., S.M.M., A.F., V.F.S., I.P., V.D., N.Y., A.G., Z.U., V.P., L.S., Y.H., M.T., A.P., Z.A., and E.K. All authors have read and agreed to the published version of the manuscript.

Acknowledgments: We gratefully acknowledge support from Liza Villas and Gerben Rienk for making the COSI project possible. We also acknowledge the leadership of the principal investigators from Ireland (Cecily Kelleher), Kyrgyzstan (Gulmira Aitmurzaeva), Romania (Constanta Huidimac Petrescu), and Tajikistan (Zulfiya Abdurrahmonova). The authors alone are responsible for the views expressed in this article and they do not necessarily represent the views, decisions or policies of the institutions with which they are affiliated.

References

1. Park, M.H.; Falconer, C.; Viner, R.M.; Kinra, S. The impact of childhood obesity on morbidity and mortality in adulthood: A systematic review. *Obes. Rev.* **2012**, *13*, 985–1000. [CrossRef] [PubMed]

2. Wijnhoven, T.M.; van Raaij, J.M.; Spinelli, A.; Starc, G.; Hassapidou, M.; Spiroski, I.; Rutter, H.; Martos, E.; Rito, A.I.; Hovengen, R.; et al. WHO European Childhood Obesity Surveillance Initiative: Body mass index and level of overweight among 6-9-year-old children from school year 2007/2008 to school year 2009/2010. *BMC Public Health* **2014**, *14*, 806. [CrossRef]
3. Afshin, A.; Sur, P.J.; Fay, K.A.; Cornaby, L.; Ferrara, G.; Salama, J.S.; Mullany, E.C.; Abate, K.H.; Abbafati, C.; Abebe, Z. Health effects of dietary risks in 195 countries, 1990–2017: A systematic analysis for the Global Burden of Disease Study 2017. *Lancet* **2019**, *393*, 1958–1972. [CrossRef]
4. Freemark, M. Determinants of Risk for Childhood Obesity. *N. Engl. J. Med.* **2018**, *379*, 1371–1372. [CrossRef] [PubMed]
5. Freemark, M. Childhood obesity in the modern age: Global trends, determinants, complications, and costs. In *Pediatric Obesity*; Springer: Berlin/Heidelberg, Germany, 2018; pp. 3–24.
6. WHO. *WHO European Childhood Obesity Surveillance Initiative: Report of the Fourth Round of Data Collection (2015–2017)*; WHO: Geneva, Switzerland, 2020.
7. WHO. The Double Burden of Malnutrition. Available online: https://www.who.int/nutrition/double-burden-malnutrition/en/#:~{}:text=Double%20burden%20of%20malnutrition,populations%2C%20and%20across%20the%20lifecourse (accessed on 1 June 2020).
8. Djordjic, V.; Jorga, J.; Radisavljevic, S.; Milanovic, I.; Bozic, P.; Ostojic, S.M. Thinness in young schoolchildren in Serbia: Another case of the double burden of malnutrition? *Public Health Nutr.* **2018**, *21*, 877–881. [CrossRef] [PubMed]
9. Global Burden of Disease Collaborators Health effects of overweight and obesity in 195 countries over 25 years. *N. Engl. J. Med.* **2017**, *377*, 13–27. [CrossRef]
10. WHO. World Health Organization Global Monitoring Framework for NCDs: Target 7: Halt the Rise in Obesity. Available online: https://www.who.int/nmh/ncd-tools/target7/en/ (accessed on 1 June 2020).
11. United Nations. Sustainable Development Goals. Available online: https://sustainabledevelopment.un.org/?menu=1300 (accessed on 28 June 2020).
12. Sachs, J.; Schmidt-Traub, G.; Kroll, C.; Lafortune, G.; Fuller, G. *Sustainable Development Report 2019*; Bertelsmann Stiftung and Sustainable Development Solutions Network (SDSN): New York, NY, USA, 2019; Volume 2.
13. Mikkilä, V.; Räsänen, L.; Raitakari, O.T.; Pietinen, P.; Viikari, J. Longitudinal changes in diet from childhood into adulthood with respect to risk of cardiovascular diseases: The Cardiovascular Risk in Young Finns Study. *Eur. J. Clin. Nutr.* **2004**, *58*, 1038–1045. [CrossRef]
14. WHO. *Increasing Fruit and Vegetable Consumption to Reduce the Risk of Noncommunicable Diseases*; World Health Organization: Geneva, Switzerland, 2014.
15. WHO. *Diet, Nutrition and the Prevention of Chronic Diseases: Report of a Joint WHO/FAO Expert Consultation*; WHO Technical Report Series, No. 916; World Health Organization: Geneva, Switzerland, 2003.
16. WHO. *Guideline: Sugars Intake for Adults and Children*; World Health Organization: Geneva, Switzerland, 2015.
17. Mozaffarian, D.; Fahimi, S.; Singh, G.M.; Micha, R.; Khatibzadeh, S.; Engell, R.E.; Lim, S.; Danaei, G.; Ezzati, M.; Powles, J.; et al. Global sodium consumption and death from cardiovascular causes. *N. Engl. J. Med.* **2014**, *371*, 624–634. [CrossRef]
18. Malik, V.S.; Pan, A.; Willett, W.C.; Hu, F.B. Sugar-sweetened beverages and weight gain in children and adults: A systematic review and meta-analysis. *Am. J. Clin. Nutr.* **2013**, *98*, 1084–1102. [CrossRef]
19. Moynihan, P.J.; Kelly, S.A.M. Effect on caries of restricting sugars intake: Systematic review to inform WHO guidelines. *J. Dent. Res.* **2014**, *93*, 8–18. [CrossRef]
20. Wijnhoven, T.M.; van Raaij, J.; Breda, J. *WHO European Childhood Obesity Surveillance Initiative. Implementation of Round 1 (2007/2008) and Round 2 (2009/2010)*; WHO Regional Office for Europe: Copenhagen, Denmark, 2014.
21. Council for International Organizations of Medical Sciences, Council for International Organizations of Medical Sciences, World Health Organization. *International Ethical Guidelines for Biomedical Research Involving Human Subjects*; World Health Organization: Geneva, Switzerland, 2002.
22. Wijnhoven, T.M.; van Raaij, J.M.; Spinelli, A.; Rito, A.I.; Hovengen, R.; Kunesova, M.; Starc, G.; Rutter, H.; Sjoberg, A.; Petrauskiene, A.; et al. WHO European Childhood Obesity Surveillance Initiative 2008: Weight, height and body mass index in 6-9-year-old children. *Pediatr. Obes.* **2013**, *8*, 79–97. [CrossRef] [PubMed]

23. WHO. *European Childhood Obesity Surveillance Initiative: Overweight and Obesity among 6–9-year-old Children. Report of the Third Round of Data Collection 2012–2013*; WHO: Geneva, Switzerland, 2018.
24. WHO. Healthy Diet: Key Facts. Available online: https://www.who.int/news-room/fact-sheets/detail/healthy-diet (accessed on 29 June 2020).
25. United Nations. Statistical Division Standard Country or Area Codes for Statistical Use (M49). Available online: https://unstats.un.org/unsd/methodology/m49/ (accessed on 6 August 2020).
26. Monzani, A.; Ricotti, R.; Caputo, M.; Solito, A.; Archero, F.; Bellone, S.; Prodam, F. A systematic review of the association of skipping breakfast with weight and cardiometabolic risk factors in children and adolescents. What should we better investigate in the future? *Nutrients* **2019**, *11*, 387. [CrossRef] [PubMed]
27. Inchley, J.; Currie, D.B.; Budisavljevic, S.; Torsheim, T.; Jåstad, A.; Cosma, A.; Kelly, C.; Arnarsson, Á. *Spotlight on Adolescent Health and Well-Being: Findings from the 2017/2018 Health Behaviour in School-Aged Children (HBSC) Survey in Europe and Canada*; WHO Regional Office for Europe: Copenhagen, Denmark, 2020.
28. Vereecken, C.; Pedersen, T.P.; Ojala, K.; Krølner, R.; Dzielska, A.; Ahluwalia, N.; Giacchi, M.; Kelly, C. Fruit and vegetable consumption trends among adolescents from 2002 to 2010 in 33 countries. *Eur. J. Public Health* **2015**, *25*, 16–19. [CrossRef]
29. Rosi, A.; Paolella, G.; Biasini, B.; Scazzina, F.; Alicante, P.; De Blasio, F.; dello Russo, M.; Paolella, G.; Rendina, D.; Rosi, A. Dietary habits of adolescents living in North America, Europe or Oceania: A review on fruit, vegetable and legume consumption, sodium intake, and adherence to the Mediterranean Diet. *Nutr. Metab. Cardiovasc. Dis.* **2019**, *29*, 554–560. [CrossRef] [PubMed]
30. Scaglioni, S.; De Cosmi, V.; Ciappolino, V.; Parazzini, F.; Brambilla, P.; Agostoni, C. Factors Influencing Children's Eating Behaviours. *Nutrients* **2018**, *10*, 706. [CrossRef] [PubMed]
31. Smith, R.; Kelly, B.; Yeatman, H.; Boyland, E. Food marketing influences children's attitudes, preferences and consumption: A systematic critical review. *Nutrients* **2019**, *11*, 875. [CrossRef] [PubMed]
32. Micha, R.; Karageorgou, D.; Bakogianni, I.; Trichia, E.; Whitsel, L.P.; Story, M.; Penalvo, J.L.; Mozaffarian, D. Effectiveness of school food environment policies on children's dietary behaviors: A systematic review and meta-analysis. *PLoS ONE* **2018**, *13*, e0194555. [CrossRef]
33. European Commission. School Fruit, Vegetables and Milk Scheme. Available online: https://ec.europa.eu/info/food-farming-fisheries/key-policies/common-agricultural-policy/market-measures/school-fruit-vegetables-and-milk-scheme (accessed on 25 May 2020).
34. WHO. Nutrition-Friendly Schools Initiative (NFSI). Available online: https://www.who.int/nutrition/topics/nutrition_friendly_schools_initiative/en/ (accessed on 25 May 2020).
35. U.S. Department of Agriculture. School Breakfast Program. Available online: https://www.fns.usda.gov/sbp/school-breakfast-program (accessed on 26 May 2020).
36. WHO. *Taxes on Sugary Drinks: Why Do It?* World Health Organization: Geneva, Switzerland, 2017.
37. Colchero, M.A.; Rivera-Dommarco, J.; Popkin, B.M.; Ng, S.W. In Mexico, Evidence of Sustained Consumer Response two Years after Implementing a Sugar-Sweetened Beverage Tax. *Health Aff. (Millwood)* **2017**, *36*, 564–571. [CrossRef]
38. van Raaij, J.; Hendriksen, M.; Verhagen, H. Potential for improvement of population diet through reformulation of commonly eaten foods. *Public Health Nutr.* **2009**, *12*, 325–330. [CrossRef]
39. Goiana-da-Silva, F.; Cruz, E.S.D.; Gregorio, M.J.; Miraldo, M.; Darzi, A.; Araujo, F. The future of the sweetened beverages tax in Portugal. *Lancet Public Health* **2018**, *3*, e562. [CrossRef]
40. Griffith, R.; O'Connell, M.; Smith, K. The Importance of Product Reformulation Versus Consumer Choice in Improving Diet Quality. *Economica* **2017**, *84*, 34–53. [CrossRef]
41. Macgregor, G.A.; Hashem, K.M. Action on sugar–lessons from UK salt reduction programme. *Lancet* **2014**, *383*, 929–931. [CrossRef]
42. Cairns, G.; Angus, K.; Hastings, G.; Caraher, M. Systematic reviews of the evidence on the nature, extent and effects of food marketing to children. A retrospective summary. *Appetite* **2013**, *62*, 209–215. [CrossRef] [PubMed]
43. WHO. *Monitoring and Restricting Digital Marketing of Unhealthy Products to Children and Adolescents*; World Health Organization Regional Office for Europe: Copenhagen, Denmark, 2019.
44. WHO. *Noncommunicable Diseases Progress Monitor*; World Health Organization: Geneva, Switzerland, 2017.
45. Hodder, R.K.; O'Brien, K.M.; Tzelepis, F.; Wyse, R.J.; Wolfenden, L. Interventions for increasing fruit and

vegetable consumption in children aged five years and under. *Cochrane Database Syst. Rev.* **2018**, *2018*, CD008552. [CrossRef]
46. Mazarello Paes, V.; Hesketh, K.; O'Malley, C.; Moore, H.; Summerbell, C.; Griffin, S.; Van Sluijs, E.M.F.; Ong, K.K.; Lakshman, R. Determinants of sugar-sweetened beverage consumption in young children: A systematic review. *Obes. Rev.* **2015**, *16*, 903–913. [CrossRef]
47. Kairey, L.; Matvienko-Sikar, K.; Kelly, C.; McKinley, M.C.; O'Connor, E.M.; Kearney, P.M.; Woodside, J.V.; Harrington, J.M. Plating up appropriate portion sizes for children: A systematic review of parental food and beverage portioning practices. *Obes. Rev.* **2018**, *19*, 1667–1678. [CrossRef]
48. WHO. *Report of the Commission on Ending Childhood Obesity*; World Health Organization: Geneva, Switzerland, 2016.
49. Crockett, R.A.; King, S.E.; Marteau, T.M.; Prevost, A.T.; Bignardi, G.; Roberts, N.W.; Stubbs, B.; Hollands, G.J.; Jebb, S.A. Nutritional labelling for healthier food or non-alcoholic drink purchasing and consumption. *Cochrane Database Syst. Rev.* **2018**, 2, CD009315. [CrossRef]
50. Monsivais, P.; Aggarwal, A.; Drewnowski, A. Are socio-economic disparities in diet quality explained by diet cost? *J. Epidemiol. Community Health* **2012**, *66*, 530–535. [CrossRef]
51. Spinelli, A.; Buoncristiano, M.; Kovacs, V.A.; Yngve, A.; Spiroski, I.; Obreja, G.; Starc, G.; Pérez, N.; Rito, A.I.; Kunešová, M. Prevalence of severe obesity among primary school children in 21 European countries. *Obes. Facts* **2019**, *12*, 244–258. [CrossRef]
52. Pérez-Rodrigo, C.; Artiach Escauriaza, B.; Artiach Escauriaza, J.; Polanco Allúe, I. Dietary assessment in children and adolescents: Issues and recommendations. *Nutr. Hosp.* **2015**, *31* (Suppl. 3), 76–83. [CrossRef]
53. Medin, A.C.; Hansen, B.H.; Astrup, H.; Ekelund, U.; Frost Andersen, L. Validation of energy intake from a web-based food recall for children and adolescents. *PLoS ONE* **2017**, *12*, e0178921. [CrossRef] [PubMed]
54. Cheung, K.L.; Peter, M.; Smit, C.; de Vries, H.; Pieterse, M.E. The impact of non-response bias due to sampling in public health studies: A comparison of voluntary versus mandatory recruitment in a Dutch national survey on adolescent health. *BMC Public Health* **2017**, *17*, 276. [CrossRef] [PubMed]
55. Berg, C.; Jonsson, I.; Conner, M.T.; Lissner, L. Sources of bias in a dietary survey of children. *Eur. J. Clin. Nutr.* **1998**, *52*, 663–667. [CrossRef] [PubMed]

9

Is the Perceived Fruit Accessibility Related to Fruit Intakes and Prevalence of Overweight in Disadvantaged Youth

Narae Yang and **Kirang Kim** *

Department of Food Science and Nutrition, College of Natural Sciences, Dankook University, Dandae-ro, Dongnam-gu, Cheonan-si, Chungnam 31116, Korea; skfo2581@daum.net

* Correspondence: kirangkim@dankook.ac.kr.

Abstract: Background: Few investigations have studied the relationship between home and school food environments, fruit intakes, and prevalence of overweight in children and adolescents from disadvantaged backgrounds. This study aimed to determine whether food environments for fruit intake at household and school levels affect fruit intakes and risk of overweight among children and adolescents with low household income. Methods: Students (n = 3148) in Seoul, Korea completed questionnaires pertaining to select aspects of their food environments, frequency of fruit intakes, and weight status. Chi-square tests and logistic regressions evaluated associations between the aforementioned variables. Results: Participants consumed fruit an average of 0.77 times per day, though its frequency increased when fruit accessibility was perceived positively. The percentage of overweight participants was 23.5% for boys and 22.8% for girls. Generally, fruit intake frequency was linked to a lower prevalence of overweight. Regular provision of fruit in school lunches was associated with a reduced risk of overweight among elementary school girls (odds ratio (OR): 0.52, 95% confidence interval (CI): 0.30–0.92), and having someone at home to prepare fruit was associated with a reduced risk of overweight in elementary school boys (OR: 0.64, 95% CI: 0.43–0.94) and girls (OR: 0.63, 95% CI: 0.43–0.93). Conclusions: The frequency of fruit intake was low among disadvantaged youth. Increasing access to fruit in their food environments appears to enhance consumption and lower the risk of overweight, especially for elementary school girls.

Keywords: food environment; fruit; children; adolescents; obesity; overweight; home; school

1. Introduction

The epidemic of pediatric overweight and obesity has expanded steadily over the past few decades, currently reaching more than 370 million children worldwide [1]. Consequences of early excess adiposity include a heightened risk of psychological problems such as depression, low self-esteem, and disordered eating in the immediate term, as well as cardiovascular disease and various cancers upon adulthood [2–5]. Adult obesity, implemented in child obesity, makes it difficult to lose weight [6]. Therefore, it is important to prevent obesity in childhood [6]. The prevalence of obesity among children and adolescents has increased in Asia [7]. Although the rising trends of body mass index (BMI) have flattened in high-income countries, the prevalence of obesity is still high in worldwide [7].

Obesity has been explained with reduced intakes of healthy foods and unhealthy eating behaviors [8–11]. Especially fruit, which are rich in water and fiber, to enhance satiety, and low in energy density [12], have been known to prevent obesity, coronary heart disease, stroke, cardiovascular disease, total cancer, and all-cause mortality [13–16]. Obesity prevention interventions that take into account healthy food intake, such as fruit, are needed. For effective obesity intervention, it is important to identify the relationship between eating healthy foods and obesity and to find the main determinants that affect obesity. Previous intervention methods for eating healthy foods to prevent obesity have focused on individual behavior changes. However, individual level interventions fundamentally could not change the obesogenic environment, which have been reported to have little effect on long-term improvement [17,18]. In recent years, the ecological model has been applied to promote health in the public health sector. The multilevel interventions that take an account for both individual and environmental factors have been paid attention for effective behavior change. Among environmental factors, food environments include political, economic, social, physical, and natural environment factors which affect accessibility, availability, and affordability of foods [19,20]. The food environments have been known as an important factor related to food choice and dietary intakes [19,20]. For children and adolescents, the household is the first physical and social environment to learn about food intake [21], and the school is responsible for their lunches and another setting to make them eat healthy food [21]. Thus, for effective intervention, factors at household and school levels that affect the availability and accessibility of foods as well as at the individual level should be included [22].

It has been reported that the food environment has a greater effect on health and nutritional status in the vulnerable group than in the general group [23], but most of the studies have been conducted on the general group [24], and there is a dearth of research exploring how food environments at home and school affect fruit intakes and risk of overweight among disadvantaged children and adolescents. Therefore, research is needed to determine how the food environments of vulnerable children is related to healthy food intake and obesity. For this study, we surveyed low socioeconomic status youth to determine how select aspects of their food environments associate with consumption of fruit and weight status. Therefore, the objective of this study was to investigate whether food environments at household and school levels affect fruit intakes and risk of overweight among disadvantaged children and adolescents.

2. Methods

2.1. Study Population

Participants were recruited in 2015 from the Community Childcare Center, located in Seoul, Korea. They provide welfare services (e.g., protection, education, and meals) after school to youth from disadvantaged backgrounds (e.g., beneficiaries of national basic livelihood or single-parent families, etc.) [25]. During this time, the Community Childcare Center participated in the Healthy Fruit Basket Program, which aims to prevent the development of chronic diseases by providing access to fresh fruits [25,26]. In total, 4154 students (mean age; elementary school: 10.4 y, middle and high school: 14.3 y) were recruited; however, only 3148 were included in the final analyses because they supplied information for all the variables of interest and were of an eligible weight status (i.e., normal and overweight) [27,28]. The Institutional Review Board approved this study, and all participants gave written informed consent and assent (DKU 2015-10-016).

2.2. Weight Status

Height and weight were measured by a trained measurer at the public health centers or the Community Childcare Centers using a nationally certified weight and height scale. BMI was calculated as weight (kg) divided by height squared (m^2). According to the 2007 Korean National Growth Charts for children and adolescents [29], classification of normal weight was defined as having a body weight between the fifth and eighty-fourth percentiles, based on one's gender and age; classification of overweight was defined as having a body weight in the eighty-fifth percentile or above, or BMI 25 kg/m^2 or greater, based on one's gender and age.

2.3. Fruit Intakes

Fruit frequency questionnaires examined fruit intakes from the month preceding study enrollment. Scoring ranged from 0 (never) to 9 (3+ times per day). All responses were converted into times per day and collapsed into two categories (<0.5 times per day vs. ≥0.5 times per day) to determine the association with overweight.

2.4. Food Environments

Participants were asked five questions about their food environments, adapted from those employed in a previous investigation [30]. Here, three dimensions of the physical environment were evaluated: (1) Availability of fruit at home, (2) accessibility of fruit at home (i.e., is there someone who prepares fruit for children to eat?), and (3) accessibility of fruit at school (i.e., does the school provide fruit twice a week?). For the social environment, questions inquired about the habit of frequently eating fruit among parents and friends. Responses for the questions ranged from 1 (strongly disagree) to 5 (strongly agree), and all were collapsed into categories of disagree (strongly disagree, disagree), neutral, and agree (agree, strongly agree).

2.5. Statistical Analysis

Chi-square tests assessed the distribution of participants' general characteristics, the food environment, and weight status according to the frequency of fruit intakes and aspects of the food environment. T-tests evaluated differences in the frequency of fruit intakes by sex and grade level. An analysis of variance and Scheffe's post-hoc test determined differences between the food environments. Logistic regressions analyzed the effects of fruit intakes and food environments on weight status, showing odds ratios (ORs), 95% confidence intervals (95% CI). All analyses were performed by SPSS Statistics (v. 23.0); $p \leq 0.05$ was considered statistically significant.

3. Results

General characteristics of the participants are shown in Table 1. Overall, 49.0% were boys and 71.5% were in elementary school. The percentage of overweight for boys and girls was 23.5% and 22.8%, respectively. The percentage of overweight for elementary school, and middle and high school students was 24.3% and 20.4%, respectively. There was a significant difference of weight status between grades, and the percentage of overweight was high in elementary school students.

Table 1. General characteristics of subjects [1].

	All (n = 3148)	Normal Weight (n = 2419)	Overweight (n = 729)	p [2]
Sex				
Boys	1542 (49.0)	1179 (76.5)	363 (23.5)	0.617
Girls	1606 (51.0)	1240 (77.2)	366 (22.8)	
Grade				
Elementary school	2251 (71.5)	1705 (75.7)	546 (24.3)	0.021
Middle and high school	897 (28.5)	714 (79.6)	183 (20.4)	
Sex, grade				
Boys				
Elementary school	1061 (68.8)	797 (75.1)	264 (24.9)	0.065
Middle and high school	481 (31.2)	382 (79.4)	99 (20.6)	
Girls				
Elementary school	1190 (74.1)	908 (76.3)	282 (23.7)	0.142
Middle and high school	416 (25.9)	332 (79.8)	84 (20.2)	

[1] Qualitative variables are presented as n (%). [2] p-values for differences between the weight statuses were obtained by a chi-square test.

Table 2 details aspects of the participants' food environments. Overall, 59.5% to 63.2% of participants responded positively (i.e., affirmed the availability of fruit at home, a regular provision of fruit in school lunches, having someone at home to prepare fruit for them, and a family habit of frequently eating fruit). Between the sexes, girls perceived their food environments more positively than boys ($p < 0.001$). Between the grade levels, elementary school students perceived their food environments more positively than middle and high school students ($p < 0.001$).

Table 2. Select aspects of participants' food environments [1].

	All	Sex		Grade	
		Boys	Girls	Elementary School	Middle and High School
		Availability of fruit at home			
Disagree	458 (14.5)	238 (15.4)	220 (13.7)	313 (13.9)	145 (16.2)
Neutral	816 (25.9)	441 (28.6)	375 (23.3)	557 (24.7)	259 (28.9)
Agree	1874 (59.5)	863 (56.0)	1011 (63.0)	1381 (61.4)	493 (55.0)
p [2]		<0.001		0.004	
		Regular provision of fruit in school lunches			
Disagree	259 (8.2)	155 (10.1)	104 (6.5)	145 (6.4)	114 (12.7)
Neutral	959 (30.5)	504 (32.7)	455 (28.3)	624 (27.7)	335 (37.3)
Agree	1930 (61.3)	883 (57.3)	1047 (65.2)	1482 (65.8)	448 (49.9)
p [2]		<0.001		<0.001	
		Having someone at home to prepare fruit			
Disagree	439 (13.9)	226 (14.7)	213 (13.3)	295 (13.1)	144 (16.1)
Neutral	718 (22.8)	393 (25.5)	325 (20.2)	471 (20.9)	247 (27.5)
Agree	1991 (63.2)	923 (59.9)	1068 (66.5)	1485 (66.0)	506 (56.4)
p [2]		<0.001		<0.001	
		Family habit of eating fruit frequently			
Disagree	282 (9.0)	143 (9.3)	139 (8.7)	193 (8.6)	89 (9.9)
Neutral	954 (30.3)	518 (33.6)	436 (27.1)	618 (27.5)	336 (37.5)
Agree	1912 (60.7)	881 (57.1)	1031 (64.2)	1440 (64.0)	472 (52.6)
p [2]		<0.001		<0.001	
		Friends' habit of eating fruit frequently			
Disagree	544 (17.3)	299 (19.4)	245 (15.3)	364 (16.2)	180 (20.1)
Neutral	1378 (43.8)	710 (46.0)	668 (41.6)	936 (41.6)	442 (49.3)
Agree	1226 (38.9)	533 (34.6)	693 (43.2)	951 (42.2)	275 (30.7)
p [2]		<0.001		<0.001	

[1] Values are presented as absolute numbers and percentages. [2] p-values for differences between sexes or grade levels, obtained by a chi-square test.

Table 3 shows the relationship between aspects of participants' food environments and frequency of fruit intakes. Regardless of sex or grade level, fruit intakes differed according to how one's food environment was perceived. Here, the group who perceived their food environments positively was found to consume fruit 0.87 to 0.95 times per day, whereas the group who perceived their food environments negatively was found to consume fruit 0.42 to 0.67 times per day ($p < 0.001$). Interestingly, there were no differences in fruit intakes between sexes when they shared the same perception about their food environments. However, when both grade levels responded positively about their food environments, consumption of fruit was found to be higher among elementary school students. For groups displaying a negative or neutral perception, frequency of fruit intakes was comparable.

Table 3. Relationship between aspects of participants' food environments and frequency of fruit intakes [1].

	All	Sex		Grade	
		Boys	Girls	Elementary School	Middle and High School
All	0.77 ± 0.17	0.74 ± 0.02 ^{a}	0.80 ± 0.02 ^{b}	0.85 ± 0.02 ^{a}	0.59 ± 0.02 ^{b}
p [2]		0.036		<0.001	
Availability of fruit at home					
Disagree	0.47 ± 0.03 ^{a}	0.46 ± 0.04 ^{a}	0.49 ± 0.04 ^{a}	0.51 ± 0.04 ^{a}	0.39 ± 0.03 ^{a}
Neutral	0.55 ± 0.02 ^{a}	0.54 ± 0.03 ^{a}	0.55 ± 0.03 ^{a}	0.60 ± 0.03 ^{ab}	0.44 ± 0.03 ^{a}
Agree	0.95 ± 0.02 ^{b}	0.92 ± 0.03 ^{b}	0.96 ± 0.03 ^{b}	1.03 ± 0.03 ^{c}	0.71 ± 0.03 ^{b}
p [2]	<0.001	<0.001		<0.001	
Regular provision of fruit in school lunches					
Disagree	0.65 ± 0.05 ^{a}	0.62 ± 0.06 ^{a}	0.69 ± 0.08 ^{ab}	0.64 ± 0.07 ^{acd}	0.66 ± 0.06 ^{ad}
Neutral	0.62 ± 0.02 ^{a}	0.62 ± 0.03 ^{a}	0.63 ± 0.03 ^{a}	0.70 ± 0.03 ^{a}	0.47 ± 0.03 ^{cd}
Agree	0.87 ± 0.02 ^{b}	0.83 ± 0.03 ^{b}	0.89 ± 0.03 ^{b}	0.93 ± 0.02 ^{b}	0.64 ± 0.03 ^{ad}
p [2]	<0.001	<0.001		<0.001	
Having someone at home to prepare fruit					
Disagree	0.60 ± 0.04 ^{a}	0.55 ± 0.05 ^{a}	0.64 ± 0.05 ^{a}	0.67 ± 0.05 ^{ae}	0.43 ± 0.03 ^{ad}
Neutral	0.53 ± 0.02 ^{a}	0.52 ± 0.03 ^{a}	0.55 ± 0.04 ^{a}	0.58 ± 0.03 ^{ac}	0.44 ± 0.03 ^{cd}
Agree	0.90 ± 0.02 ^{b}	0.88 ± 0.03 ^{b}	0.91 ± 0.03 ^{b}	0.97 ± 0.02 ^{b}	0.70 ± 0.03 ^{e}
p [2]	<0.001	<0.001		<0.001	
Family habit of eating fruit frequently					
Disagree	0.42 ± 0.04 ^{a}	0.42 ± 0.05 ^{a}	0.43 ± 0.05 ^{a}	0.46 ± 0.05 ^{ab}	0.33 ± 0.03 ^{ab}
Neutral	0.54 ± 0.02 ^{a}	0.55 ± 0.03 ^{a}	0.53 ± 0.03 ^{a}	0.59 ± 0.03 ^{bc}	0.45 ± 0.03 ^{ab}
Agree	0.94 ± 0.02 ^{b}	0.91 ± 0.03 ^{b}	0.97 ± 0.03 ^{b}	1.01 ± 0.02 ^{d}	0.72 ± 0.03 ^{c}
p [2]	<0.001	<0.001		<0.001	
Friends' habit of eating fruit frequently					
Disagree	0.67 ± 0.03 ^{a}	0.63 ± 0.04 ^{a}	0.71 ± 0.05 ^{ab}	0.75 ± 0.04 ^{a}	0.49 ± 0.03 ^{bd}
Neutral	0.67 ± 0.02 ^{a}	0.68 ± 0.03 ^{a}	0.67 ± 0.03 ^{a}	0.73 ± 0.03 ^{a}	0.56 ± 0.03 ^{bd}
Agree	0.93 ± 0.03 ^{b}	0.89 ± 0.04 ^{bc}	0.96 ± 0.04 ^{c}	1.00 ± 0.03 ^{c}	0.69 ± 0.04 ^{ad}
p [2]	<0.001	<0.001		<0.001	

[1] Values are fruit intake per day, presenting as means ± standard errors. [2] p-values for differences between sexes or grade levels, obtained by ANOVA; letters (^{a,b,c,d,e}) indicate significant differences between groups (Scheffe's post-hoc test, $p < 0.05$).

Table 4 shows the relationship between aspects of participants' food environments, frequency of fruit intakes, and weight status. The fruit intake frequency was not related to weight status in total subjects but as classified by grade; the lower intake frequency was shown in overweight groups of elementary school students. In terms of fruit environments and overweight, regular provision of fruit in school lunches and having a person at home to prepare fruit were negatively correlated to an overweight status for all participants. A low frequency of fruit intakes was associated with an overweight status among elementary school students. The proportion of overweight students was lower among those who perceived their food environment at school positively compared to those who did not ($p = 0.044$), especially for girls ($p = 0.047$) and elementary school students ($p = 0.005$). In addition, the proportion of overweight students was lower among those who had someone at home to prepare fruit compared to those who did not ($p < 0.001$), notably again for girls ($p = 0.007$) and elementary school students ($p = 0.001$).

Table 4. Relationship between aspects of participants' food environments, frequency of fruit intakes, and weight status [1].

	All		Sex				Grade			
			Boys		Girls		Elementary School		Middle and High School	
	Normal Weight	Over Weight	Normal Weight	Over Weight	Normal Weight	Over Weight	Normal Weight	Over Weight	Normal Weight	Over Weight
Fruits intakes per day										
<0.5	1194 (49.4)	378 (51.9)	610 (51.7)	191 (52.6)	584 (47.1)	187 (51.1)	771 (45.2)	274 (50.2)	423 (59.2)	104 (56.8)
≥0.5	1225 (50.6)	351 (48.1)	569 (48.3)	172 (47.4)	656 (52.9)	179 (48.9)	934 (54.8)	272 (49.8)	291 (40.8)	79 (43.2)
p [2]	0.238		0.770		0.179		0.043		0.554	
Food environments										
Availability of fruit at home										
Disagree	348 (14.4)	110 (15.1)	181 (15.4)	57 (15.7)	167 (13.5)	53 (14.5)	232 (13.6)	81 (14.8)	116 (16.2)	29 (15.8)
Neutral	629 (26.0)	187 (25.7)	335 (28.4)	106 (29.2)	294 (23.7)	81 (22.1)	420 (24.6)	137 (25.1)	209 (29.3)	50 (27.3)
Agree	1442 (59.6)	432 (59.3)	663 (56.2)	200 (55.1)	779 (62.8)	232 (63.4)	1053 (61.8)	328 (60.1)	389 (54.5)	104 (56.8)
p [2]	0.892		0.929		0.768		0.713		0.838	
Regular provision of fruit in school lunches										
Disagree	187 (7.7)	72 (9.9)	115 (9.8)	40 (11.0)	72 (5.8)	32 (8.7)	99 (5.8)	46 (8.4)	88 (12.3)	26 (14.2)
Neutral	723 (29.9)	236 (32.4)	380 (32.2)	124 (34.2)	343 (27.7)	112 (30.6)	454 (26.6)	170 (31.1)	269 (37.7)	66 (36.1)
Agree	1509 (62.4)	421 (57.8)	684 (58.0)	199 (54.8)	825 (66.5)	222 (60.7)	1152 (67.6)	330 (60.4)	357 (50.0)	91 (49.7)
p [2]	0.044		0.535		0.047		0.005		0.775	
Having someone at home to prepare fruit										
Disagree	310 (12.8)	129 (17.7)	160 (13.6)	66 (18.2)	150 (12.1)	63 (17.2)	204 (12.0)	91 (16.7)	106 (14.8)	38 (20.8)
Neutral	539 (22.3)	179 (24.6)	297 (25.2)	96 (26.4)	242 (19.5)	83 (22.7)	342 (20.1)	129 (23.6)	197 (27.6)	50 (27.3)
Agree	1570 (64.9)	421 (57.8)	722 (61.2)	201 (55.4)	848 (68.4)	220 (60.1)	1159 (68.0)	326 (59.7)	411 (57.6)	95 (51.9)
p [2]	<0.001		0.055		0.007		0.001		0.135	
Family habit of eating fruit frequently										
Disagree	211 (8.7)	71 (9.7)	107 (9.1)	36 (9.9)	104 (8.4)	35 (9.6)	141 (8.3)	52 (9.5)	70 (9.8)	19 (10.4)
Neutral	730 (30.2)	224 (30.7)	393 (33.3)	125 (34.4)	337 (27.2)	99 (27.0)	454 (26.6)	164 (30.0)	276 (38.7)	60 (32.8)
Agree	1478 (61.1)	434 (59.5)	679 (57.6)	202 (55.6)	799 (64.4)	232 (63.4)	1110 (65.1)	330 (60.4)	368 (51.5)	104 (56.8)
p [2]	0.629		0.780		0.778		0.141		0.339	
Friends' habit of eating fruit frequently										
Disagree	421 (17.4)	123 (16.9)	233 (19.8)	66 (18.2)	188 (15.2)	57 (15.6)	275 (16.1)	89 (16.3)	146 (20.4)	34 (18.6)
Neutral	1051 (43.4)	327 (44.9)	541 (45.9)	169 (46.6)	510 (41.1)	158 (43.2)	697 (40.9)	239 (43.8)	354 (49.6)	88 (48.1)
Agree	947 (39.1)	279 (38.3)	405 (34.4)	128 (35.3)	542 (43.7)	151 (41.3)	733 (43.0)	218 (39.9)	214 (30.0)	61 (33.3)
p [2]	0.796		0.798		0.702		0.415		0.652	

[1] Values are presented as absolute numbers and percentages. [2] p-values for differences between sexes and grade levels, obtained by a chi-square test.

Table 5. Relationship between aspects of participants' food environments and odds of being overweight.

	Boys				Girls			
	Elementary School		Middle and High School		Elementary School		Middle and High School	
	OR [1] (95% CI)	Adjusted OR [2] (A95% CI)	OR (95% CI)	Adjusted OR (A95% CI)	OR (95% CI)	Adjusted OR (A95% CI)	OR (95% CI)	Adjusted OR (A95% CI)
	Availability of fruit at home							
Disagree	1.00	1.00	1.00	1.00	1.00	1.00	1.00	1.00
Neutral	0.87 (0.56–1.35)	0.87 (0.56–1.34)	1.41 (0.69–2.90)	1.41 (0.69–2.88)	1 (0.63–1.60)	1.02 (0.64–1.62)	0.61 (0.29–1.29)	0.61 (0.29–1.27)
Agree	0.8 (0.54–1.19)	0.79 (0.53–1.18)	1.44 (0.74–2.80)	1.41 (0.72–2.77)	1 (0.67–1.50)	1.08 (0.72–1.63)	0.77 (0.40–1.48)	0.7 (0.36–1.37)
p-trend [3]	0.278	0.246	0.342	0.392	0.988	0.652	0.701	0.464
	Regular provision of fruit in school lunches							
Disagree	1.00	1.00	1.00	1.00	1.00	1.00	1.00	1.00
Neutral	0.87 (0.52–1.47)	0.87 (0.52–1.47)	0.98 (0.49–1.96)	1 (0.50–1.99)	0.72 (0.39–1.30)	0.72 (0.40–1.31)	0.66 (0.30–1.44)	0.71 (0.32–1.55)
Agree	0.71 (0.43–1.16)	0.7 (0.43–1.15)	1.01 (0.52–1.98)	1.01 (0.52–1.98)	0.52 (0.30–0.92)	0.54 (0.31–0.95)	0.7 (0.34–1.46)	0.71 (0.34–1.49)
p-trend [3]	0.081	0.075	0.939	0.963	0.005	0.01	0.527	0.492
	Having someone at home to prepare fruit							
Disagree	1.00	1.00	1.00	1.00	1.00	1.00	1.00	1.00
Neutral	0.76 (0.49–1.19)	0.76 (0.49–1.19)	0.85 (0.44–1.64)	0.85 (0.45–1.64)	0.95 (0.60–1.50)	0.93 (0.59–1.47)	0.56 (0.27–1.16)	0.55 (0.27–1.14)
Agree	0.64 (0.43–0.94)	0.63 (0.42–0.93)	0.72 (0.40–1.32)	0.7 (0.38–1.29)	0.63 (0.43–0.93)	0.65 (0.44–0.96)	0.57 (0.30–1.05)	0.51 (0.27–0.96)
p-trend [3]	0.023	0.019	0.275	0.223	0.004	0.009	0.122	0.06
	Family habit of eating fruit frequently							
Disagree	1.00	1.00	1.00	1.00	1.00	1.00	1.00	1.00
Neutral	1.16 (0.69–1.93)	1.15 (0.68–1.92)	0.63 (0.29–1.36)	0.63 (0.29–1.36)	0.81 (0.48–1.37)	0.82 (0.49–1.38)	1.08 (0.45–2.58)	1.03 (0.43–2.46)
Agree	0.83 (0.51–1.36)	0.81 (0.49–1.33)	1.01 (0.48–2.12)	1.00 (0.47–2.13)	0.78 (0.49–1.25)	0.84 (0.52–1.36)	1.09 (0.47–2.50)	0.96 (0.41–2.25)
p-trend [3]	0.097	0.081	0.301	0.346	0.357	0.649	0.879	0.835
	Friends' habit of eating fruit frequently							
Disagree	1.00	1.00	1.00	1.00	1.00	1.00	1.00	1.00
Neutral	1.06 (0.72–1.56)	1.06 (0.72–1.56)	1.26 (0.69–2.31)	1.25 (0.69–2.29)	1.06 (0.70–1.59)	1.04 (0.69–1.58)	0.86 (0.45–1.65)	0.85 (0.44–1.63)
Agree	1.02 (0.69–1.52)	1.02 (0.69–1.51)	1.31 (0.67–2.57)	1.29 (0.65–2.54)	0.84 (0.56–1.27)	0.86 (0.57–1.31)	1.13 (0.59–2.17)	1.07 (0.55–2.08)
p-trend [3]	0.962	0.977	0.459	0.496	0.204	0.302	0.586	0.699

[1] Odds ratios (ORs) were derived from logistic regression models. [2] Adjusted ORs adjusted for fruit intake frequency and were derived from logistic regression models. [3] *p*-values for trends.

Table 5 shows the relationship between aspects of participants' food environments and odds of being overweight, unadjusted and adjusted for fruit intake frequency. For boys, those who had someone at home to prepare fruit were unlikely to be overweight (OR = 0.64, 95% CI = 0.43–0.94, *p-trend* = 0.023), and these results remained significant after adjusting for frequency of fruit intakes (OR = 0.63, 95% CI = 0.420.93, *p-trend* = 0.019). For elementary school girls, regular provision of fruit in school lunches (OR = 0.52, 95% CI = 0.30–0.92, *p-trend* = 0.005) and having someone at home to prepare fruit for them (OR = 0.63, 95% CI = 0.43–0.93, *p-trend* = 0.004) were negatively related to an overweight status, even after adjusting for frequency of fruit intakes (OR = 0.54, 95% CI = 0.31–0.95, *p-trend* = 0.01 for regular provision of fruit in school lunches; OR = 0.65, 95% CI = 0.44–0.96, *p-trend* = 0.009 for having someone at home to prepare fruit). Among middle and high school girls, having someone at home to prepare fruit was significantly associated with a lower risk of being overweight after adjusting for frequency of fruit intakes (OR = 0.51, 95% CI = 0.27–0.96, *p-trend* = 0.06).

4. Discussion

Because of the prominent influence that food environments exert on an individual's tendency toward obesity, we explored the relationship between aspects of the home and school food environments, fruit intakes, and overweight status among disadvantaged children and adolescents. We found that the frequency of fruit intakes increased when participants perceived their food environments positively, and this was associated with a reduced prevalence of overweight. In particular, regular provision of fruit in school lunches and having someone at home to prepare fruit was associated with a healthier body weight among elementary school students and girls.

Fruit was consumed an average of 0.77 times per day by our participants, which was below the recommended level of the Dietary Reference Intake for Koreans of at least twice per day [31]. According to the Korea National Health and Nutrition Examination Survey [32], low-income families consume less fruit than medium-income families (100.1 vs. 135.2 g/day). In this study, frequency of fruit intake varied according to a participant's perception of their food environment, with higher rates of consumption among those who responded positively. These results provide evidence that food environments to increase fruit intakes would play an important role in fruit consumption.

Previously, review papers and meta-analyses have shown that increasing the availability and accessibility of fruits and vegetables for children at school is effective at preventing obesity [33,34]. In this study, regular provision of fruit in school lunches was positively related to fruit intakes among elementary school students, but not middle and high school students. These findings do not align with those from a related investigation in the United States, wherein high school students who received fruits and vegetables from The Fresh Fruit and Vegetable Program were likely to eat fruit more often than those who did not (59.1% vs. 40.9%) [35]. Given that middle and high school students appear to have more established eating habits, it may be necessary to provide fruit at a higher frequency in order to enhance intakes [35,36]. The school lunch service in Korea could provide fruits as a dessert within the school budget, but the current frequency of provision of fruit at school lunch would not be enough to meet the consumption of fruit for the disadvantaged middle and high school students in Korea. Therefore, additional funding for more frequent provision of fruit at school lunch should be needed to increase their fruit consumption.

Regarding the food environment at home, having someone to prepare fruit for students was found to relate favorably to fruit intakes and weight status. This result was consistent with those from other studies reporting that social support for healthy food intakes aides in the prevention of obesity among vulnerable children [37,38]. A few reasons might explain this. First, caregivers give children fruit in a form that allows them to eat it easily. Several studies have shown that providing fruit in a ready-to-eat form or making it visible to children promotes fruit intakes [39,40]. Because the process of washing, cutting, and peeling fruit has been described as an impediment to consumption, providing or storing it in an accessible form may help children eat fruit more frequently [40,41]. Indeed, analyses from the Healthy Habits randomized trial [42] revealed that the frequency of fruit provision from a parent positively impacted their children's fruit intakes after 12 months. Second, caregivers could promote fruit intakes simply by encouraging their children [43]. Considering that participants in our study hailed from disadvantaged backgrounds, it is unlikely that their caregivers purchase much fruit for them or monitor their intakes at home. Thus, incorporating the Healthy Fruit Basket Program into all Community Childcare Centers and related institutions nationwide may help these individuals increase fruit intakes and attenuate risk of overweight or obesity [25,26].

It is well established that availability of food in the home is a key determinant of consumption among children and adolescents [44–46], and our analyses confirmed this phenomenon for fruit, in particular. Additionally, we observed that a family's habit of eating fruit frequently was connected to high fruit intakes across all participants, similar to findings from other publications [39,42,43].

Interestingly, this investigation detected no difference in fruit intakes between sexes sharing the same perception about their food environments. However, with respect to the grade levels, elementary school students were found to consume fruit more frequently than middle or high school students when their food environment was perceived positively. Childhood is a period of social modeling, as individuals learn how to interact with their environments and behave appropriately [11,47,48]. Hence, the benefits of food environments on fruit intakes may apply more strongly to children than adolescents. For another explanation, a recent study of adults with low socioeconomic position found that self-efficacy on fruit and vegetable consumption was more strongly associated with fruit and vegetable consumption than perceived food environments, which implies the importance of capacity building to partially overcome the poor food environment [49]. As several studies have shown the positive effect of nutritional education on fruit and vegetable intakes [50–52], nutritional education intervention should be included for adolescents with negative perception of food environment who especially have low self-efficacy to increase their fruit and vegetable intakes.

When we examined the relationship between fruit intakes and weight status, a high frequency (>0.5 times per day) was tied to a lower prevalence of overweight in girls. According to systematic reviews, consumption of fruit as a means to prevent pediatric obesity did not always produce consistent results in terms of gender or amount (38,39). For example, one investigation noted that eating fruit more than twice a day was only protective against obesity in boys [53], and another showed that excessive fruit intakes actually engendered obesity [54]. Heeding our results and those from earlier studies, consumption of fruit alone may not be adequate to prevent obesity. Specifically, our investigation found that the effects of some aspects of the food environment on the prevalence of obesity remained significant after adjusting for fruit intake frequency, and a related study observed a positive link between parental concern for their children's diet and fitness practices ($r = 0.552$, $p < 0.001$) [55]. It could suggest that the home environment supporting children to eat fruits could also support other behaviors that can prevent obesity in children, such as encouraging exercise. Further research exploring caretakers' interest in their children's health will provide a more holistic understanding of how environments moderate their risk of obesity.

The present study had several limitations and strengths. Concerning limitations, this was a cross-sectional study, so any causal associations between food environments, fruit intakes, and overweight status have yet to be determined. In addition, the questionnaire evaluating fruit availability and accessibility in the home and school food environments was not validated, although it had been employed in a previous study [30]. Moreover, we did not collect information pertaining to other confounders of overweight, which could offer deeper insight into factors underlying the present findings [25,26]. Granted, this was a highly homogenous cohort since all participants were recruited from the Community Childcare Center, so it is unlikely they possessed any remarkable characteristics that would alter our results. Nonetheless, future studies examining a more diverse population are needed to confirm the relationship between the food environment and risk of obesity by adjusting the confounding factor. Despite limitations, these results provide evidence that food environments play an important role in overweight prevention as well as fruit consumption among underprivileged Asian children and adolescents, using a relatively large sample size.

5. Conclusions

This study found that the frequency of fruit intakes was generally low among children and adolescents from disadvantaged backgrounds; however, those who perceived their food environments positively consumed more fruit and were less likely to be overweight than those who perceived them negatively. Noteworthily, regular provision of fruit in school lunches and having someone at home to prepare fruit were predictive of a high frequency of fruit intakes and lower prevalence of overweight, and these discoveries were most apparent among elementary school students and girls. On the whole, our findings demonstrate that augmenting access to fruit within any realm of the food environment is associated with increased consumption and healthier body weights for low-income youth. Going forward, the school lunch service in Korea could consider increasing fruit servings since current provisions are not sufficient for enabling disadvantaged middle and high school students to meet the dietary guidelines. In addition, a nation-wide program to increase fruit consumption at the Community Childcare Center where they usually spend time would be essential to improve their health.

Author Contributions: K.K. conceived and designed the study; N.Y. analyzed the data and wrote the first draft of the paper; K.K. supervised the data analysis and revised the draft paper. All authors have read and agreed to the published version of the manuscript.

References

1. Di Cesare, M.; Sorić, M.; Bovet, P.; Miranda, J.J.; Bhutta, Z.; Stevens, G.A.; Laxmaiah, A.; Kengne, A.P.; Bentham, J. The epidemiological burden of obesity in childhood: A worldwide epidemic requiring urgent action. *BMC Med.* **2019**, *17*, 1–20. [CrossRef]
2. Rankin, J.; Matthews, L.; Cobley, S.; Han, A.; Sanders, R.; Wiltshire, H.D.; Baker, J.S. Psychological consequences of childhood obesity: Psychiatric comorbidity and prevention. *Adolesc. Health Med. Ther.* **2016**, *7*, 125–146. [CrossRef]
3. Sagar, R.; Gupta, T. Psychological Aspects of Obesity in Children and Adolescents. *Indian J. Pediatr.* **2018**, *85*, 554–559. [CrossRef]
4. Anthropometric Measures during Infancy and Childhood and the Risk of Developing Cardiovascular Disease or Diabetes Mellitus Type 2 in Later Life: A Systematic Review 2015. Available online: https://www.who.int/maternal_child_adolescent/documents/singh-anthropometry-ncd-infants-children-2015.pdf?ua=1 (accessed on 27 August 2020).
5. Preventing and Managing the Global Epidemic—WHO Technical Report Series. Available online: https://www.who.int/nutrition/publications/obesity/WHO_TRS_894/en/ (accessed on 27 August 2020).
6. Dehghan, M.; Akhtar-Danesh, N.; Merchant, A.T. Childhood obesity, prevalence and prevention. *Nutr. J.* **2005**, *4*, 1–8. [CrossRef]
7. Bentham, J.; Di Cesare, M.; Bilano, V.; Bixby, H.; Zhou, B.; Stevens, G.A.; Riley, L.M.; Taddei, C.; Hajifathalian, K.; Lu, Y.; et al. Worldwide trends in body-mass index, underweight, overweight, and obesity from 1975 to 2016: A pooled analysis of 2416 population-based measurement studies in 128·9 million children, adolescents, and adults. *Lancet* **2017**, *390*, 2627–2642. [CrossRef]
8. Poti, J.; Braga, B.; Quin, B. Ultra-processed food intake and obesity: What really matters for health—Processing or nutrient content? *Curr. Obes. Rep.* **2018**, *6*, 420–431. [CrossRef]
9. Huang, J.-Y.; Qi, S.-J. Childhood obesity and food intake. *World J. Pediatr.* **2015**, *11*, 101–107. [CrossRef]
10. Epstein, L.H.; Paluch, R.A.; Beecher, M.D.; Roemmich, J.N. Increasing healthy eating vs. reducing high energy-dense foods to treat pediatric obesity. *Obesity* **2008**, *16*, 318–326. [CrossRef]
11. Ricotti, R.; Caputo, M.; Prodam, F. Chapter 9—Mediterranean diet, nutrition transition, and cardiovascular risk factor in children and adolescents. In *The Mediterranean Diet: An Evidence-Based Approach*, 2nd ed.; Preedy, V.R., Watson, R.R., Eds.; Academic Press: Cambridge, MA, USA, 2020; pp. 89–95, ISBN 978-0-12-818649-7.

12. Rolls, B.J.; Ello-Martin, J.A.; Tohill, B.C. What Can Intervention Studies Tell Us about the Relationship between Fruit and Vegetable Consumption and Weight Management? *Nutr. Rev.* **2004**, *62*, 1–17. [CrossRef]
13. Aune, D.; Giovannucci, E.; Boffetta, P.; Fadnes, L.T.; Keum, N.N.; Norat, T.; Greenwood, D.C.; Riboli, E.; Vatten, L.J.; Tonstad, S. Fruit and vegetable intake and the risk of cardiovascular disease, total cancer and all-cause mortality-A systematic review and dose-response meta-analysis of prospective studies. *Int. J. Epidemiol.* **2017**, *46*, 1029–1056. [CrossRef]
14. Hebden, L.; O'Leary, F.; Rangan, A.; Singgih Lie, E.; Hirani, V.; Allman-Farinelli, M. Fruit consumption and adiposity status in adults: A systematic review of current evidence. *Crit. Rev. Food Sci. Nutr.* **2017**, *57*, 2526–2540. [CrossRef]
15. Stamler, J.; Dolecek, T. Chapter 13. Relation of food and nutrient intakes to body mass in the special intervention and usual care groups in the Multiple Risk Factor Intervention Trial. *Am. J. Clin. Nutr.* **1997**, *65*, 366S–373S. [CrossRef]
16. Buijsse, B.; Feskens, E.J.M.; Schulze, M.B.; Forouhi, N.G.; Wareham, N.J.; Sharp, S.; Palli, D.; Tognon, G.; Halkjaer, J.; Tjønneland, A.; et al. Fruit and vegetable intakes and subsequent changes in body weight in European populations: Results from the project on Diet, Obesity, and Genes (DiOGenes). *Am. J. Clin. Nutr.* **2009**, *90*, 202–209. [CrossRef]
17. Kamath, C.C.; Vickers, K.S.; Ehrlich, A.; McGovern, L.; Johnson, J.; Singhal, V.; Paulo, R.; Hettinger, A.; Erwin, P.J.; Montori, V.M. Behavioral interventions to prevent childhood obesity: A systematic review and metaanalyses of randomized trials. *J. Clin. Endocrinol. Metab.* **2008**, *93*, 4606–4615. [CrossRef]
18. Swinburn, B.; Egger, G.; Raza, F. The Development and Application of a Framework for Identifying and Prioritizing Environmental Interventions for Obesity. *Dissecting Obesog. Environ.* **1999**, *29*, 563–570.
19. Rideout, K.; Mah, C.; Minaker, L. *Food Environments: An Introduction for Public Health Practice*; National Collaborating Centre for Environmental Health British Columbia Centre for Disease Control: Vancouver, BC, Canada, 2015.
20. Rosenkranz, R.R.; Dzewaltowski, D.A. Model of the home food environment pertaining to childhood obesity. *Nutr. Rev.* **2008**, *66*, 123–140. [CrossRef]
21. Chan, K.; Prendergast, G.; Grønhøj, A.; Bech-Larsen, T. The role of socializing agents in communicating healthy eating to adolescents: A cross-cultural study. *J. Int. Consum. Mark.* **2011**, *23*, 59–74. [CrossRef]
22. Food and Health in Europe: A New Basis for Action. Available online: https://www.who.int/nutrition/publications/Food_and_health_Europe%20_newbasis_for_%20action.pdf (accessed on 27 August 2020).
23. Lytle, L.A. Measuring the Food Environment. State of the Science. *Am. J. Prev. Med.* **2009**, *36*, 1–18. [CrossRef]
24. Micha, R.; Karageorgou, D.; Bakogianni, I.; Trichia, E.; Whitsel, L.P.; Story, M.; Peñalvo, J.L.; Mozaffarian, D. Effectiveness of school food environment policies on children's dietary behaviors: A systematic review and meta-analysis. *PLoS ONE* **2018**, *13*, 1–27. [CrossRef]
25. Ministry of Health and Welfare. *2015 Community Child Centers Support Program Manual*; Ministry of Health and Welfare: Sejong, Korea, 2015; p. 19.
26. Ministry of Health and Welfare; Korea Health Promotion Institute. *Healthy Fruit Basket Program Manual*; Korea Health Promotion Institute: Sejong, Seoul, 2013; p. 9.
27. Aarestrup, J.; Gamborg, M.; Ulrich, L.G.; Sørensen, T.I.A.; Baker, J.L. Childhood body mass index and height and risk of histologic subtypes of endometrial cancer. *Int. J. Obes.* **2016**, *40*, 1096–1102. [CrossRef]
28. Nogueira, L.; Stolzenberg-Solomon, R.; Gamborg, M.; Sørensen, T.I.; Baker, J.L. Childhood Body Mass Index and Risk of Adult Pancreatic Cancer. *Curr. Dev. Nutr.* **2017**, *1*, e001362. [CrossRef]
29. Korea Centers for Disease Control and Prevention; Committee for the Development of Growth Standard for Korean Children and Adolescents; Korean Pediatric Society. *2007 Korean Children and Adolescents Growth Standard (Commentary for the Development of 2007 Growth Chart)*; Korea Centers for Disease Control and Prevention: Cheongju, Korea, 2007; pp. 93–104.
30. Story, M.; Kaphingst, K.M.; Robinson-O'Brien, R.; Glanz, K. Creating Healthy Food and Eating Environments: Policy and Environmental Approaches. *Annu. Rev. Public Health* **2008**, *29*, 253–272. [CrossRef]
31. The Ministry of Health and Welfare; The Korean Nutrition Society. *Dietary Reference Intakes for Koreans 2015*; The Korean Nutrition Society: Sejong, Korea, 2015; pp. 958–959.

32. The Ministry of Health and Welfare; Korea Centers for Disease Control and Prevention. *Korea Health Statistics 2018: Korea National Health and Nutrition Examination Survey (KNHANES VII-3)*; Korea Centers for Disease Control and Prevention: Sejong, Korea, 2020.
33. Pineda, E.; Swinburn, B.; Sassi, F. Effective school food environment interventions for the prevention of childhood obesity: Systematic review and meta-analysis. *Lancet* **2019**, *394*, S77. [CrossRef]
34. Bere, E.; Klepp, K.I.; Øverby, N.C. Free school fruit: Can an extra piece of fruit every school day contribute to the prevention of future weight gain? A cluster randomized trial. *Food Nutr. Res.* **2014**, *58*, 1–5. [CrossRef]
35. Davis, E.M.; Cullen, K.W.; Watson, K.B.; Konarik, M.; Radcliffe, J. A Fresh Fruit and Vegetable Program Improves High School Students' Consumption of Fresh Produce. *J. Am. Diet. Assoc.* **2009**, *109*, 1227–1231. [CrossRef]
36. Ridberg, R.A.; Bell, J.F.; Merritt, K.E.; Harris, D.M.; Young, H.M.; Tancredi, D.J. Effect of a fruit and vegetable prescription program on children's fruit and vegetable consumption. *Prev. Chronic Dis.* **2019**, *16*, 1–13. [CrossRef]
37. Story, M. School-based approaches for preventing and treating obesity. *Int. J. Obes.* **1999**, *23*, S43–S51. [CrossRef]
38. Heredia, N.I.; Ranjit, N.; Warren, J.L.; Evans, A.E. Association of parental social support with energy balance-related behaviors in low-income and ethnically diverse children: A cross-sectional study. *BMC Public Health* **2016**, *16*, 1–12. [CrossRef]
39. Ray, C.; Roos, E.; Brug, J.; Behrendt, I.; Ehrenblad, B.; Yngve, A.; Te Velde, S.J. Role of free school lunch in the associations between family-environmental factors and children's fruit and vegetable intake in four European countries. *Public Health Nutr.* **2013**, *16*, 1109–1117. [CrossRef]
40. Wyse, R.; Campbell, E.; Nathan, N.; Wolfenden, L. Associations between characteristics of the home food environment and fruit and vegetable intake in preschool children: A cross-sectional study. *BMC Public Health* **2011**, *11*, 938. [CrossRef]
41. McMorrow, L.; Ludbrook, A.; Macdiarmid, J.I.; Olajide, D. Perceived barriers towards healthy eating and their association with fruit and vegetable consumption. *J. Public Health* **2017**, *39*, 330–338. [CrossRef]
42. Wyse, R.; Wolfenden, L.; Bisquera, A. Characteristics of the home food environment that mediate immediate and sustained increases in child fruit and vegetable consumption: Mediation analysis from the Healthy Habits cluster randomised controlled trial. *Int. J. Behav. Nutr. Phys. Act.* **2015**, *12*, 1–9. [CrossRef]
43. Pearson, N.; Biddle, S.J.H.; Gorely, T. Family correlates of fruit and vegetable consumption in children and adolescents: A systematic review. *Public Health Nutr.* **2009**, *12*, 267–283. [CrossRef]
44. Yee, A.Z.H.; Lwin, M.O.; Ho, S.S. The influence of parental practices on child promotive and preventive food consumption behaviors: A systematic review and meta-analysis. *Int. J. Behav. Nutr. Phys. Act.* **2017**, *14*, 1–14. [CrossRef]
45. Befort, C.; Kaur, H.; Nollen, N.; Sullivan, D.K.; Nazir, N.; Choi, W.S.; Hornberger, L.; Ahluwalia, J.S. Fruit, vegetable, and fat intake among non-hispanic black and non-hispanic white adolescents: Associations with home availability and food consumption settings. *J. Am. Diet. Assoc.* **2006**, *106*, 367–373. [CrossRef]
46. Spurrier, N.J.; Magarey, A.A.; Golley, R.; Curnow, F.; Sawyer, M.G. Relationships between the home environment and physical activity and dietary patterns of preschool children: A cross-sectional study. *Int. J. Behav. Nutr. Phys. Act.* **2008**, *5*, 1–12. [CrossRef]
47. Goslin, D.A. *Handbook of Socialization Theory and Research*, 4th ed.; Rand McNally: Chicago, IL, USA, 1969; pp. 213–262, ISBN 0528686801.
48. Schmitt, R. The Stages of Moral Development: A Basis for an Educational Concept? *Int. Rev. Educ.* **1980**, *26*, 207–216.
49. de Menezes, M.C.; Diez Roux, A.V.; Souza Lopes, A.C. Fruit and vegetable intake: Influence of perceived food environment and self-efficacy. *Appetite* **2018**, *127*, 249–256. [CrossRef]
50. Wagner, M.G.; Rhee, Y.; Honrath, K.; Blodgett Salafia, E.H.; Terbizan, D. Nutrition education effective in increasing fruit and vegetable consumption among overweight and obese adults. *Appetite* **2016**, *100*, 94–101. [CrossRef]
51. Honrath, K.; Wagner, M.G.; Rhee, Y. Does Nutrition Education with Fruit and Vegetable Supplementation Increase Fruit and Vegetable Intake and Improve Anthropometrics of Overweight or Obese People of Varying Socioeconomic Status? *Ecol. Food Nutr.* **2018**, *57*, 32–49. [CrossRef]

52. Clark, R.L.; Famodu, O.A.; Holásková, I.; Infante, A.M.; Murray, P.J.; Olfert, I.M.; McFadden, J.W.; Downes, M.T.; Chantler, P.D.; Duespohl, M.W.; et al. Educational intervention improves fruit and vegetable intake in young adults with metabolic syndrome components. *Nutr. Res.* **2019**, *62*, 89–100. [CrossRef]
53. Santiago, S.; Zazpe, I.; Martí, A.; Cuervo, M.; Martínez, J.A. Gender differences in lifestyle determinants of overweight prevalence in a sample of Southern European children. *Obes. Res. Clin. Pract.* **2013**, *7*, e391–e400. [CrossRef]
54. Field, A.E.; Gillman, M.W.; Rosner, B.; Rockett, H.R.; Colditz, G.A. Association between fruit and vegetable intake and change in body mass index among a large sample of children and adolescents in the United States. *Int. J. Obes.* **2003**, *27*, 821–826. [CrossRef]
55. Attorp, A.; Scott, J.E.; Yew, A.C.; Rhodes, R.E.; Barr, S.I.; Naylor, P.J. Associations between socioeconomic, parental and home environment factors and fruit and vegetable consumption of children in grades five and six in British Columbia, Canada. *BMC Public Health* **2014**, *14*, 1–9. [CrossRef]

10

Effects of the Preschool-Based Family-Involving DAGIS Intervention Program on Children's Energy Balance-Related Behaviors and Self-Regulation Skills

Carola Ray [1,2,*], Rejane Figuereido [1,3], Henna Vepsäläinen [2], Reetta Lehto [1,2], Riikka Pajulahti [1,2], Essi Skaffari [1,2], Taina Sainio [1,4], Pauliina Hiltunen [1,2], Elviira Lehto [1,4], Liisa Korkalo [2], Katri Sääksjärvi [4], Nina Sajaniemi [4,5], Maijaliisa Erkkola [2] and Eva Roos [1,2,6]

1 Folkhälsan Research Center, Topeliuksenkatu 20, FI-00250 Helsinki, Finland; rejane.fig@gmail.com (R.F.); reetta.lehto@folkhalsan.fi (R.L.); riikka.pajulahti@helsinki.fi (R.P.); essi.skaffari@helsinki.fi (E.S.); taina.sainio@helsinki.fi (T.S.); pauliina.hiltunen@folkhalsan.fi (P.H.); elviira.lehto@helsinki.fi (E.L.); eva.roos@folkhalsan.fi (E.R.)

2 Department of Food and Nutrition, University of Helsinki, P.O. Box 66, FI-00014 Helsinki, Finland; henna.vepsalainen@helsinki.fi (H.V.); liisa.korkalo@helsinki.fi (L.K.); maijaliisa.erkkola@helsinki.fi (M.E.)

3 Clinicum, Faculty of Medicine, University of Helsinki, FI-00014 Helsinki, Finland

4 Department of Teacher Education, University of Helsinki, P.O. Box 9, FI-00100 Helsinki, Finland; katri.saaksjarvi@helsinki.fi (K.S.); nina.sajaniemi@helsinki.fi (N.S.)

5 School of Applied Educational Science and Teacher Education, Philosophical Faculty, University of Eastern Finland, P.O. Box 111, FI-80101 Joensuu, Finland

6 Department of Public Health, Clinicum, P.O. Box 63, University of Helsinki, FI-00014 Helsinki, Finland

* Correspondence: carola.ray@folkhalsan.fi.

Abstract: The study examines the effects of a preschool-based family-involving multicomponent intervention on children's energy balance-related behaviors (EBRBs) such as food consumption, screen time and physical activity (PA), and self-regulation (SR) skills, and whether the intervention effects differed among children with low or high parental educational level (PEL) backgrounds. The Increased Health and Wellbeing in Preschools (DAGIS) intervention was conducted as a clustered randomized controlled trial, clustered at preschool level, over five months in 2017–2018. Altogether, 802 children aged 3–6 years in age participated. Parents reported children's consumption of sugary everyday foods and beverages, sugary treats, fruits, and vegetables by a food frequency questionnaire, and screen time by a 7-day diary. Physical activity was assessed by a hip-worn accelerometer. Cognitive and emotional SR was reported in a questionnaire by parents. General linear mixed models with and without repeated measures were used as statistical methods. At follow-up, no differences were detected in EBRBs or SR skills between the intervention and control group, nor did differences emerge in children's EBRBs between the intervention and the control groups when stratified by PEL. The improvement in cognitive SR skills among low PEL intervention children differed from low PEL control children, the significance being borderline. The DAGIS multicomponent intervention did not significantly affect children's EBRBs or SR. Further sub-analyses and a comprehensive process evaluation may shed light on the non-significant findings.

Keywords: energy balance-related behaviors; self-regulation skills; preschoolers; children; randomized controlled trial; intervention effects; parental educational level; intervention mapping; multicomponent intervention

1. Introduction

Young children's food intake, screen time, and physical activity (PA), commonly referred to as energy balance-related behaviors (EBRBs) [1], are of importance since they can predict the future weight status and health of children [2–4]. A socio-economic status (SES) gradient exists already in preschoolers' EBRBs; those with low SES family backgrounds tend to have less healthy EBRBs such as higher intake of sugary foods or beverages and excessive screen time [5–7].

Home and an early childhood education and care center, hereafter preschool, are the settings where three to six-year-olds spend most of their time, and it is therefore important that these environments promote healthy EBRBs including sufficient PA and fruit and vegetable (FV) consumption [8–10]. Reviews have concluded that EBRB interventions should be conducted at preschools and homes simultaneously in order to be successful [11,12]. Preschool-based family-involving interventions have been reported to be promising [12–15], although some studies show no effects on EBRBs [12,14,16]. This has raised discussion on intervention design and implementation in families [12]. When designing interventions for the general population, they should reach and show higher effects on those needing it most, namely those with low SES backgrounds [5,17]. To date, knowledge of the equity effectiveness of EBRB interventions among children is sparse [18,19]. Promoting several EBRBs simultaneously is challenging, as the aim can be to both promote healthy behaviors and discourage unhealthy behaviors. Strategies can differ, a review concluding that promoting PA among young children is successful when focusing on the preferred behavior, rather than focusing on decreasing sedentary time such as lying or sitting down [20].

Strengthening children's self-regulation (SR) skills in parallel to promoting children's healthy EBRBs could be an effective strategy in interventions [21,22]. Self-regulation is a multidimensional concept, briefly described as the capacity of a goal-directed behavior to regulate actions, emotions, and cognitions [23]. Cognitive SR skills refer to executive functioning such as self-monitoring to plan and proceed toward long-term goals [24–26], whereas emotional SR skills refers to capacities such as being able to recognize one's own feelings and staying calm in stressful situations [24,25]. Associations between children's SR skills and less favorable EBRBs and weight status have been found [21,22,24,25]. The Head Start study tested the strategy of strengthening young children's SR skills alongside promoting their healthy EBRBs [27]. The intervention included four arms: intervening on EBRBs and SR skills; intervening on EBRBs; intervening on SRs skills; and no intervention. Effects were seen in lower sugar-sweetened beverage consumption in the study arm promoting EBRBs and SR skills compared with the other arms [27].

The Increased Health and Wellbeing in Preschools (DAGIS) intervention aimed to promote preschoolers' (aged 3–6 years) healthy EBRBs and SR skills. The assumption was that there would be greater effects on children from families with low parental educational levels (PEL), also assuming a reduction in any health gaps between children with low and high PEL backgrounds [28]. The intervention development process was guided by the Intervention Mapping (IM) framework [29] and the process is described elsewhere [28]. A cross-sectional study served as the needs assessment [7,28], and based on these findings, there were three main aims: to reduce children's screen time; to reduce the consumption of sugary everyday foods and beverages; and to increase vegetable consumption. In these three behaviors, the needs assessment showed less favorable behaviors among children with low PEL background [28]. To promote alternatives to the reductions, additional aims were to increase fruit and berry consumption and total PA (light, moderate, and vigorous intensity) [28]. In addition, the intervention aimed to strengthen children's SR skills. Activities were planned to suit families with low PEL backgrounds.

In Finland, 78–86% of three to six year-olds attend municipality-driven preschools [30]. Therefore, preschools offer a good setting for interventions. As screen time and sugary food and beverage consumption occurs mostly at home [31], homes were considered as an equally important intervention setting. The developed program lasted 23 weeks, and was divided into five themes: SR skills; PA; fruit and vegetables; screen time; and sugary foods and beverages. Each theme was in focus for four to five weeks.

In this study, we aimed: (1) to evaluate the effects of a preschool-based family intervention on children's EBRBs and SR skills, and (2) to evaluate whether effects were stronger among children with low PEL background than among those with high PEL background.

2. Materials and Methods

The DAGIS intervention study is a preschool-level clustered randomized controlled trial (RCT) aimed to promote preschoolers' healthy EBRBs and SR skills so that those from low SES background would benefit most from the program. The study was conducted between September 2017 and May 2018 including baseline and follow-up measurements [28]. Early educators delivered the program and all included activities to all preschoolers independently of their participation in the study. Prospective trial registration number: ISRCTN57165350 (the 8th of January 2015).

2.1. Recruitment

We aimed to invite municipalities that had a high number of preschools and had a large variety in educational and income levels among inhabitants as well as being located within a convenient distance from the Helsinki region. Municipalities invited were selected by comparing municipality statistics from southern and western Finland [32], and excluded municipalities that were already part of the previous comprehensive DAGIS survey in 2015–2016 [7]. Power calculations prior to the recruitment for the intervention were based on the DAGIS survey results; specifically, we used the average (about 1.7 times/week for all and about 2 times/week for low PEL group) and standard deviations of children's sugary food and beverage consumption frequency [7]. Based on those values, we decided to aim at a decrease of 0.74 times/day in sugary foods and beverages consumption frequency. To detect a change of 0.74 times/day less sugary foods and beverages, the required sample size was calculated to be 432 children, considering an attrition rate of 70% (Fpower macro, SAS version 9.4.). The significance level was set at 5% and the power at 80%.

Altogether, seven municipalities were invited to participate in the study, and an oral presentation on the study was offered. Five municipalities had an oral presentation; two of these municipalities chose to participate. One municipality decided that all of its preschools ($n = 29$, preschool managers $n = 19$) would participate, whereas the other municipality allowed its preschool managers to make the decision individually, as such, the managers of three preschools chose to participate. We decided that these 32 preschools and 1702 eligible preschoolers were sufficient for our study (Figure 1).

Researchers visited each preschool to inform early educator professionals about the project and their role in the project. The recruitment phase lasted 1–2 weeks, and families returned informed consents (or refusals to participate) to preschools in sealed envelopes. Thereafter, the researchers returned to preschools to distribute the baseline research material for early educators, parents, and children.

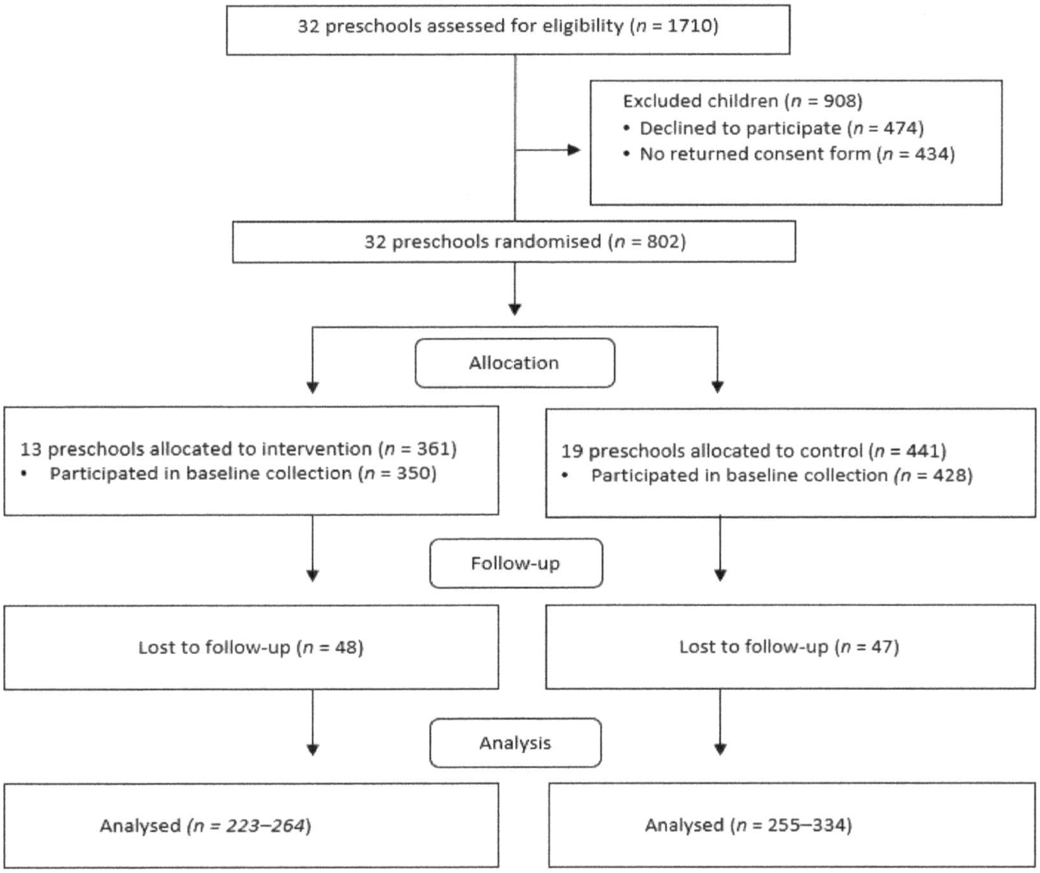

Figure 1. Flow chart in the Increased Health and Wellbeing in Preschools (DAGIS) intervention study, in accordance with the Consolidated Standards of Reporting Trials (CONSORT) 2010 statement [33].

2.2. Ethical Issues

The DAGIS intervention study received ethics approval from the Helsinki Ethics Review Board in humanities and social and behavioral sciences (22/2017; 16 May 2017). Early education professionals were informed about the study through site visits. The early educators' questionnaire stated that participation was voluntary and that the early educators had the option to withdraw at any stage of the study. Early educators gave their consent by filling in the questionnaire. Families returned written informed consent, and thereafter, the questionnaires were delivered.

2.3. Data Collection and Measurements

The baseline data collection occurred in four waves over five weeks and the follow-up data collection in three waves over five weeks. Data collection in waves was necessary due to the limited number of accelerometers available for measuring children's PA. Research staff visited each preschool to instruct early educators and left printed screen time diaries for families, study questionnaires for families who had requested paper copies, and accelerometers for children. These materials were picked up from preschools one week later. However, most parents requested that their questionnaires be sent electronically by sending the parent's main questionnaire as a personal link and the food frequency questionnaire link by email.

2.3.1. Measurements

Screen time was assessed by a printed screen time diary. In the diary, parents recorded their child's use of screens outside preschool time whenever the child used a screen for more than 10 min in a row. Screen use was recorded separately for different screens: TV, DVD, computer, tablet, or cell phone. The screen time diary was a slightly modified version from a previous validated diary [34], as the original did not include portable screens and questions about screen contexts. The screen time diary has shown good reproducibility [35]. Screen time was calculated for children who presented data for at least three weekdays, and one weekend day. Total screen time (min/day) was calculated as a weighted mean: (5 × weekday mean + 2 × weekend mean)/7.

Children's PA was assessed by a hip-worn accelerometer, the ActiGraph wGT3X-BT (ActiGraph, LLC, Pensacola, FL, USA), 24 h/day over seven consecutive days, and parents kept a screen time diary over the same days. A 15-s epoch length was used for data derived from accelerometers, and more than ten minutes of consecutive zeroes was set as non-wearing time [36]. In the analyses, the cut-off points of Evenson et al. [37] for children aged 5–15 years were used, which means that total PA including light, moderate, and vigorous intensity PA is defined as more than 100 counts/min. Inclusion criteria for the child's PA data to be in the analyses were that there were data for at least four days, of which one was a weekend day. In addition, each day needed to have 600 min or more of awake wearing time. The mean total PA (min/day) was used in the analyses.

The original 47-item food frequency questionnaire (FFQ) was designed for the DAGIS survey to particularly measure the consumption frequencies of vegetables and fruits as well as sugary foods and beverages [38]. It has shown acceptable validity for ranking food group consumption compared with 3-day food records [38], and testing the reproducibility of the items has yielded acceptable results [35]. In the DAGIS intervention, the FFQ was expanded into a 51-item FFQ that included six food groups (vegetables, fruit, and berries; dairy products; fish meat and eggs; cereal products; beverages; and other foods such as sweets and snacks). A link to the electronic 51-item FFQ was sent to all parents and hard copies were sent to those who did not fill in the electronic version. Parents reported how many times during the past week the child had consumed foods outside preschool hours. The FFQ included three answer options: not at all, times per week, and times per day. The instruction was to either tick the 'not at all' box or to write a number in one of the other columns. The FFQ was intentionally restricted to not cover municipality-provided foods and beverages consumed during preschool hours because parents would not have been able to reliably report these foods.

The three food consumption frequency variables ('sugary everyday foods and beverages', 'sugary treats', and 'fruit and vegetables (FV)') were formed by summing up the consumption frequencies (times/week). The sugary everyday foods and beverages variable included flavored yogurt and quark; puddings; sugar-sweetened cereals and muesli; berry, fruit, and chocolate porridge with added sugar; berry and fruit soups with added sugar; soft drinks; flavored and sweetened milk- and plant-based beverages; and sugar-sweetened juices. The sugary treats variable included ice cream, chocolate, sweets, cakes, cupcakes, sweet rolls, Danish pastries, pies and other sweet pastries, and sweet biscuits and cereal bars. The FV variable included fresh vegetables, cooked and canned vegetables, fresh fruit, and fresh and frozen berries.

Children's SR skills were assessed with 10 items derived from the Child Social Behavior Questionnaire, previously used in the Millennium Cohort Study on 3-year-olds [26]. Five items assessed cognitive skills and five items emotional SR skills. Each statement had three response options: disagree; agree to some extent; and fully agree. The mean points for each sub-dimension were calculated and used in the analyses. The internal consistency reliability as Cronbach's alphas was 0.68 for cognitive and 0.78 for emotional SR skills.

2.3.2. Parental Educational Level

The parent filling in the guardian's questionnaire reported his/her own highest educational achievement and the education of a partner living in the same household. The six answer options were categorized as follows: low educational level (comprising comprehensive school, vocational school, or high school); middle educational level (bachelor's degree or college); and high educational level (master's degree or licentiate/doctor). The highest educational level among parents was used as the parental educational level (PEL) variable in the analyses. In four cases, the highest education was not the education level of the mother or the father of the child, but that of a spouse living in the same household.

2.3.3. Confounding Factors

The parent reported the date of birth and gender of the participating child. In the statistical analysis, adjustments were made for the child's gender and age at baseline (continuous) for the categorical variable PEL and for the municipality.

2.4. Randomization, the Intervention, and the Program Content

Randomization was made at the preschool manager-level, separately for the two municipalities by an online randomization program (https://www.randomlists.com/team-generator). Preschools were divided into small and large preschools before randomization. After the baseline measurements, preschools were informed whether they had been randomized into the intervention (n = 13) or control (n = 19) group (Figure 1).

In intervention preschools, all early educators received program training. The training was split into a longer training session after the baseline measurements and a shorter training session around the middle of the 23-week program, in all, approximately 8 h [28]. Throughout the intervention, two researchers engaged with early educators conducting the program by email. Basically, the program at preschools was based on the international MindUp™ program [39]. Healthy EBRBs promoting strategies and methods were added to the existing ones in the program, and a program for families was developed [28]. The program was run in both preschools and homes and divided into five themes, all of which lasted 4–5 weeks: SR skills; physical activity; fruit and vegetables; screen time; and sugary foods and beverages. SR skills along with each EBRB were emphasized throughout the program in the preschool activities. SR skills were promoted by brain breaks, which were a few minutes' calming down and breathing sessions three times per day, led by early educators. In addition, early educators were trained to teach children to recognize and reflect on different feelings. In the family activities, focus was set on the children's EBRBs, and on how parents, by acting as role models and changing the availability and accessibility of the home environment, could influence their children's EBRBs. The methods used for families were, among others, information letters, emails containing videos or articles, bingos related to EBRBs, and two fairy tales written for the project. For each of the five themes, preschools arranged one activity afternoon. Early educators received the instructions and needed materials for the activities at the program training sessions. The activity afternoons were conducted as a workshop for children and parents to which all families were invited. An activity afternoon could consist of a working sheet about vegetable eating habits and favorite vegetables, or a vegetable tasting session that children and parents conducted together. Materials that were produced during the afternoons were expected to be displayed at the preschool, so that families could see each other's works. The early educators in the control preschools received training for the program after the intervention was finished.

2.5. Statistical Analyses

Differences between the participants' characteristics and the two groups (intervention/control) at baseline were analyzed by the Chi-square test (categorized variables) and t-test (continuous variables). Our main outcomes were total screen time (min/day), total PA (min/day), two variables related to sugar consumption (sugary everyday foods and beverages, and sugary treats, as times/week), total FV consumption frequency (times/week), and SR skills (cognitive and emotional dimensions, as scores). As a first step, a simple model was used to show the comparison between the intervention and control groups. To evaluate this, we used the general linear mixed models adjusted for baseline value of the outcome. This first model was used as a simple description of the results at follow-up. As a second step, a more complete and appropriate model was used with the major interest to evaluate the results between follow-up and baseline for the control and intervention groups. For this aim we used the linear mixed models with repeated measures for all outcomes, taking into account the interaction between the two groups and two time-points of baseline and follow-up. In the mixed models, normal distribution was visually checked. The preschool unit was used as a random effect in order to adjust for variability between the preschools. All aforementioned analyses were adjusted for child's gender, age at baseline, municipality, and PEL. Furthermore, accelerometer wearing time was included as an adjustment variable in the analyses where PA was the outcome. We also evaluated linear mixed models with three-level interactions: groups (intervention and control), time-points (baseline and post-intervention), and PEL. For these models, the results for the comparison between the two groups and time-points were presented as stratified by PEL group. In all analyses, multiple imputation was applied for independent variables with missing values. The number of children included in the analysis of each dependent variable and the missing values are presented in Supplementary Table S1 and the complete results for the linear mixed models with repeated measures and the respective effect size for interaction is presented in Supplementary Table S3.

All analyses were based on the intention-to-treat principle so that all randomized participants were included in the analysis in their randomized intervention group. General statistical analysis was performed and tables created using SPSS version 25. Mixed models, effect size for models' interaction, and multiple imputation analysis were conducted in R version 3.4.3 using the lme4, MuMIn, and MICE packages, respectively. For all analyses, a 5% statistical significance level was adopted.

3. Results

The average age of children in the study was 5.24 (±1.06) and 5.14 (±1.04) years for the control and intervention groups, respectively. Even though most characteristics were similar in the groups, a higher percentage of children with high educational level parents were found in the control group (26%) than in the intervention group (18%) (Table 1).

Table 1. Children's characteristics by the control and intervention group at baseline (n = 802).

		Control		Intervention		p-Value
		n	Mean ± SD *	n	Mean ± SD *	
Child's Age [c]		**441**	**5.24 ± 1.06**	**360**	**5.14 ± 1.04**	**0.060 [a]**
		n	%	n	%	
Child's gender	girl	203	46.0%	172	47.8%	0.496 [b]
	boy	238	54.0%	188	52.2%	
Parental educational level [d]	low	116	29.9%	109	35.4%	<0.001 [b]
	middle	169	43.6%	143	46.4%	
	high	103	26.5%	56	18.2%	
Municipality	Salo	357	81.0%	306	84.8%	0.040 [b]
	Riihimäki	84	19.0%	55	15.2%	

* SD, standard deviation; [a] comparison using t-test; [b] comparison using Chi-square test; [c] one missing value for age; [d] low educational level (comprehensive school, vocational school, or high school), middle (bachelor's degree or college), high (master's degree or licentiate/doctor).

Table 2 shows the descriptive results for children's EBRBs and SR skills according to the intervention and control group, at baseline and at follow-up, whereas the corresponding results according to PEL are presented in Supplementary Table S2. Children had about the same daily screen time in the intervention and control groups at baseline (Table 2), but low PEL children had higher screen time than the other groups (Supplementary Table S2). The FV consumption at baseline was higher in the high PEL groups than in the other groups (Supplementary Table S2).

Table 3 shows the comparison between the intervention and control groups at follow-up adjusted for respective baseline outcome values. Figures 2 and 3 present the mean of the main outcomes (descriptive values from Table 2) at the baseline and follow-up for the intervention and control groups, and for the PEL subgroups of the intervention group.

Table 2. Descriptors for children's EBRBs and self-regulation skills by control and intervention group.

EBRBs and SR Skills *	Baseline				Follow-Up			
	Control		Intervention		Control		Intervention	
	n	Mean ± SD **	*n*	Mean ± SD **	*n*	Mean ± SD **	*n*	Mean ± SD **
Total screen time (min/day)	370	84.87 ± 43.45	303	87.27 ± 44.06	325	88.84 ± 42.47	261	85.37 ± 41.34
Total physical activity [a] (min/day)	335	412.68 ± 48.40	282	405.66 ± 48.61	270	418.02 ± 45.34	210	414.42 ± 50.42
Sugary everyday food and beverages (times/week)	307	9.70 ± 6.89	293	10.53 ± 7.84	241	10.21± 8.96	200	9.76 ± 6.88
Sugary treats (times/week)	318	5.86 ± 3.99	299	5.77 ± 3.21	236	7.00 ± 5.34	192	6.99 ± 5.34
Fruit and vegetables (times/week)	323	21.79 ± 10.67	298	22.06 ± 13.12	258	22.26 ± 11.38	200	23.22 ± 13.39
Cognitive SR skills (scale 1–3)	383	2.31 ± 0.39	313	2.27 ± 0.43	324	2.32 ± 0.41	256	2.34 ± 0.43
Emotional SR skills (scale 1–3)	383	2.26 ± 0.51	313	2.25 ± 0.52	324	2.25 ± 0.51	256	2.29 ± 0.53

* EBRBs, energy balance-related behaviors; SR, self-regulation. ** SD, standard deviation.

Table 3. Comparison of EBRBs and SR skills between intervention and control, and changes within the groups *.

Children's EBRBs and SR Skills	General Linear Mixed Model [c]			Linear Mixed Models with Repeated Measures					
	Comparison between Intervention and Control Group at Follow-Up [c]			Change between Follow-Up and Baseline in Control Group			Change between Follow-Up and Baseline in Intervention Group		
		(95% C.I.)	*p*-Value	diff F–B	(95% C.I.)	*p*-Value	diff F–B	(95% C.I.)	*p*-Value
Total screen time (min/day) [a]	−4.20	(−9.86; 1.46)	0.146	4.46	(0.48; 8.44)	0.028	−1.42	(−5.86; 3.01)	0.529
Total physical activity (min/day) [b]	−0.56	(−6.65; 5.53)	0.858	23.77	(18.57; 28.97)	<0.001	27.30	(21.74; 32.86)	<0.001
Sugary food and beverage (times/week) [a]	−0.57	(−2.09; 0.96)	0.466	0.51	(−0.42; 1.43)	0.285	−0.79	(−1.77; 0.19)	0.112
Sugary treats (times/week) [a]	−0.13	(−1.03; 0.78)	0.781	1.20	(0.62; 1.77)	<0.001	1.28	(0.67; 1.90)	<0.001
Fruit and vegetables (times/week) [a]	1.43	(−0.64; 3.49)	0.176	−0.37	(−1.63; 0.89)	0.565	1.21	(−0.18; 2.61)	0.088
Cognitive SR skills (scale 1–3) [a]	0.02	(−0.04; 0.08)	0.505	0.01	(−0.03; 0.05)	0.574	0.06	(0.01; 0.11)	0.011
Emotional SR skills (1–3) [a]	−0.03	(−0.04; 0.10)	0.405	0.004	(−0.04; 0.05)	0.858	0.04	(−0.02; 0.09)	0.195

* (n = 645–737, estimates, and their 95% confidence intervals (C.I.); [a] models adjusted for gender, age, municipality, and parental educational level; [b] models adjusted for gender, age, municipality, parental educational level, and accelerometer wear time; [c] models adjusted for gender, age, municipality, parental educational level, (accelerometer wear time in PA as behavior), and baseline value of the outcome.

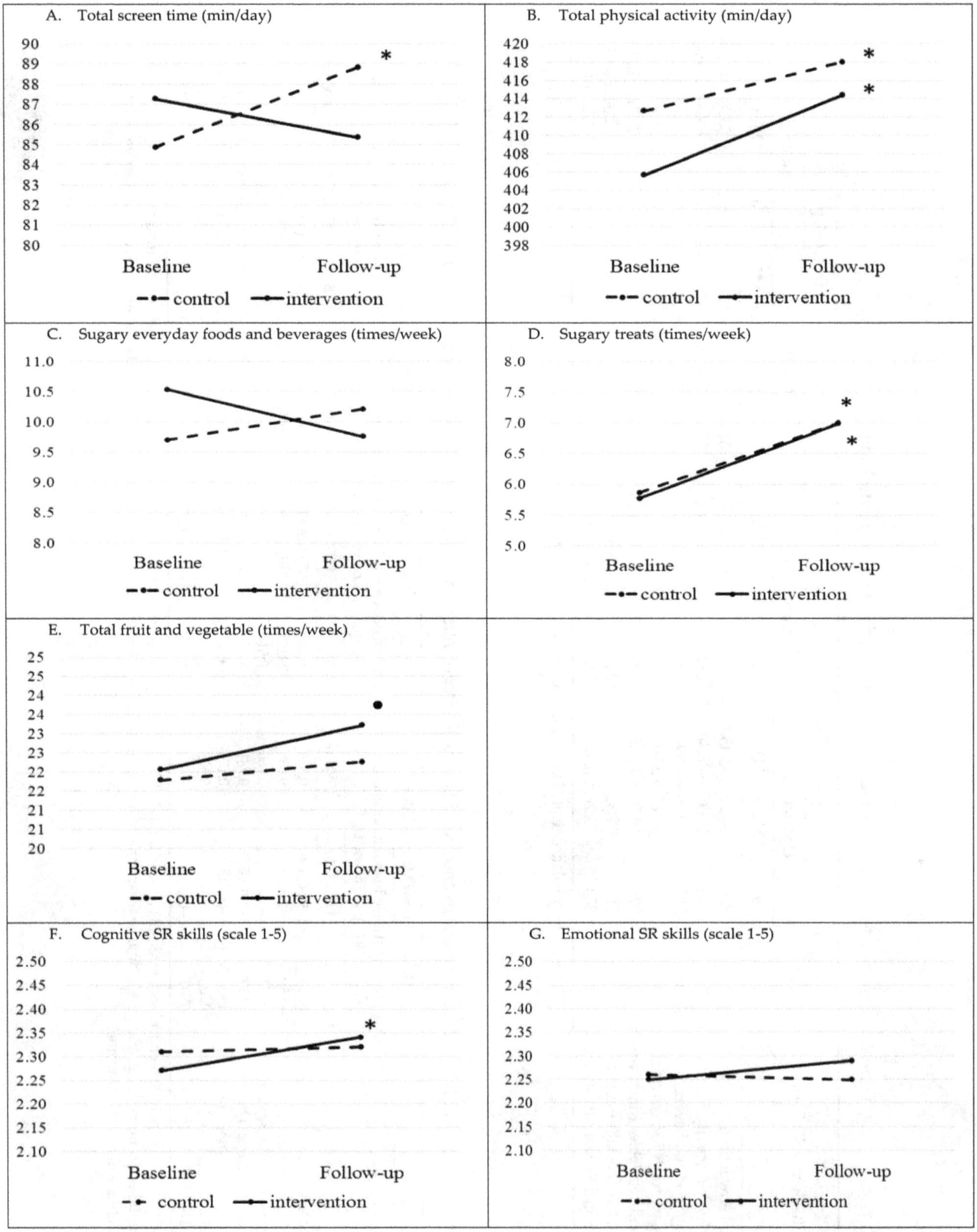

Figure 2. Children's EBRBs (heading (**A–E**)) and SR skills (headings (**F,G**)) at the baseline and follow-up in the intervention and control groups (means). For exact mean values, please see Table 2 (* p-value < 0.05, • p-value < 0.01 for the difference between the follow-up and baseline within the group).

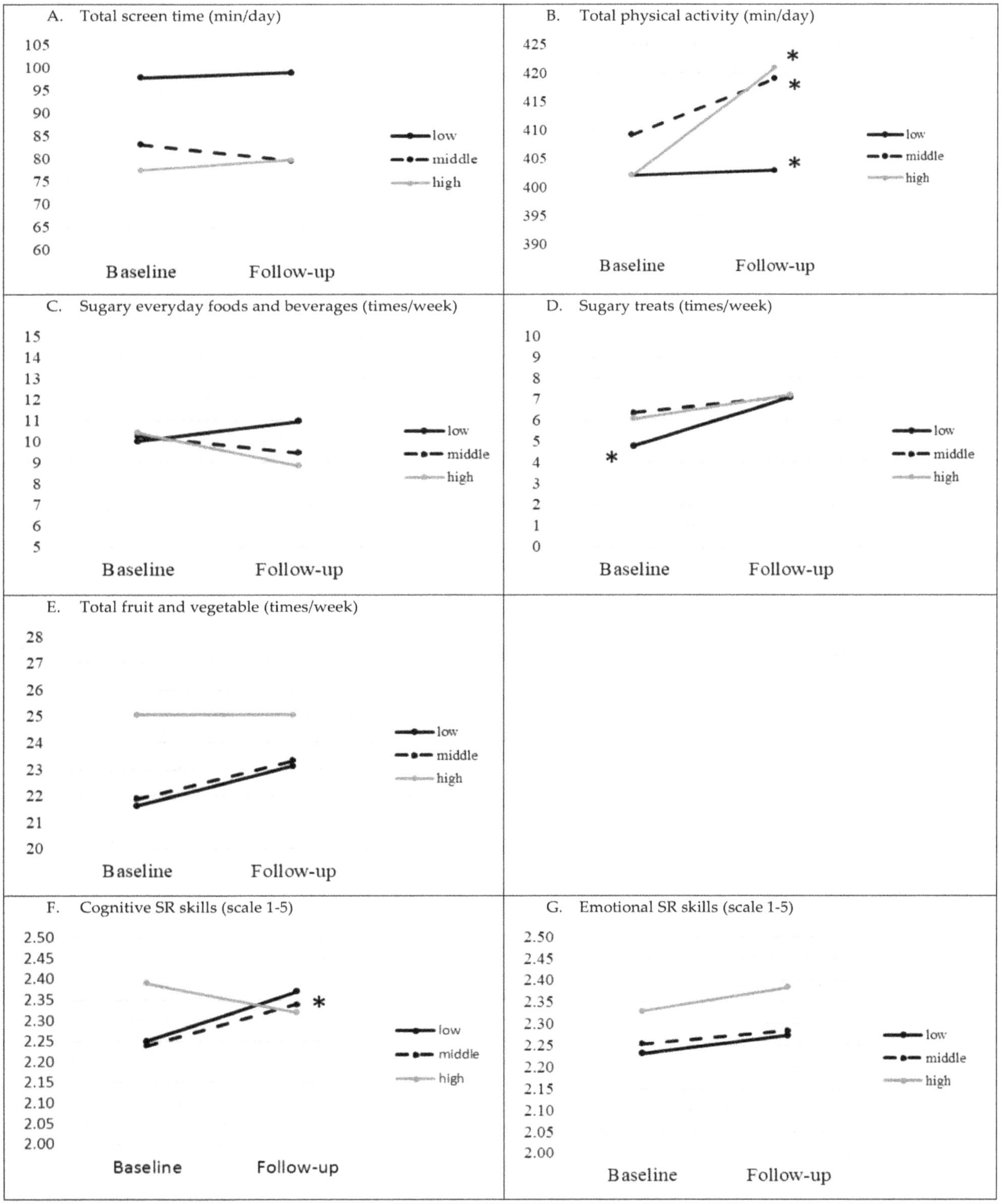

Figure 3. Children's EBRBs (headings (**A–E**)) and SR skills (headings (**F**,**G**)) within the intervention group separated by highest parental educational level (PEL) (means). For exact mean values, please see Supplementary Table S2 (* p-value < 0.05 for difference between follow-up and baseline within the group).

There were no significant differences detected in follow-up between the intervention and control groups for children's total screen time, total PA, consumption frequencies of sugary everyday foods and beverages, sugary treats, and FV, and cognitive and emotional SR skills (Table 3).

The results between the baseline and follow-up within the control and intervention groups differed for some EBRBs and SR skills (Table 3, see means in Figure 2). In the intervention group, the change between baseline and follow-up in total screen time was not significant, whereas there was a significant increase, approximately 4.5 min/day, in screen time in the control group ($p = 0.028$, Table 3, Figure 2A). The control group significantly increased in total PA on average by 24 min/day ($p < 0.001$), and the intervention group had a significant increase of 27 min/day ($p < 0.001$, Table 3 and Figure 2B). There was an increase in sugary treat consumption frequency in both groups ($p < 0.001$ in both groups, Table 3). In the intervention group, there was a trend, albeit not significant ($p = 0.088$), where FV consumption frequency increased (Table 3, Figure 2E). A positive significant change in points in cognitive SR skills was observed in the intervention group ($p = 0.011$, Table 3, Figure 2F).

Similar comparisons of children's EBRBs and SRs skills at follow-up stratified by PEL and the comparison between baseline and follow-up for intervention and control groups stratified by PEL are presented in Table 4. To illustrate the results within the separate PEL intervention groups, figures are presented with the mean of main outcomes at baseline and follow-up (Figure 3).

No significant differences were found when examining EBRBs and SR skills stratified by PEL (Table 4). In follow-up, there was a borderline significant result in cognitive SR skills when comparing low PEL intervention and control groups ($p = 0.051$).

Within the groups, the low PEL control group decreased their cognitive SR skills (borderline significance, $p = 0.052$). The total PA increased significantly within all intervention and control groups when stratified by PEL ($p < 0.001$ for all subgroups, Table 4, Figure 3B). The sugary treat consumption frequency increased within low PEL control and intervention groups ($p < 0.001$ in both groups), and in the middle PEL control group ($p = 0.027$, Table 4, Figure 3D). Cognitive SR skills strengthened in the middle PEL intervention group ($p = 0.038$, Table 4, Figure 3F).

Table 4. Comparison between the intervention and control group by parental educational level and changes within groups *.

Children's EBRBs and SR Skills	PEL	General Mixed Model: Comparison between Intervention and Control Group at Follow-Up [c]			Linear Mixed Models with Repeated Measures: Comparison between Follow-Up and Baseline in Control Group			Linear Mixed Models with Repeated Measures: Comparison between Follow-Up and Baseline in Intervention Group		
			(95% C.I.)	p-Value	diff F-B	(95% C.I.)	p-Value	diff F-B	(95% C.I.)	p-Value
Total screen time (min/day) [a]	low	−1.69	(−12.30; 8.92)	0.753	1.95	(−5.74; 9.64)	0.619	−3.42	(−11.23; 4.40)	0.391
	middle	−7.88	(−16.60; 0.84)	0.076	4.05	(−1.87; 9.98)	0.179	−2.00	(−8.57; 4.57)	0.551
	high	−3.73	(−16.13; 8.66)	0.553	7.65	(−0.10; 15.39)	0.053	2.95	(−6.86; 12.76)	0.555
Total physical activity (min/day) [b]	low	−7.17	(−24.15; 9.80)	0.404	21.41	(11.82; 31.00)	<0.001	22.10	(12.89; 31.32)	<0.001
	middle	1.86	(−11.90; 15.63)	0.787	26.61	(19.56; 33.66)	<0.001	30.89	(22.96; 38.83)	<0.001
	high	−0.77	(−19.96; 18.42)	0.937	21.10	(12.08; 30.13)	<0.001	27.66	(16.37; 38.95)	<0.001
Sugary foods and beverages (times/week) [a]	low	−0.15	(−2.70; 2.41)	0.909	0.83	(−1.07; 2.74)	0.392	0.10	(−1.71; 1.92)	0.911
	middle	−1.08	(−3.08; 0.93)	0.286	0.61	(−0.75; 1.96)	0.380	−0.88	(−2.26; 0.50)	0.210
	high	−1.34	(−4.14; 1.45)	0.344	0.09	(−1.64; 1.81)	0.920	−1.91	(−4.12; 0.31)	0.092
Sugary treats (times/week) [a]	low	−0.79	(−2.86; 1.29)	0.454	2.17	(0.97; 3.37)	<0.001	2.22	(1.15; 3.29)	<0.001
	middle	0.52	(−1.19; 2.22)	0.545	0.93	(0.10; 1.75)	0.027	0.74	(−0.17; 1.65)	0.109
	high	−0.07	(−2.32; 2.18)	0.954	0.89	(−0.18; 1.96)	0.103	1.02	(−0.34; 2.38)	0.140
Fruit and vegetables (times/week) [a]	low	2.99	(−1.00; 6.98)	0.141	−0.14	(−2.75; 2.47)	0.915	1.51	(−0.98; 3.99)	0.235
	middle	0.59	(−2.56; 3.74)	0.710	0.37	(−1.49; 2.23)	0.695	1.43	(−0.61; 3.48)	0.169
	high	1.03	(−3.30; 5.37)	0.638	−1.68	(−3.96; 0.60)	0.149	0.31	(−2.74; 3.36)	0.841
Cognitive SR skills (scale 1–3) [a]	low	0.11	(0.00; 0.21)	0.051	−0.11	(−0.22; 0.00)	0.052	0.04	(−0.08; 0.15)	0.513
	middle	0.001	(−0.09; 0.09)	0.987	−0.03	(−0.13; 0.06)	0.468	0.10	(0.01; 0.20)	0.038
	high	−0.06	(−0.18; 0.07)	0.380	0.04	(−0.09; 0.18)	0.536	−0.04	(−0.18; 0.09)	0.543
Emotional SR skills (scale 1–3) [a]	low	0.01	(−0.12; 0.13)	0.921	−0.02	(−0.11; 0.08)	0.750	0.03	(−0.07; 0.12)	0.563
	middle	0.05	(−0.05; 0.15)	0.313	−0.02	(−0.09; 0.05)	0.547	0.04	(−0.04; 0.12)	0.286
	high	0.01	(−0.13; 0.16)	0.861	0.07	(−0.02; 0.16)	0.141	0.03	(−0.09; 0.15)	0.611

* Estimates and their 95% confidence intervals (C.I.); [a] models adjusted for gender, age in years, municipality, and parental educational level; [b] models adjusted for gender, age in years, municipality, parental educational level, and accelerometer wear time; [c] models gender, age in years, municipality, parental educational level, (accelerometer wear time in PA as behavior), and for baseline value of outcome.

4. Discussion

We detected no differences in EBRBs or SR skills between the intervention and the control group in our preschool-based family-involving RCT. Furthermore, changes in children's EBRBs according to PEL did not differ between the intervention and control groups at follow-up, although a borderline significant result emerged in low PEL children in the intervention group, improving their cognitive SR skills compared with the corresponding control group ($p = 0.051$).

A possible reason for not detecting significant intervention effects might be that the goals set were unrealistic (0.74 times/day decrease in sugary foods and beverages), or it would have required a higher number of children. Our study was a complex multicomponent intervention of relatively short duration. Each of the five program themes were focused on for 4–5 weeks, which could have been too short a duration for changes to occur. Therefore, further evaluation of the effects is needed. Furthermore, the analysis did not show stronger intervention effects in low PEL children. Still, cognitive SR skills strengthened in the low PEL intervention group compared with the low PEL control group, and the results bordered on statistical significance. Within the low PEL control group, cognitive SR skills decreased; also here the results did border to reach statistical significance. However, a significant improvement in cognitive SR skills occurred among middle PEL intervention children. Since the above-mentioned increases in cognitive SR points when comparing control and intervention group were small, these results might lack practical implication. The Head Start intervention showed improvements in SR skills and a decrease in sugar-sweetened drink consumption in the group that received the intervention promoting both EBRBs and SR skills, compared with the other three groups [27]. Although the aims of that study and ours were similar, the results are not totally comparable. The age group in Head Start was slightly older (4–9 years), and SR skills were measured by another instrument. In both studies, activities to strengthen SR skills were mainly conducted in preschools, whereas parents were the main target when promoting healthy EBRBs. It was discussed that parents might not have been sufficiently engaged, which may have led to null results regarding the children's EBRBs, which may also be the case in the DAGIS.

Within the intervention and control group, several significant changes occurred in the EBRBs. The control group increased their screen time by approximately 4.5 min/day, whereas no changes were detected within the intervention group. For the control group, it had about a 30 min/week higher screen time, which might eventually harm energy balance, weight status, and development of SR skills. The results of the control children followed the trend that screen time increases with age among young children [40]. The ToyBox study also did not reveal an overall positive effect on screen time [16], nevertheless when including a process evaluation, a reduction in computer/video games time was shown [14]. Subgroup analyses in ToyBox showed less TV time during weekends in the intervention girls [16], and subgroup analyses should also be considered in the DAGIS study.

The total PA increased in the control and intervention group. A recently published European study reported that moderate-to-vigorous PA increased from the age group of 2–3 years to 4–5 years, and further to 6–7 years [41]. The trend might explain the results in the DAGIS. Moreover, the follow-up occurred in spring, when there are more daylight hours than at the baseline in autumn. Studies have revealed that the higher the temperature and the more daylight present, the higher the level of PA among children [42,43]. The municipality, in which all preschools participated, simultaneously runs a training program for all early educators aimed at increasing preschool PA, which has increased all children's preschool PA independently of intervention status. Previous interventions have reported no effects on children's PA [44–46], and discussion has ensued on whether short durations such as six weeks of promoting PA are sufficient to detect an increase in children's PA [16,47].

The follow-up results for sugary everyday food and beverage consumption outside preschool hours did not differ between the intervention and control groups. The reduction was mainly supposed to happen at home, as these foods are seldom served at Finnish preschools [31]. The program implementation in families might have been weak, leading to no changes. This needs to be further studied by analyzing the processes in the intervention. We found an increase in sugary treat consumption in both the control and intervention low PEL groups (Supplementary Table S2), but no changes in the middle or high intervention groups. It seems that as children grow older, the consumption increases, especially in low PEL groups, which might lead to a greater gap between the PEL groups. The change in FV consumption did not differ between the intervention and control groups. However, while the control group had a stable consumption of FV at both time-points, the consumption frequency in the intervention group increased by 1.3 times/week. Similarly, some intervention studies have shown improvements in FV consumption [48], although a systematic review concluded that multicomponent FV interventions have provided low evidence of increasing FV consumption [49].

When developing the DAGIS intervention, the focus was set on understanding the low educational level context and how to, by means of a universal intervention, reach those with low PEL backgrounds [28]. One strategy was to produce easy-to-read materials as the ToyBox intervention study discussed that the lack of significant results for children's food consumption might have been due to the intervention materials being insufficiently tailored to those with low education levels [13]. The DAGIS logic model of change included primary outcomes, which were seen as the most important determinants for explaining socio-economic differences in children's EBRBs. The main primary outcomes (i.e., adults role modeling and changes in the environment in availability and accessibility of, for example, foods and screens), should be examined next. It is more likely to see changes in these due to the relatively short duration of the intervention. Generally, it has been concluded that availability and accessibility (foods, screens) in the home environment would be of great importance for children's health behaviors in low PEL families [13].

As this study includes the intention-to-treat effect analysis, it was assumed that all intervention preschools and families conducted the program in the same manner and at the same intensity. Further analysis including fidelity and implementation degree of the program will yield a deeper understanding of the effects. The importance of the implementation degree has been discussed in conjunction with null results in multicomponent interventions [50].

The DAGIS intervention study had limitations that should be acknowledged. The short intervention time, in all, five months, was a limitation, but the project as a whole needed to be conducted during a preschool year. Previous discussion has questioned whether a short time period is adequate for children to change their EBRBs [13,44]. In addition, children's baseline consumption of FV, mean three times/day outside preschool time, was fairly high, which sets challenges for achieving an increase. Furthermore, reliably measuring food consumption is challenging. However, reproducibility and validity of our parental FFQ have been tested [36,38]. Still, the FFQ reflects the foods eaten during the last week outside preschool time and does not allow for analysis of whether food consumption changed at preschool. The 10-item questionnaire assessing two dimensions of children's SR skills had three answer categories, which might not have been sensitive enough to capture changes. Many instruments are available to assess children's SR skills, but no consensus exists on their validity in evaluating this multidimensional concept [51]. Finally, the sample size might not have been sufficiently large to detect significant results. The power calculations were conducted based on means and standard deviations from the DAGIS cross-sectional survey [7]. Some dissimilarities exist between these two studies such as the number of preschools and municipalities and the proportion of low PEL families participating, which might have led to an underpowered study.

A strength of the study is that the study development was guided by the IM framework [28], which enabled systematic planning. The logic model of change was formed on the best existing knowledge, and on a comprehensive evaluation of the Finnish preschool-family context [10,28]. This enables further systematic evaluations of the processes. The fairly high response rate of families, 47%, and having all preschools from one municipality participating including diverse preschools as well as diverse families can be seen as a strength. The high response rate indicates a lower selection bias among the participants. In addition, slightly more than 30% of the participating families had low education levels. It is often seen as a challenge that the less educated tend not to participate in intervention studies [52].

The study also included a combination of instruments such as the accelerometer for assessing PA, a validated screen time diary, and a validated FFQ for robust assessment [35,38].

The fairly new approach of simultaneously strengthening children's SR skills and promoting their EBRBs can be seen as a strength and also as a risk. To the best of our knowledge, this approach has been evaluated in one other study [27], where it was discussed that the next step should be integrating SR skill promotion into the EBRB context. In the DAGIS study, this can be seen as a strength as the program enhanced SR skills, while simultaneously promoting EBRBs by adding more materials to the existing program. The materials and methods for the program also underwent pretesting [28].

5. Conclusions

The DAGIS intervention study aimed to promote preschoolers' EBRBs and SR skills through a preschool-based family-involving intervention conducted as a clustered RCT. We detected no significant differences in the preschoolers' EBRBs between the intervention and control groups at follow up. No differences at follow-up between the PEL groups were found, except for the cognitive SR skills, where a borderline significant result emerged between low PEL control and intervention group. Within the middle PEL intervention group, there was an increase in cognitive SR skills. Even though the intervention did not achieve its goal and the aims were not attained, further analyses should examine whether changes can be seen in the determinants of children's EBRBs, especially those of importance for children with low PEL. In addition, a thorough process evaluation may provide insight into the non-significant findings.

Supplementary Materials: The following are available online at Table S1: Number of children and missing values in each outcome, Table S2: Descriptors for study outcomes by the control and intervention groups and by parental educational level (PEL), Table S3: Adjusted differences and their 95% confidence interval (C.I.) between intervention and control group separated for baseline and follow-up; and adjusted differences between follow-up and baseline for each study group.

Author Contributions: Conceptualization, C.R., R.F., and E.R; Investigation, C.R., H.V., R.L., R.P., E.S., T.S., P.H., E.L., and L.K.; Formal analysis, R.F.; Data Curation, R.L.; Writing—Original Draft Preparation, C.R. and R.F.; Writing—Review & Editing C.R., R.F., H.V., R.L., R.P., E.S., T.S., P.H., E.L., L.K., K.S., N.S., M.E., and E.R.; Visualization, R.F.; Project Administration, C.R., Funding Acquisition, N.S., M.E., and E.R. All authors have read and agreed to the published version of the manuscript.

Acknowledgments: The authors thank the preschools, the preschool personnel, and the families for their participation in the DAGIS study, and the research staff for the data collection. The authors thank the collaborating partners of the DAGIS study for providing assistance in designing the DAGIS study.

References

1. Kremers, S.P.J.; de Bruijn, G.J.; Visscher, T.L.S.; van Mechelen, W.; de Vries, N.K.; Brug, J. Environmental Influences on Energy Balance-Related Behaviors: A Dual-Process View. *Int. J. Behav. Nutr. Phys. Act.* **2006**, *3*, 1–10. [CrossRef] [PubMed]
2. World Health Organization. *Report of the Comission on Ending Childhood Obesity*; WHO: Geneva, Switzerland, 2016.
3. Halfon, N.; Larson, K.; Slusser, W. Associations between Obesity and Comorbid Mental Health, Developmental, and Physical Health Conditions in a Nationally Representative Sample of US Children Aged 10 to 17. *Acad. Pediatr.* **2013**, *13*, 6–13. [CrossRef] [PubMed]
4. Reilly, J.J.; Methven, E.; Mcdowell, Z.C.; Hacking, B.; Alexander, D.; Stewart, L.; Kelnar, C.J.H. Health Consequences of Obesity. *Arch. Dis. Child.* **2003**, *88*, 748–752. [CrossRef] [PubMed]

5. Mantziki, K.; Vassilopoulos, A.; Radulian, G.; Borys, J.-M.; Du Plessis, H.; Gregorio, M.J.; Graca, P.; De Henauw, S.; Handjiev, S.; Visscher, T. Inequities in Energy-Balance Related Behaviours and Family Environmental Determinants in European Children: Baseline Results of the Prospective EPHE Evaluation Study. *BMC Public Health* **2015**, *15*, 1203. [CrossRef]
6. Fernandez-Alvira, J.; Mouratidou, T.; Bammann, K.; Hebestreit, A.; Barba, G.; Sieri, S.; Reisch, L.; Eiben, G.; Hadjigeorgiou, C.; Kovacs, E.; et al. Parental Education and Frequency of Food Consumption in European Children: The IDEFICS Study. *Public Health Nutr.* **2013**, *16*, 487–498. [CrossRef]
7. Lehto, E.; Ray, C.; Vepsäläinen, H.; Korkalo, L.; Lehto, R.; Kaukonen, R.; Suhonen, E.; Nislin, M.; Nissinen, K.; Skaffari, E.; et al. Increased Health and Wellbeing in Preschools (DAGIS) Study—Differences in Children's Energy Balance-Related Behaviors (EBRBs) and in Long-Term Stress by Parental Educational Level. *Int. J. Environ. Res. Public Health* **2018**, *15*, 2313. [CrossRef]
8. Gubbels, J.S.; Van Kann, D.H.H.; de Vries, N.K.; Thijs, C.; Kremers, S.P.J. The next Step in Health Behavior Research: The Need for Ecological Moderation Analyses—An Application to Diet and Physical Activity at Childcare. *Int. J. Behav. Nutr. Phys. Act.* **2014**, *11*, 52. [CrossRef]
9. Gubbels, J.S.; Stessen, K.; Van De Kolk, I.; De Vries, N.K.; Thijs, C.; Kremers, S.P.J. Energy Balance-Related Parenting and Childcare Practices: The Importance of Meso-System Consistency. *PLoS ONE* **2018**, *13*, e0203689. [CrossRef]
10. Määttä, S.; Lehto, R.; Nislin, M.; Ray, C.; Erkkola, M.; Sajaniemi, N.; Roos, E. Increased Health and Well-Being in Preschools (DAGIS): Rationale and Design for a Randomized Controlled Trial Health Behavior, Health Promotion and Society. *BMC Public Health* **2015**, *15*, 1–10. [CrossRef]
11. Biddle, S.J.H.; Petrolini, I.; Pearson, N. Interventions Designed to Reduce Sedentary Behaviours in Young People: A Review of Reviews. *Br. J. Sports Med.* **2014**, *48*, 182–186. [CrossRef]
12. Black, A.P.; D'Onise, K.; McDermott, R.; Vally, H.; O'Dea, K. How Effective Are Family-Based and Institutional Nutrition Interventions in Improving Children's Diet and Health? A Systematic Review. *BMC Public Health* **2017**, *17*, 1–19. [CrossRef] [PubMed]
13. Pinket, A.S.; De Craemer, M.; Huybrechts, I.; De Bourdeaudhuij, I.; Deforche, B.; Cardon, G.; Androutsos, O.; Koletzko, B.; Moreno, L.A.; Socha, P.; et al. Multibehavioural Interventions with a Focus on Specific Energy Balance-Related Behaviours Can Affect Diet Quality in Preschoolers from Six European Countries: The Toybox-Study. *Nutrients* **2017**, *9*, 479. [CrossRef] [PubMed]
14. Latomme, J.; Cardon, G.; De Bourdeaudhuij, I.; De Craemer, M.; Iotova, V.; Koletzko, B.; Socha, P.; Moreno, L.; Androutsos, O.; Manios, Y. Effect and Process Evaluation of a Kindergarten-Based, Family-Involved Intervention with a Randomized Cluster Design on Sedentary Behaviour in 4- to 6- Year Old European Preschool Children: The ToyBox-Study. *PLoS ONE* **2017**, *12*, e0172730. [CrossRef] [PubMed]
15. Duncan, S.; Stewart, T.; McPhee, J.; Borotkanics, R.; Prendergast, K.; Zinn, C.; Meredith-Jones, K.; Taylor, R.; McLachlan, C.; Schofield, G. Efficacy of a Compulsory Homework Programme for Increasing Physical Activity and Improving Nutrition in Children: A Cluster Randomised Controlled Trial. *Int. J. Behav. Nutr. Phys. Act.* **2019**, *16*, 80. [CrossRef] [PubMed]
16. De Craemer, M.; De Decker, E.; Verloigne, M.; De Bourdeaudhuij, I.; Manios, Y.; Cardon, G. The Effect of a Cluster Randomised Control Trial on Objectively Measured Sedentary Time and Parental Reports of Time Spent in Sedentary Activities in Belgian Preschoolers: The ToyBox-Study. *Int. J. Behav. Nutr. Phys. Act.* **2016**, *13*, 1–17. [CrossRef]
17. Marmot, M. Proportionate universalism. In *The Health Gap—The Challenge of an Unequal World*; Bloomsbury Publishing: London, UK, 2015; pp. 279–289.
18. Wijtzes, A.I.; Van De Gaar, V.M.; Van Grieken, A.; De Kroon, M.L.A.; Mackenbach, J.P.; Van Lenthe, F.J.; Jansen, W.; Raat, H. Effectiveness of Interventions to Improve Lifestyle Behaviors among Socially Disadvantaged Children in Europe. *Eur. J. Public Health* **2017**, *27*, 240–247. [CrossRef]
19. Love, R.E.; Adams, J.; van Sluijs, E.M.F. Equity Effects of Children's Physical Activity Interventions: A Systematic Scoping Review. *Int. J. Behav. Nutr. Phys. Act.* **2017**, *14*, 134. [CrossRef]
20. Downing, K.L.; Hnatiuk, J.A.; Hinkley, T.; Salmon, J.; Hesketh, K.D. Interventions to Reduce Sedentary Behaviour in 0–5-Year-Olds: A Systematic Review and Meta-Analysis of Randomised Controlled Trials. *Br. J. Sports Med.* **2018**, *52*, 314–321. [CrossRef]
21. Aparicio, E.; Canals, J.; Arija, V.; De Henauw, S.; Michels, N. The Role of Emotion Regulation in Childhood Obesity: Implications for Prevention and Treatment. *Nutr. Res. Rev.* **2016**, *29*, 17–29. [CrossRef]

22. Miller, A.L.; Lumeng, J.C. Pathways of Association from Stress to Obesity in Early Childhood. *Obesity* **2018**, *26*, 1117–1124. [CrossRef]
23. Nigg, J.T. Annual Research Review: On the Relations among Self-Regulation, Self-Control, Executive Functioning, Effortful Control, Cognitive Control, Impulsivity, Risk-Taking, and Inhibition for Developmental Psychopathology. *J. Child. Psychol. Psychiatry* **2017**, *58*, 361–383. [CrossRef] [PubMed]
24. Seeyave, D.M.; Coleman, S.; Appugliese, D.; Corwyn, R.F.; Bradley, R.H.; Davidson, N.S.; Kaciroti, N.; Lumeng, J.C. Ability to Delay Gratification at Age 4 Years and Risk of Overweight at Age 11 Years. *Arch. Pediatr. Adolesc. Med.* **2009**, *163*, 303–308. [CrossRef] [PubMed]
25. Liang, J.; Matheson, B.E.; Kaye, W.H.; Boutelle, K.N. Neurocognitive Correlates of Obesity and Obesity-Related Behaviors in Children and Adolescents. *Int. J. Obes.* **2014**, *38*, 494–506. [CrossRef] [PubMed]
26. Anderson, S.; Sacker, A.; Whitaker, R.; Kelly, Y. Self-Regulation and Household Routines at Age Three and Obesity at Age Eleven: Longitudinal Analysis of the UK Millennium Cohort Study. *Int. J. Obes.* **2017**, *41*, 1459–1466. [CrossRef]
27. Lumeng, J.C.; Miller, A.L.; Horodynski, M.A.; Brophy-Herb, H.E.; Contreras, D.; Lee, H.; Sturza, J.; Kaciroti, N.; Peterson, K.E. Improving Self-Regulation for Obesity Prevention in Head Start: A Randomized Controlled Trial. *Pediatrics* **2017**, *139*, e20162047. [CrossRef]
28. Ray, C.; Kaukonen, R.; Lehto, E.; Vepsäläinen, H.; Sajaniemi, N.; Erkkola, M.; Roos, E. Development of the DAGIS Intervention Study: A Preschool-Based Family-Involving Study Promoting Preschoolers' Energy Balance-Related Behaviours and Self-Regulation Skills. *BMC Public Health* **2019**, *19*, 1670. [CrossRef]
29. Eldredge, L.K.B.; Markham, C.M.; Ruiter, R.A.C.; Fernandez, M.E.; Parcel, G.S. *Planning Health Promotion Programs—An Intervention Mapping Approach*, 4th ed.; Jossey-Bass: San Fransisco, CA, USA, 2016.
30. Säkkinen, S.; Kuoppala, T. *Varhaiskasvatus 2017 (Children's Day Care 2018)*; National Institute of Health and Welfare: Helsinki, Finland, 2018. Available online: http://urn.fi/URN:NBN:fi-fe2018100937865 (accessed on 24 August 2020).
31. Korkalo, L.; Nissinen, K.; Skaffari, E.; Vepsäläinen, H.; Lehto, R.; Kaukonen, R.; Koivusilta, L.; Sajaniemi, N.; Roos, E.; Erkkola, M. The Contribution of Preschool Meals to the Diet of Finnish Preschoolers. *Nutrients* **2019**, *11*, 1531. [CrossRef]
32. National Institute for Health and Welfare. The Welfare Compass for Monitoring Regional Welfare. Available online: https://www.hyvinvointikompassi.fi/en/web/hyvinvointikompassi/etusivu (accessed on 21 March 2019).
33. Schulz, K.F.; Altman, D.G.; Moher, D. CONSORT 2010 Statement: Updated Guidelines for Reporting Parallel Group Randomised Trials. *BMJ* **2010**, *340*, c332. [CrossRef]
34. Wen, L.; van der Ploeg, H.; Kite, J.; Cashmore, A.; Rissel, C. A Validation Study of Assessing Physical Activity and Sedentary Behavior in Children Aged 3 to 5 Years. *Pediatr. Exerc. Sci.* **2010**, *22*, 408–420. [CrossRef]
35. Määttä, S.; Vepsäläinen, H.; Lehto, R.; Erkkola, M.; Roos, E.; Ray, C. Reproducibility of Preschool Personnel and Guardian Reports on Energy Balance-Related Behaviors and Their Correlates in Finnish Preschool Children. *Children* **2018**, *5*, 144. [CrossRef]
36. Cliff, D.; Okely, A.; Smith, L.; McKeen, K. Relationships between Fundamental Movement Skills and Objectively Measured Physical Activity in Preschool Children. *Pediatr. Exerc. Sci.* **2009**, *21*, 436–449. [CrossRef] [PubMed]
37. Evenson, K.; Catellier, D.; Gill, K.; McMurray, R. Calibration of Two Objective Measures of Physical Activity for Children. *J. Sports Sci.* **2008**, *26*, 1557–1565. [CrossRef] [PubMed]
38. Korkalo, L.; Vepsäläinen, H.; Ray, C.; Skaffari, E.; Lehto, R.; Hauta-alus, H.; Nissinen, K.; Meinilä, J.; Erkkola, M.; Roos, E. Parents' Reports of Preschoolers' Diets: Relative Validity of a Food Frequency Questionnaire and Dietary Patterns. *Nutrients* **2019**, *11*, 159. [CrossRef] [PubMed]
39. Maloney, J.E.; Lawlor, M.S.; Shonert-Reichl, K.A.; Whitehead, J. A universal, mindfulness-based social and emotional learning (SEL) Program designed to be implemented in schools by regular classroom teachers. In *Handbook of Mindfulness in Education—Integrating Theory into Practice*; Shonert-Reichl, K.A., Roeser, R.W., Eds.; Springer: New York, NY, USA, 2016; pp. 313–334.
40. Carson, V.; Lee, E.Y.; Hesketh, K.D.; Hunter, S.; Kuzik, N.; Predy, M.; Rhodes, R.E.; Rinaldi, C.M.; Spence, J.C.; Hinkley, T. Physical Activity and Sedentary Behavior across Three Time-Points and Associations with Social Skills in Early Childhood. *BMC Public Health* **2019**, *19*, 1–8. [CrossRef] [PubMed]

41. Steene-Johannessen, J.; Hansen, B.; Dalene, K.; Kolle, E.; Northstone, K.; Møller, N.; Grøntved, A.; Wedderkopp, N.; Kriemler, S.; Page, A.; et al. Variations in Accelerometry Measured Physical Activity and Sedentary Time across Europe—Harmonized Analyses of 47,497 Children and Adolescents. *Int. J. Behav. Nutr. Phys. Act.* **2020**, *17*, 38. [CrossRef] [PubMed]
42. Brusseau, T.A. The Intricacies of Children's Physical Activity. *J. Hum. Kinet.* **2015**, *47*, 269–275. [CrossRef] [PubMed]
43. Harrison, F.; Goodman, A.; van Sluijs, E.M.F.; Andersen, L.B.; Cardon, G.; Davey, R.; Janz, K.F.; Kriemler, S.; Molloy, L.; Page, A.S.; et al. Weather and Children's Physical Activity; How and Why Do Relationships Vary between Countries? *Int. J. Behav. Nutr. Phys. Act.* **2017**, *14*, 74. [CrossRef]
44. De Craemer, M.; Verloigne, M.; De Bourdeaudhuij, I.; Androutsos, O.; Iotova, V.; Moreno, L.; Koletzko, B.; Socha, P.; Manios, Y.; Cardon, G.; et al. Effect and Process Evaluation of a Kindergarten-Based, Family-Involved Cluster Randomised Controlled Trial in Six European Countries on Four- to Six-Year-Old Children's Steps per Day: The ToyBox-Study. *Int. J. Behav. Nutr. Phys. Act.* **2017**, *14*, 116. [CrossRef]
45. Bellows, L.; Davies, P.; Anderson, J.; Kennedy, C. Effectiveness of a Physical Activity Intervention for Head Start Preschoolers: A Randomized Intervention Study. *Am. J. Occup. Ther.* **2013**, *67*, 28–36. [CrossRef]
46. Reilly, J.; Kelly, L.; Montgomery, C.; Williamson, A.; Fisher, A.; McColl, J.; Lo Conte, R.; Paton, J.; Grant, S. Physical Activity to Prevent Obesity in Young Children: Cluster Randomised Controlled Trial. *BMJ Open* **2006**, *333*, 1041. [CrossRef]
47. Buscemi, J.; Odoms-Young, A.; Stolley, M.R.; Schiffer, L.; Blumstein, L.; Clark, M.H.; Berbaum, M.L.; McCaffrey, J.; Braunschweig, C.; Fitzgibbon, M.L. Comparative Effectiveness Trial of an Obesity Prevention Intervention in EFNEP and SNAP-ED: Primary Outcomes. *Nutrients* **2019**, *11*, 1012. [CrossRef] [PubMed]
48. Rios, L.M.; Serrano, M.M.; Aguilar, A.J.; Chacón, L.B.; Neria, C.R.; Monreal, L.A. Promoting Fruit, Vegetable and Simple Water Consumption among Mothers and Teachers of Preschool Children: An Intervention Mapping Initiative. *Eval. Program Plann.* **2019**, *76*, 101675. [CrossRef] [PubMed]
49. Wolfenden, L.; Barnes, C.; Jones, J.; Finch, M.; Wyse, R.; Kingsland, M.; Tzelepis, F.; Grady, A.; Hodder, R.; Booth, D.; et al. Strategies to Improve the Implementation of Healthy Eating, Physical Activity and Obesity Prevention Policies, Practices or Programmes within Childcare Services. *Cochrane Database Syst. Rev.* **2020**, *2*, CD011779. [CrossRef] [PubMed]
50. Steenbock, B.; Buck, C.; Zeeb, H.; Rach, S.; Pischke, C.R. Impact of the Intervention Program "JolinchenKids-Fit and Healthy in Daycare" on Energy Balance Related-Behaviors: Results of a Cluster Controlled Trial. *BMC Pediatr.* **2019**, *19*, 432. [CrossRef] [PubMed]
51. Halle, T.G.; Darling-Churchill, K.E. Review of Measures of Social and Emotional Development. *J. Appl. Dev. Psychol.* **2016**, *45*, 8–18. [CrossRef]
52. Prevo, L.; Kremers, S.; Jansen, M. Small Successes Make Big Wins: A Retrospective Case Study towards Community Engagement of Low-SES Families. *Int. J. Environ. Res. Public Health* **2020**, *17*, 612. [CrossRef]

11

Salt Reduction Strategies in Portuguese School Meals, from Pre-School to Secondary Education—The Eat Mediterranean Program

Ana Isabel Rito [1,2,*], Sofia Mendes [2,3], Mariana Santos [1,3], Francisco Goiana-da-Silva [4], Francesco Paolo Cappuccio [5], Stephen Whiting [6], Ana Dinis [7], Carla Rascôa [7], Isabel Castanheira [1], Ara Darzi [4] and João Breda [6]

1. WHO Collaborating Centre on Nutrition and Childhood Obesity—National Institute of Health Dr. Ricardo Jorge (INSA, IP), 1649-016 Lisbon, Portugal; Mariana.Coelho@insa.min-saude.pt (M.S.); isabel.castanheira@insa.min-saude.pt (I.C.)
2. Centre for Studies and Research in Social Dynamics and Health (CEIDSS), 1649-016 Lisbon, Portugal; sofiamendes@ceidss.com
3. National School of Public Health, NOVA University of Lisbon, 1600-560 Lisbon, Portugal
4. Centre for Health Policy, Institute of Global Health Innovation, Imperial College London, London SW7 2AZ, UK; franciscogoianasilva@gmail.com (F.G.-d.-S.); a.darzi@imperial.ac.uk (A.D.)
5. University of Warwick, WHO Collaborating Centre for Nutrition, Warwick Medical School, Coventry CV2 2DX, UK; f.p.cappuccio@warwick.ac.uk
6. WHO European Office for the Prevention and Control of Noncommunicable Diseases, 125009 Moscow, Russia; whitings@who.int (S.W.); rodriguesdasilvabred@who.int (J.B.)
7. Regional Health Administration of Lisbon and Tagus Valley (ARSLVT), 1700-179 Lisbon, Portugal; ana.dinis@arslvt.min-saude.pt (A.D.); carla.rascoa@arslvt.min-saude.pt (C.R.)

* Correspondence: ana.rito@insa.min-saude.pt.

Abstract: High sodium (salt) consumption is associated with an increased risk of developing non-communicable diseases. However, in most European countries, Portugal included, sodium intake is still high. This study aimed to assess the sodium content of school meals before and after the Eat Mediterranean (EM) intervention—a community-based program to identify and correct nutritional deviations through the implementation of new school menus and through schools' food handlers training. EM (2015–2017) was developed in 25 schools (pre to secondary education) of two Portuguese Municipalities, reaching students aged 3–21 years old. Samples of the complete meals (soup + main course + bread) from all schools were collected, and nutritional quality and laboratory analysis were performed to determine their nutritional composition, including sodium content. Overall, there was a significant decrease (−23%) in the mean sodium content of the complete school meals, which was mainly achieved by the significant reduction of 34% of sodium content per serving portion of soup. In conclusion, EM had a positive effect on the improvement of the school meals' sodium content, among the participant schools. Furthermore, school setting might be ideal for nutrition literacy interventions among children, for flavors shaping, and for educating towards less salty food acceptance.

Keywords: community-based program; childhood obesity; school meals; salt intake; sodium consumption

---

1. Introduction

Given the well-established evidence that excessive sodium consumption (1 g of sodium per 100 g represents 2.5 g of salt per 100 g) is linked to an increased risk of developing non-communicable diseases (NCD) [1], a reduction in population's sodium consumption has been a key focus of both the international and national policy agendas. Reducing salt intake in the general population is not only a practical action that can prevent adverse health outcomes—such as increased blood pressure—but it is also a feasible and cost-effective strategy to reduce the growing burden of NCDs and reduce health-care costs for governments and individuals [2].

The World Health Organization (WHO) recommends a population reduction in salt intake as one of the 'best buys' or cost-effective actions that should be prioritized to tackle the global burden of NCDs [3–5]. Targets of a daily salt intake lower than 5 g for adults and 2 g for children have been recommended [6]. In addition, WHO Member States have agreed to work towards the global target of a 30% relative reduction in mean population intake of salt by 2025 relative to 2010 levels. It is crucial that this target is met in order to achieve the overall goal of a 25% reduction in premature mortality from NCDs by 2025 [2].

The overall number of countries implementing a national salt reduction strategy more than doubled from 2010 to 2015. However, despite the remarkable efforts and actions that have since been taken, more needs to be done. Data from 2013 revealed that population salt consumption in most European countries ranged from around 7 g/day (Bulgaria, Cyprus, Germany, and Latvia) to 13 g/day (Czech Republic) [7,8].

Among all dietary habits, excessive salt intake has the most adverse outcomes. The average daily intake of salt per capita among the Portuguese population is 10.7 g [9], which is double the level recommended by WHO (<5 g) [6]. Portugal ranks the highest among European countries regarding salt intake, with excessive intake reported in 63.2% of women and 88.9% of men [10]. The problem also affects younger groups, as research shows that most children and adolescents exceed daily recommendations [11–13].

Excessive salt intake is associated with an increased risk of obesity—partially due to poor diets that are high in both energy and salt, such as regular consumption of breakfast cereals [14] and highly processed foods [10]. Another reason for this association may be that consumption of salty foods stimulates thirst and increases fluid intake, thereby increasing the consumption of sugar-sweetened beverages, which can further fuel obesity [15]. This scenario is of particular interest in Portugal, where the prevalence of childhood overweight has been among the highest in Europe, affecting around one in three children [16]. It is, therefore, urgent to tackle this issue, as even small reductions in salt consumption can bring great health benefits to children by reducing the risk of developing cardiovascular diseases—the leading cause of death and disability in Portugal and worldwide [17,18].

The Portuguese "National Program for the Promotion of Healthy Eating" [19], in line with internationally recommended interventions [20], strongly advocates for the implementation of strategies to reduce dietary salt intake in children by providing information and education on healthy eating as well as the strengthening of consumer protections, particularly by reducing the salt content of school meals.

Several attempts have been made to reach children in schools to encourage healthier eating habits and improve the nutritional quality of the food served to them. These interventions can potentially impact all children of school age, irrespective of their ethnicity or socioeconomic group [21–25]. Primary and secondary schools serve at least one meal every day and can also determine the types of food and beverages that are available or served at schools (i.e., schools' cafeterias and vending machines). Schools can positively impact eating behaviors and promote healthier eating [26–28], for example, by deploying nutrition education classes.

School is a key setting to deliver health education to children, promote healthy lifestyles and social equality, and to ensure access to nutritionally balanced meals, regardless of the family's socioeconomic status [29]. In Portugal, municipalities are responsible for providing school meals (lunch) for pre-school and primary schools as well as for the management [30] of the menu. During secondary education, the supply of school meals is supported by the Directorate General of Education Institutions (DGEstE) [31], except for schools with their own cooking facilities. In Portugal, a set of guidelines for the school food supply has been established, which includes limits on the salt content of the school meal's components—bread, soup, and the main dish [31].

Assuming that lunch represents 30% of the total energy value [32] and considering the WHO recommendation [6], 1.5 g of salt should be the maximum level in this meal. In Portugal, little is known about the nutritional composition of the complete school meal. The amount of different nutrients in food samples can be measured through laboratory analyses, using standardized techniques recommended by international organizations [33]. In the few studies that have been conducted to estimate sodium content of school meals in Portugal, mean salt content has ranged from 2.83 and 3.82 g [34–36], which clearly should be reduced.

Eat Mediterranean—A Program for Eliminating Dietary Inequalities in Schools (EM) [37], was a European Economic Area (EEA) Grant funded project developed as a Portuguese community-based intervention (2015 to 2017) through a multi-sectorial approach involving health, education, and political stakeholders. The program's goal was to reduce nutritional inequalities among school-aged children through the promotion of the Mediterranean diet. The program comprised a comprehensive approach both at the individual level (child and family) and at the group/community level (nutritional education sessions at schools and improvement of school food environments). One of the objectives and key priority areas in the implementation of EM at the community level was to evaluate and improve the nutritional quality of food available in school meals. Within the school food environment, the EM program proposed a qualitative and quantitative (laboratory) analysis and evaluation of the nutritional adequacy of school meals. The aim was to identify nutritional deviations, according to international/national recommendations [29,31,38,39] and correct them by modifying the food composition of school meals through both training of the schools' food handlers and through the development and implementation of new menus.

2. Materials and Methods

2.1. Program and Participant Schools

The EM program was implemented over two school years (2015/2016 (Y1) to 2016/2017 (Y2)) in two Portuguese municipalities: Santarém and Alpiarça. In total, 25 individual public schools and 5773 students (3–21 years old), from pre-school to secondary education, participated in EM.

The entities responsible for the supply of school meals in both pre-schools and primary schools were Santarém Municipality (17 schools) and Alpiarça Municipality (three schools). For secondary schools, DGEstE supplied meals to four schools, while one had their own cooking service.

The specific evaluation and intervention on nutritional adequacy of served school meals (lunch) were organized in three phases:

- Evaluation (Y1): 386 school menus were analyzed qualitatively. Thirty-nine school meal samples were collected from 10 kitchens that served all 25 Schools for analysis during the period between March and June 2016. A report on qualitative and quantitative nutritional adequacy of school meals was presented to school communities.
- Intervention (Y1/Y2): From July 2016 to March 2017, a working group was established to discuss the results of the report from the evaluation phase and to develop a new proposal for school menus. The working group included public health professionals, nutritionists, a municipal food engineer, school cooks, teachers, and parents. The new school menus were developed according to the WHO recommendations [29,38] and national guidelines [32,40], and these were implemented in all participant schools. Additionally, training was provided for the schools' food handlers in order to implement the new changes. During the intervention period, nutritionists from the working group closely followed and guided every step of the process, including food preparation, cooking and serving of the meals while, at the same time, providing training to the food handlers. The training covered topics, such as food safety, cooking methods, and portion guidance (for example, to estimate the amount of salt that could be added to food, a standard measuring spoon or cup was introduced for all food handlers to use). Additionally, technical

sheets of the new menus were developed, and their implementation was conducted under the supervision of members of the working group.

- Post-intervention (Y2): A new set of 39 school meal samples was collected from the same kitchens from April to June 2017, and a qualitative and quantitative evaluation of the changes was performed.

Ethical approval was granted by Lisbon and Tagus Valley Regional Health Administration Ethical Committee (089.CES/INV/2015).

2.2. Food Samples and Sample Preparation

Food samples were collected from all 10 kitchens that served meals to the 25 schools. Of the 10 kitchens, nine served meals at their own schools, so samples were collected at the moment of serving. One school was served by transporting meals from a central kitchen outside the city. In this case, food samples were collected at the school immediately prior to serving.

The samples consisted of the food portions that were served to children at lunchtime. Each food sample consisted of three main items: bread, soup, and the main course (including salad or cooked vegetables and one piece of fruit). These were collected during both evaluation and post-intervention phases in a total of 39 samples in each phase. In one of the schools (school B), it was not possible to analyze the bread samples, as they were not sent to the laboratory. The meal items were weighed on a Mettler-Toledo PB3002-S/FACT (Mettler-Toledo, Inc., Columbus, OH) laboratory scale, with an accuracy of 0.01 g. Samples were collected using latex gloves, placed in sterile polythene bags, and alphabetically coded to maintain confidentiality. The samples were transported to the laboratory, refrigerated, homogenized, and milled using a high-speed grinder, a knife mill Grindomix GM 200; Retsch, Haan, Germany equipped with titanium knives to prevent contamination. The prepared samples were stored in vacuum bags at the freezing temperature (−20 °C) until processing.

2.3. Laboratory Analysis and Interpretation

The analysis was performed in accordance with the methodology recommended by the Official Methods of Analysis of AOAC International [33], under quality assurance conditions complying with the requirements described in standard EN ISO/IEC 17025: 2005 [41]. For sodium determination, the samples were analyzed in triplicate using an inductively-coupled plasma optical emission spectrometer, ICP OES, model iCAP 6000, Thermo Fisher Scientific, Madison, WI, USA for the determination of sodium (Na) content. There are several common sources of sodium in food, including from salt added during preparation or during processing, as well as from the sodium in seasoning (e.g., sodium phosphate, sodium bicarbonate, MSG mono-glutamate, etc.). However, this study assumed that all sodium in food was in the form of sodium chloride and equivalents, so all results were expressed in terms of "salt".

The salt content in g/100 g of food was calculated by the formula: salt (g) = sodium (g) × 2.5 [41]. Considering a school meal (lunch) makes up 30% of the daily total energy intake [32], 1.5 g of salt was the reference value used in the present study (according to the WHO recommendation of salt intake [6]: $0.30 \times 5 = 1.5$ g).

2.4. Statistical Analysis

Data sets were produced using Microsoft Excel® spreadsheets, and statistical analyses were performed using IBM SPSS® statistics for Windows, version 22.0, Armonk, NY, USA [42]. Results were reported as mean (+ standard deviation). Non-parametric tests for comparing means were carried out for paired samples. A significance level of $\alpha = 0.05$ was considered statistically significant.

3. Results

The quantitative analysis of the school menus found that the standardized serving portions collected during the evaluation phase and the post-intervention phase were similar. Regarding the reduction in sodium and salt equivalent of the individual meal components, there was a 34% reduction per serving portion of soup. There were no significant changes in sodium and salt equivalent per serving portion of bread or per serving portion of the main course. In the complete meal, including the three components, there was a 23% reduction in sodium and salt equivalent per serving portion (Table 1).

Table 1. Sodium and salt content of school meals components (soup, main course, and bread) and of the complete meal (all components) analyzed at the evaluation and the post-intervention phases of the eat Mediterranean program.

		Serving Portion (g) [(a)]		Sodium (g/Serving Portion)			Salt (g/Serving Portion) [(b)]		
	n	Evaluation	Post-Intervention	Evaluation	Post-Intervention	*p*-Value	Evaluation	Post-Intervention	*p*-Value
Soup	10	227.10 ± 30.24	220.30 ± 37.08	0.59 ± 0.12	0.39 ± 0.24	0.017 Change 0.20~34%	1.48 ± 0.29	0.98 ± 0.59	0.017 Change 0.49~34%
Main course	10	262.30 ± 51.71	269.80 ± 61.28	0.68 ± 0.21	0.60 ± 0.25	0.169	1.70 ± 0.54	1.50 ± 0.63	0.169
Bread	9	46.00 ± 14.80	46.56 ± 16.08	0.19 ± 0.09	0.18 ± 0.11	0.441	0.48 ± 0.21	0.45 ± 0.27	0.514
Complete meal	10	-	-	1.50 ± 0.30	1.16 ± 0.45	0.028 Change 0.34~23%	3.75 ±0.40	2.90 ± 1.12	0.047 Change 0.85~23%

[(a)] There were no statistically significant differences between serving portions (g) ($p > 0.05$); [(b)] The salt content was calculated by the formula: salt (g) = sodium (g) × 2.5 [35].

Changes in the mean salt content of the complete school meal in grams (g) at evaluation and at the post-intervention phase are shown, for individual schools and for all schools combined, in Figure 1. For all schools except for two (B and J), there was a decrease in salt content between the two time-points.

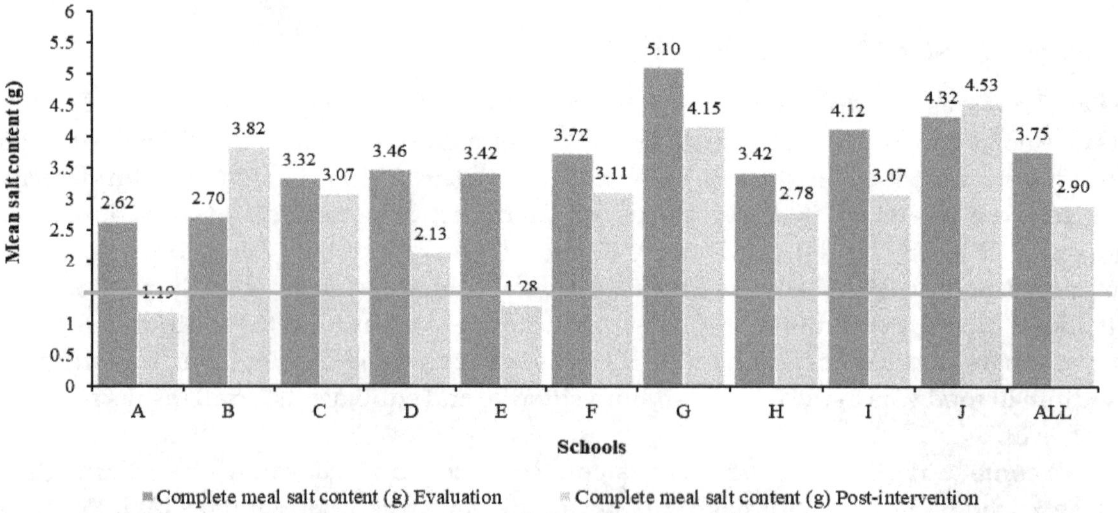

Figure 1. Mean salt content (g) of the complete school meals analyzed at the evaluation phase and the post-intervention phase of the eat Mediterranean program and its adequacy regarding the reference value (maximum 1.5 g of salt/meal), by the school.

4. Discussion

While community-based programs designed to improve the nutritional quality of school meals have been shown to be effective previously [43,44], EM was one of the first programs in Portugal to address qualitative and nutritional laboratory analysis together. Through a multidisciplinary approach targeting the school food environment, a key objective of the program was to improve the nutritional composition of school meals served to young people during lunchtime. In Portugal, addressing the quality of school meals is an important way to promote healthy diets as at least one meal is offered every day, and at pre- and primary education levels, almost every child has lunch at school [45].

The qualitative assessment of the 386 school menus has been presented elsewhere [46]. As part of evaluating EM, this study focused on identifying the nutritional deviations of sodium and salt equivalent content of school meals from international and national recommendations [29,31,38,39] and aimed to correct them by modifying the nutritional composition of school meals. This was done through training of the schools' food handlers and the development and implementation of new menus. The results showed that EM had a positive effect on the improvement of the school meals' salt content among the participating schools, achieving an overall reduction of 23% of the salt content of school meals served at lunchtime.

At the beginning of the EM program, the mean salt content of school meals was 3.75 g of salt per meal. These findings were similar to those reported in previous Portuguese studies [34–36], as well as in studies from other countries that assessed the salt content in school meals served in canteens [47]. Interventions as part of the EM program led to a significant reduction ($p < 0.05$) of salt content (from 3.75 g to 2.90 g of salt per meal, i.e., ~23%); however, it was still far from the reference value of lunch salt content (1.5 g of salt), and it was estimated that it would need to be met to achieve recommended salt consumption levels.

Looking separately at each component of the meal, the main dish was the component with the highest contribution to the salt content of the whole meal. This was also found in the study conducted by Barbosa et al. 2018 [48] in Portuguese University Canteens, in which it was suggested that one possible explanation for this result was the presence of intrinsic sodium in foods, such as meat and fish, which is higher than the sodium intrinsically present in vegetables used for soups [49]. However, we found a significant reduction in the salt content of soup from 1.48 g per serving portion before the intervention to 0.98 g per serving portion after the intervention (~34% reduction).

The values for lunch salt content, after EM intervention, are yet slightly higher than those reported by other Portuguese studies [50,51]. According to the Portuguese 2018 guidelines for menus and school canteens [31], the maximum value that can be added to soups and main dishes during the cooking process is 0.2 g of iodized salt. In addition, it is recommended that salt be replaced by glasswort or aromatic herbs. Regarding the serving of bread included in the school meals, according to the recommendations for Portuguese school meals [31], it should be one small piece of bread of 25 g for pre-school and primary school and 45 g for elementary and secondary school, with a maximum salt composition of 1%, meaning 0.25 g and 0.45 g of salt per serving of bread, respectively. As there was no intervention targeted at reducing bread provided during school meals, this study observed that, despite the level of education, the mean serving of bread was around 45 g, and the salt content of bread per serving, both before and after the intervention, was above the guidelines (0.46 g–0.49 g). In Portugal, there is a culture of always serving bread at mealtime, which is reflected in the official guidelines [31]. It could be suggested that if there was a non-mandatory offer of bread at school meals, at least for young children, and if carbohydrate intake recommendations were met through foods with less salt, a further reduction on overall salt intake could have been observed through this action alone.

There were several challenges in the implementation of the EM program. One of these was to reduce the amount of salt added by cooks while preparing the meals, as while the technical guidance clearly requires that the amount of salt added during meal preparation be accurately measured, several cooks still opted to measure by "hand". This was also described by Gonçalves et al. [52], who found that the amount of added salt was influenced by the taste of the cook, even though many food handlers acknowledged that they did not taste the food before adding salt. That study also pointed out that food handlers were aware of the health problems associated with excessive salt intake as well as the recommended salt intake values, but they mentioned that the greatest difficulty in salt reduction was the opinion and acceptance of the consumers toward less salt in foods [52]. Such limitations reinforce the importance of educating both consumers and food handlers so that programs aiming at reducing the salt content in school meals and other settings can be more effective.

Action to reduce salt consumption is urgent, including among younger populations, in order to reduce the risk of developing cardiovascular diseases. The offer of high sodium meals in a school environment can contribute to individuals acquiring long-term poor eating habits, including increased consumption of processed food, which is already a pattern in Portuguese children [10]. Additionally, emerging evidence suggests dietary sodium intake may be associated with obesity, both through pathophysiological mechanisms and through the induction of thirst and increased consumption of high energy drinks [53–57], enhancing the need to address and tackle this public health issue.

The improvement of the menus introduced by the EM program has shown that it is possible to successfully reduce the salt content of school lunches through existing mechanisms. To ensure school meals are nutritionally adequate, it is essential that trained cooking staff and all responsible parties strictly comply with the technical sheets provided. It is also crucial to continue the education of students, parents, educators, teachers, as well as the monitoring of all stages of preparing and serving meals by the cooking staff. The integrated and concerted work among health departments, research institutions, municipalities, and educational communities was a strong part of the success of the EM program.

Among the common challenges educators face when trying to reduce the amount of added salt to meals is rejection by consumers due to "lack of flavor" [52]. However, the adaptive capacity of the flavors-linked neurological system to small reductions in salt in meals has been well described [57]. Thus, school settings may be ideal not only for nutrition literacy interventions among children but also for flavors, shaping and educating towards less salty food acceptance.

One of the pitfalls of this study was the limited time frame of the intervention to carry out all the activities projected in this comprehensive program without including a post-intervention longer monitoring period. This would have been important to continuously assess the adaptation to the changes implemented in the context of the new school food environment, in particular, the acceptance/preference of less salty meals by the children.

Nonetheless, recognizing the relevance of consumer acceptance in order to obtain long-lasting changes, EM paved the way for further work towards providing healthier meals in the participating schools, including a monitoring system to assess students' acceptance of school meals changes and also regarding food waste. The training, capacity building, and nutritional education offered during the EM intervention to all school community (teachers, parents, children, food handlers, and others) would hopefully contribute to the sustainability of the progress achieved in improvements and support continuous improvements.

5. Conclusions

This study demonstrated the success of the EM program in reducing the salt content of lunch meals served in schools. School meals must be nutritious, and reinforcement of this through regular monitoring and evaluation is a key factor to ensure school food quality. In order for school meals to be nutritionally adequate, trained cooking staff and all responsible parties would need to strictly comply with the provided technical sheets. It is crucial that the health literacy of students, parents, educators, and teachers is developed through continuous education, and the monitoring process at all stages of preparing and serving meals by school food handlers is strengthened. This comprehensive program was built through a collaboration between different stakeholders (health departments and units, research institutions, municipalities, and educational communities), which was both key to its success and ensured a holistic approach towards promoting healthier behaviors.

Author Contributions: The authors' contributions are as follows: A.I.R., was part of the coordinating team of eat Mediterranean and worked in all stages of the research, such as project design, methodology, analysis and interpretation of the data, and conceptualization, preparation and writing of the original manuscript; S.M. worked on the analysis and interpretation of the data; M.S. contributed to the laboratory analysis; A.D. (Ana Dinis) and C.R. coordinated and implemented the eat Mediterranean program, worked on the project design, data collection, and interpretation of the data. A.I.R.; S.M.; M.S.; F.G.-d.-S.; F.P.C.; S.W.; A.D. (Ana Dinis); C.R.; I.C.; A.D. (Ara Darzi); J.B. contributed to the writing, review and editing. All authors have read and agreed to the published version of the manuscript.

Acknowledgments: The authors wish to acknowledge all the nutritionists, psychologists, and other health professionals, children, parents, educators, teachers, school cooking staff, and municipality technicians for their contribution on the fieldwork, as well as the following Institutions for their partnership and support: Agrupamentos de Escolas Ginestal Machado, Sá da Bandeira e de José Relvas; Hospital Distrital de Santarém; CEIDSS—Centre for Studies and Research in Social Dynamics and Health; ISCTEIUL—Instituto Universitário de Lisboa; Municipalities of Alpiarça and Santarém and Instituto Nacional de Saúde Doutor Ricardo Jorge.

References

1. World Health Organization. *Global Status Report on Noncommunicable Diseases 2014*; World Health Organization: Geneva, Switzerland, 2014.
2. World Health Organization. *Global Action Plan for the Prevention and Control of Noncommunicable Diseases 2013-2020*; World Health Organization: Geneva, Switzerland, 2013.
3. Beaglehole, R.; Bonita, R.; Horton, R.; Adams, C.; Alleyne, G.; Asaria, P.; Baugh, V.; Bekedam, H.; Billo, N.E.; Casswell, S.; et al. Priority actions for the non-communicable disease crisis. *Lancet* **2011**, *6736*, 1438–1447. [CrossRef]
4. World Health Organization. *Noncommunicable Diseases Progress Monitor, 2017*; World Health Organization: Geneva, Switzerland, 2017; Available online: http://apps.who.int/iris/bitstream/10665/258940/1/9789241513029-eng.pdf?ua=1 (accessed on 23 September 2019).
5. World Health Organization. *Tackling NCDs: 'Best Buys' and Other Recommended Interventions for the Prevention and Control of Noncommunicable Diseases*; World Health Organization: Geneva, Switzerland, 2017; Available online: https://apps.who.int/iris/handle/10665/259232 (accessed on 23 September 2019).
6. World Health Organization. *Guideline: Sodium Intake for Adults and Children*; World Health Organization: Geneva, Switzerland, 2012; Available online: https://www.who.int/publications/i/item/9789241504836 (accessed on 23 September 2019).
7. European Commission. *Survey on Member Sates' Implementation of the EU Salt Reduction Framework*; Publications Office of the European Union: Luxembourg, 2013; Available online: https://op.europa.eu/en/publication-detail/-/publication/df7ef17e-d643-4593-94b3-84bacfa7a76a (accessed on 23 September 2019).
8. World Health Organization. *Mapping Salt Reduction Initiatives in the WHO European Region*; World Health Organization: Copenhagen, Denmark, 2013; Available online: http://www.euro.who.int/en/publications/abstracts/mapping-salt-reduction-initiatives-in-the-who-european-region (accessed on 23 September 2019).
9. Polonia, J.; Martins, L.; Pinto, F.; Nazare, J. Prevalence, awareness, treatment and control of hypertension and salt intake in Portugal: Changes over a decade the PHYSA study. *J. Hypertens.* **2014**, *32*, 1211–1221. [CrossRef]
10. Lopes, C.; Torres, D.; Oliveira, A.; Severo, M.; Alarcao, V.; Guiomar, S.; Mota, J.; Teixeira, P.J.; Rodrigues, S.; Lobato, L.; et al. Inquérito Alimentar Nacional e de Atividade Física, IAN-AF 2015-2016: Relatório de resultados. Universidade do Porto, 2017. Available online: https://ian-af.up.pt/publicacoes (accessed on 26 September 2019).
11. Goncalves, C.; Abreu, S.; Padrao, P.; Pinho, O.; Graca, P.; Breda, J.; Santos, R.; Moreira, P. Sodium and potassium urinary excretion and dietary intake: A cross-sectional analysis in adolescents. *Food Nutr. Res.* **2016**, *60*. [CrossRef] [PubMed]
12. Correiacosta, L.; Cosme, D.; Nogueirasilva, L.; Morato, M.; Sousa, T.; Moura, C.; Mota, C.; Guerra, A.; Albinoteixeira, A.; Areias, J.C.; et al. Gender and obesity modify the impact of salt intake on blood pressure in children. *Pediatric Nephrol.* **2016**, *31*, 279–288. [CrossRef]
13. Sardinha, L.B.; Santos, D.A.; Silva, A.M.; Coelhoesilva, M.J.; Raimundo, A.; Moreira, H.; Santos, R.; Vale, S.; Baptista, F.; Mota, J. Prevalence of overweight, obesity, and abdominal obesity in a representative sample of Portuguese adults. *PLoS ONE* **2012**, *7*, e47883. [CrossRef] [PubMed]
14. Rito, A.I.; Dinis, A.; Rascoa, C.; Maia, A.; Martins, I.D.; Santos, M.; Lima, J.; Mendes, S.; Padrao, J.; Steinnovais, C. Improving breakfast patterns of portuguese children-an evaluation of ready-to-eat cereals according to the European nutrient profile model. *Eur. J. Clin. Nutr.* **2019**, *73*, 465–473. [CrossRef] [PubMed]
15. Ma, Y.; He, F.; MacGregor, G. High Salt Intake—Independent Risk Factor for Obesity? *Hypertension* **2015**, *66*, 843–849. [CrossRef] [PubMed]
16. Rito, A.I.; Cruz de Sousa, R.; Mendes, S.; Graça, P. *Childhood Obesity Surveillance Initiative: COSI Portugal*

2016; Instituto Nacional de Saúde Dr. Ricardo Jorge (INSA, IP): Lisbon, Portugal, 2017; Available online: http://hdl.handle.net/10400.18/4857 (accessed on 26 September 2019).

17. Programa Nacional para a Promoção da Alimentação Saudável. *Portugal Alimentação Saudável em Números 2015*; Direção-Geral da Saúde: Lisbon, Portugal, 2016; Available online: http://nutrimento.pt/activeapp/wp-content/uploads/2016/03/Relatório-Portugal-Alimentação-Saudável-em-números-2015.pdf (accessed on 27 September 2019).
18. Li, X.; Jan, S.; Yan, L.L.; Hayes, A.J.; Chu, Y.; Wang, H.; Feng, X.; Niu, W.; He, F.J.; Ma, J.; et al. Cost and cost-effectiveness of a school-based education program to reduce salt intake in children and their families in China. *PLoS ONE* **2017**, *12*. [CrossRef]
19. Ministério da Saúde, Direção Geral da Saúde. *Programa Nacional para a Promoção da Alimentação Saudável Orientações Programáticas*; Direção-Geral da Saúde: Lisbon, Portugal, 2012; Available online: http://www.dgs.pt/programas-de-saude-prioritarios.aspx (accessed on 10 October 2019).
20. World Health Organization. *The SHAKE Technical Package for Salt Reduction*; World Health Organization: Geneva, Switzerland, 2016; Available online: https://apps.who.int/iris/rest/bitstreams/1061141/retrieve (accessed on 6 January 2020).
21. Lytle, L.A.; Kubik, M.Y. Nutritional issues for adolescents. *Best Pract. Res. Clin. Endocrinol. Metab.* **2003**, *17*, 177–189. [CrossRef]
22. World Health Organization. *Diet, Nutrition and the Prevention of Chronic Diseases: Report of a Joint WHO/FAO Expert Consultation—Technical Report Series no. 916*; World Health Organization: Geneva, Switzerland, 2003; Available online: https://apps.who.int/iris/bitstream/handle/10665/42665/WHO_TRS_916.pdf;jsessionid=EBC44FFF46A59BECE4352FE155FC349C?sequence=1 (accessed on 25 October 2019).
23. French, S.A.; Stables, G. Environmental interventions to promote vegetable and fruit consumption among youth in school settings. *Prev. Med.* **2003**, *37*, 593–610. [CrossRef]
24. Flodmark, C.E.; Marcus, C.; Britton, M. Interventions to prevent obesity in children and adolescents: A systematic literature review. *Int. J. Obes.* **2006**, *30*, 579–589. [CrossRef]
25. Sharma, M. International school-based interventions for preventing obesity in children. *Obes. Rev.* **2006**, *8*, 155–167. [CrossRef]
26. Centers for Disease Control and Prevention. Guidelines for school health programs to promote lifelong healthy eating. *J. Sch. Health* **1997**, *67*, 9–26. [CrossRef] [PubMed]
27. Branca, F.; Nikogosian, H.; Lobstein, T. *The challenge of obesity in the WHO European Region and the Strategies for Response*; World Health Organization: Copenhagen, Denmark, 2007; Available online: http://www.euro.who.int/en/publications/abstracts/challenge-of-obesity-in-the-who-european-region-and-the-strategies-for-response-the (accessed on 25 October 2019).
28. Commission of the European Communities. *Green Paper—Promoting Healthy Diets and Physical Activity: A European Dimension for The Prevention of Overweight, Obesity and Chronic Diseases*; European Commission: Brussels, Belgium, 2005; Available online: https://eur-lex.europa.eu/legal-content/EN/TXT/PDF/?uri=CELEX:52005DC0637&from=EN26 (accessed on 25 October 2019).
29. World Health Organization. *Report of the Commission on Ending Childhood Obesity*; World Health Organization: Geneva, Switzerland, 2016; Available online: https://www.who.int/end-childhood-obesity/final-report/en/ (accessed on 25 October 2019).
30. Ministério da Educação e da Ciência (2015) Parte C Despacho nº8452-a/2015. Available online: https://www.dgeste.mec.pt/wp-content/uploads/2014/01/Despacho8452A2015ASE.pdf (accessed on 25 October 2019).
31. Lima, R.M. Orientações sobre ementas e refeitórios escolares. *Ministério da Educação—Direção-Geral da Educação*. 2018. Available online: http://www.dge.mec.pt/sites/default/files/Esaude/oere.pdf (accessed on 13 November 2019).
32. Institute of Medicine (US) Committee on Nutrition Standards for National School Lunch and Breakfast Programs. *School Meals: Building Blocks for Healthy Children*; National Academies Press: Washington, DC, USA, 2010.
33. Association of Official Analytical Chemists (AOAC). *International Official Methods of Analysis of AOAC International*; AOAC International: Rockville, MD, USA, 2000.
34. Paiva, I.; Pinto, C.; Queiros, L.; Meister, M.C.; Saraiva, M.; Bruno, P.; Antunes, D.; Afonso, M. Baixo valor calórico e elevado teor de sal. *Acta Médica Portuguesa* **2011**, *24*, 215–222. [PubMed]
35. Viegas, C.; Torgal, J.; Graça, P.; Martins, M. Evaluation of salt content in school meals. *Rev. Nutr.* **2015**, *28*, 165–174. [CrossRef]

36. Fontes, T.; Bento, A.; Matias, F.; Mota, C.; Nascimento, A.; Santiago, S.; Santos, M. O valor nutricional das refeições escolares. In *Boletim Epidemiológico*; INSA, IP Nº especial _ Alimentação e Nutrição: Lisboa, Portugal, 2015.
37. Eat Mediterranean Program. Available online: http://www.ceidss.com/eat-mediterranean/ (accessed on 10 December 2019).
38. World Health Organization. *School Policy Framework: Implementation of the WHO Global Strategy on Diet, Physical Activity and Health*; World Health Organization: Geneva, Switzerland, 2008; Available online: http://www.who.int/dietphysicalactivity/SPF-En.pdf (accessed on 13 November 2019).
39. SPARE—Sistema de Planeamento e Avaliação de Refeições Escolares—Elaboração, Verificação e Monitorização na ótica do Utilizador. Available online: http://www.plataformacontraaobesidade.dgs.pt:8080/SPARE2/index.php (accessed on 15 December 2019).
40. International Organization for Standardization. *General Requirements for the Competence of Testing and Calibration Laboratories*, 2nd ed.; ISO/IEC 17025:2005 (International Standard); International Organization for Standardization: Geneva, Switzerland, 2005.
41. *Regulation (EU) No 1169/2011 of the European Parliament and of the Council of 25 October 2011 on the Provision of Food Information to Consumers*; The Publications Office of the European Union: Luxembourg, 2011.
42. IBM Corp. *IBM SPSS Statistics for Windows*; Version 22.0; IBM Corp: Armonk, NY, USA, 2016.
43. Rocha, A.; Afonso, C.; Santos, M.C.; Morais, C.; Franchini, B.; Chilro, R. System of planning and evaluation of school meals. *Public Health Nutr.* **2014**, *17*, 1264–1270. [CrossRef]
44. Sancho, T.; Candeias, A.; Mendes, C.; Rego, M.; Cartaxo, L. Promoção da qualidade nutricional de refeições em estabelecimentos de educação do Algarve análise comparativa 2004/2005–2006/2007. *Rev. Nutrícias* **2008**, *8*, 1–3.
45. Rocha, A.; Ávila, H.; Barbosa, M. Caracterização da Prestação do Serviço de Refeições Escolares pelos Municípios Portugueses. *Rev. Nutrícias* **2012**, *13*, 3–8.
46. Rito, A.; Dinis, A.; Rascôa, C.; Rodrigues, S.; Stein-Novais, C.; Mendes, S.; Maia, A.; Luís, S.; Luciano, R. Nutrition Qualitative Evaluation and Improvement of School Meals in Portugal—Eat Mediterranean Program. *Acta Port. Nutr.* **2018**, *12*, 6–12. [CrossRef]
47. Ahn, S.; Park, S.; Kim, J.N.; Han, S.N.; Jeong, S.B.; Kim, H.K. Salt content of school meals and comparison of perception related to sodium intake in elementary, middle, and high schools. *Nutr. Res. Pract.* **2013**, *7*, 59–65. [CrossRef]
48. Barbosa, M.; Fernandes, A.; Gonçalves, C.; Pena, M.; Padrão, P.; Pinho, O.; Moreira, P. Sodium and Potassium Content of Meals Served in University Canteens. *Port. J. Public Health* **2018**, *35*, 27–33. [CrossRef]
49. Martins, I.; Porto, A.; Oliveira, L. Tabela de Composição de Alimentos. In *Departamento de Alimentação e Nutrição*; Instituto Nacional de Saúde Doutor Ricardo Jorge: Lisbon, Portugal, 2007.
50. Gonçalves, C.; Silva, G.; Pinho, O.; Camelo, S.; Amaro, L.; Teixeira, V.; Padrão, P.; Moreira, P. Sodium content in vegetable soups prepared outside the home: Identifying the problem. In *International Symposium on Occupational Safety and Hygiene: Book of Abstracts*; Sociedade Portuguesa de Segurança e Higiene Ocupacionais: Guimarães, Portugal, 2012.
51. Goncalves, C.; Monteiro, S.; Padrao, P.; Rocha, A.; Abreu, S.; Pinho, O.; Moreira, P. Salt reduction in vegetable soup does not affect saltiness intensity and liking in the elderly and children. *Food Nutr. Res.* **2014**, *58*, 24825. [CrossRef] [PubMed]
52. Gonçalves, C.; Pinho, O.; Padrão, P.; Santos, C.; Abreu, S.; Moreira, P. Knowledge and practices related to added salt in meals by food handlers. *Rev. Nutrícias* **2014**, *21*, 14–17.
53. Libuda, L.; Kersting, M.; Alexy, U. Consumption of dietary salt measured by urinary sodium excretion and its associated with body weight status in healthy children and adolescents. *Public Health Nutr.* **2012**, *15*, 433–441. [CrossRef] [PubMed]
54. Yoon, Y.S.; Oh, S.W. Sodium density and obesity; the Korea National Health and Nutrition Examination Survey 2007–2010. *Eur. J. Clin. Nutr.* **2013**, *67*, 141–146. [CrossRef] [PubMed]
55. Zhu, H.; Pollock, N.K.; Kotak, I.; Gutin, B.; Wang, X.; Bhagatwala, J.; Parikh, S.; Harshfield, G.A.; Dong, Y. Dietary sodium, adiposity, and inflammation in healthy adolescents. *Pediatrics* **2014**, *133*, e635–e642. [CrossRef]
56. Grimes, A.; Bolhuis, D.; He, F.; Nowson, C. Dietary sodium intake and overweight and obesity in children and adults: A protocol for a systematic review and meta-analysis. *Syst. Rev.* **2016**, *5*, 7. [CrossRef]

12

Food Consumption Patterns and Nutrient Intakes of Children and Adolescents in the Eastern Mediterranean Region

Ayoub Al-Jawaldeh [1], Mandy Taktouk [2] and Lara Nasreddine [2,*]

[1] World Health Organization (WHO), Regional Office for the Eastern Mediterranean (EMRO), Cairo 7608, Egypt; aljawaldeha@who.int
[2] Nutrition and Food Sciences Department, Faculty of Agriculture and Food Sciences, American University of Beirut, Beirut 11-0236, Lebanon; mrt07@mail.aub.edu
* Correspondence: ln10@aub.edu.lb.

Abstract: The Eastern Mediterranean Region (EMR) has witnessed significant social and economic changes that may have influenced the diet of children and adolescents, and increased the risk for obesity and malnutrition in this age group. This review aims to characterize and assess food consumption patterns and nutrient intakes amongst school-aged children (5–10 years) and adolescents (10–19 years) in countries of the EMR. Electronic databases (MedLine, PubMed, Scopus, and Google Scholar) were searched for relevant articles published between 2005 and 2020; international organizations and governmental websites were also searched. Available studies documented low intakes of fruits, vegetables and fiber, inadequate consumption of water, milk and dairy products, coupled with high intakes of fat, saturated fat, and sugar sweetened beverages, as well as a frequent consumption of energy-dense, nutrient poor foods such as sweet and savory snacks. Micronutrient inadequacies were also observed, particularly for calcium, iron, zinc and vitamins A, D, C, and folate. Acknowledging the impact that nutrition may have on building societies and transforming the lives of children, adolescents and their families, there is a crucial need for a food system approach in developing and implementing national and regional policies and interventions aimed at improving the diet of children and adolescents.

Keywords: food consumption patterns; dietary intakes; macronutrients; micronutrients; children; adolescents; Eastern Mediterranean Region; review

1. Introduction

The health and well-being of children and adolescents are essential prerequisites for achieving the Sustainable Development Goals (SDGs), particularly those focusing on poverty, health security, education and the reduction of inequalities [1]. The World Health Organization (WHO) acknowledged the importance of adequate nutrition to "enable children and adolescents to enjoy good health while playing a full role in contributing to transformative change and sustainable development", in alignment with the SDGs [2]. Good nutrition during childhood and adolescence is in fact indispensable for growth and development, health and well-being, and the prevention of obesity and several chronic diseases [3].

Unhealthy diets in childhood and adolescence are associated with immediate as well as long-term health impacts. In the short term, inadequate dietary intakes of energy, protein, or certain micronutrients will result in slower growth rates, delayed sexual maturation, lower reserves of micronutrients, and inadequate bone mass [4]. Dietary intakes of children and adolescents may also affect their risk of developing a number of health problems, such as iron deficiency and dental caries, while also lowering their resistance to infectious diseases and adversely affecting their ability to function at peak mental and physical capacity [3]. Poor diets in these critical periods of the life course are also linked with pediatric obesity and its related metabolic abnormalities, such as high blood pressure, type 2 diabetes (T2D), metabolic syndrome, sleep disturbances, orthopedic problems, and psychosocial problems [5–8], which all tend to track into adulthood [9].

Dietary practices of children and adolescents may also carry long-term health ramifications, increasing the risk for several non-communicable diseases (NCDs), and contributing significantly to the burden of preventable diseases and premature deaths [3]. In the Eastern Mediterranean region (EMR), which has witnessed over the past few decades important social, economic, and political changes [10], three of the ten leading causes of death are related to dietary factors, including ischemic heart disease, strokes, and diabetes. Urbanization, technological development, and modernization, have in fact instigated significant demographic and epidemiologic changes in most countries of the region, with parallel shifts in diet, physical activity, and body composition [11]. These shifts represent the basis of the multidimensional phenomenon of the nutrition transition, which is characterized by increases in the intakes of energy, fat, added sugars, and salt [11,12]. Some states in the region are classified as countries in advanced nutrition transition, such as the Gulf Cooperation Council (GCC) countries, the Islamic Republic of Iran, and Tunisia, while others are classified in early nutrition transition, such as Jordan, Lebanon, Egypt, Libya, and Morocco [13]. In contrast, political turmoil and economic challenges have adversely impacted the availability of food in some EMR countries such as Iraq, Pakistan, occupied Palestinian territory, and Yemen, while some states are categorized as countries in emergency and humanitarian crisis, such as Afghanistan, Somalia, and Sudan [13,14].

Amidst the threat of transitioning to high-energy, nutrient-poor diets and the parallel hazard of food insecurity, children and adolescents may be amongst the most vulnerable population groups to the ongoing societal, lifestyle, and dietary changes in countries of the region [15]. Available evidence indicates that the region harbors one of the highest rates of pediatric and adolescent obesity worldwide, while the burden of undernutrition and micronutrient deficiencies persists in many of its countries [16]. Overcoming pediatric and adolescent malnutrition in all of its forms (overnutrition, undernourishment, and micronutrient deficiencies) entails the development of evidence-based interventions and the design of related health policies to ensure the availability of and access to healthy diets. Effective planning for such interventions should be guided by accurate, up-to date and comprehensive data on food consumption patterns and nutrient intakes. The objective of this review is to characterize and assess food consumption patterns and nutrient intakes amongst school-aged children (5–10 years) and adolescents (10–19 years) in countries of the EMR. Findings from this review will characterize food consumption patterns amongst children and adolescents in the EMR and identify prevalent nutrient excesses or inadequacies. It will also contribute to the prioritization of research to address current gaps in knowledge and inform policies and interventions aimed at developing healthy eating habits in these critical periods of the lifecycle.

2. Approach

The literature search covered the EMR, which according to the WHO, includes 21 countries that comprise Afghanistan, Bahrain, Djibouti, Egypt, Iran (Islamic Republic of), Iraq, Jordan, Kuwait, Lebanon, Libyan Arab Jamahiriya, Morocco, Oman, Pakistan, Qatar, Saudi-Arabia, Somalia, Sudan, Syrian Arab Republic, Tunisia, United Arab Emirates (UAE), and Yemen [17].

Dietary intake data including food group, energy, macronutrient, and micronutrient intakes were evaluated and compared with reference intake values and/or guidelines (when available). A comprehensive literature review was conducted, including individual studies and review articles published between 2005 and 2020, which reported on dietary intakes in children and adolescents aged 5–19 years in any country of the EMR. Electronic databases (MedLine, PubMed, Scopus, and Google Scholar) were searched between 15 July 2020, and 15 August 2020. The search was restricted to the English, French, and Arabic languages, and the key terms used in the search strategy were as follows: EMR countries and/or each country alone AND "Diet" OR "Dietary" OR "Nutritional" OR "Nutrient" AND "Intake" OR "Consumption" AND "Children" OR "Child" OR "Adolescent". In addition, for the dietary intake, a narrower search was performed while including the following key terms: "Energy", "Macronutrient", "Carbohydrate", "Fat", "Saturated Fat", "trans-fat" "Protein", "Fiber", "Sugar", "Meats", "Milk", OR "Dairy", "Fruits", "Vegetables", "Candy", OR "Candies", OR "Sweets", "Chips", "Water", "Sugar Sweetened Beverage", "Juice". A parallel search strategy was also adopted for micronutrient intake (including iron, iodine, zinc, copper, calcium, sodium, thiamin, riboflavin, folate, vitamin B12, vitamin A, vitamin D, and vitamin C). The reference lists of the specific studies were also reviewed to identify additional data sources. Studies were retained if they reported on children aged 5 to 18 years; studies reporting on under-five children were excluded. The global school-based student health survey (GSHS) database [18] was also reviewed to obtain data on the consumption of fruits, vegetables, and carbonated beverages.

Data was presented separately for school-aged children (5–10 years) and adolescents (10–19 years). Food groups were classified based on the categories proposed by Keats et al. [19] in their systematic review of dietary intakes amongst adolescent girls in low and middle income countries. Accordingly, the following food categories were adopted: (1) fruits; (2) vegetables; (3) pulses (beans, peas, lentils); (4) grains; (5) dairy; (6) meat, poultry, and fish; (7) fast foods; (8) sweet snacks; (9) salty and fried snacks, and (10) sugar-sweetened beverages (SSBs). Dietary intakes were compared, when possible, with the WHO recommendations. The recommendations of the WHO for a healthy diet include the consumption of at least 400 g, or 5 portions, of fruits and vegetables/day to reduce the risk of NCDs and ensure an adequate daily intake of dietary fiber (>25 g); reducing sodium intake to less than 2 g/day (5 g of salt), total fat intake to less than 30% of energy intake (EI), reducing saturated fat (SFA) intake to less than 10% EI, and trans fat (TFA) to less than 1% EI [20], and replacing them with unsaturated fats including polyunsaturated fats (PUFAs) (6–10% EI), n-6 PUFAs (5–8% EI), and n-3 PUFAs (1–2% EI); consuming protein in the range of 10–15% EI, carbohydrates 55–75% EI, and free sugars (FS) less than 10% EI.

3. Results

3.1. Food Consumption Patterns Amongst Children and Adolescents in the EMR

3.1.1. School-Aged Children

A striking scarcity is noticed with respect to studies investigating food consumption patterns amongst school-aged children in the EMR. Many of the available studies were conducted with the aim of investigating the relationship between dietary factors and health outcome, such as dental caries [21–23], overweight [24,25], elevated blood pressure [26], or anemia [27], in small samples of children. The majority of available studies have reported on whether the child consumes a certain food group (Yes/No) or on only the frequency of intake (per day or per week), which limits the interpretability of the findings.

In the Levant, a national study conducted in Lebanon showed that fast food alone contributed to around 11.3% of daily EI, and this was coupled with a high intake of sweets and SSBs, which provided 10.8% and 6.5% EI, respectively [24]. In the GCC, a study conducted amongst children aged six years and above in the 11 regions of Bahrain (n = 496) reported that only half of the children reported daily consumption of milk and its products and one fourth reported daily consumption of fruits and vegetables [28]. In contrast, daily consumption of soft drinks was reported by 50% of the children and daily consumption of sweets and snacks was reported by 64% of girls and 47% of boys [28]. A study conducted in all the seven emirates of the UAE showed that amongst 6–8 year old children, more than 90% did not meet the MyPyramid recommendations for vegetables and milk/dairy products, 72–89% did not meet the recommendations for fruits, 49–68% did not meet the recommendations for grains, and 64–75% did not meet the recommendations for meat and beans [29]. In the Kingdom of Saudi-Arabia (KSA), a study conducted amongst 7–12 year old children in Al-Baha city indicated that, 69% and 71% of children did not report daily consumption of fruits and vegetables, respectively, and that only 0.9% met the recommended intake levels of fruits and vegetables [30]. This study also showed that 32% of children did not consume milk/dairy products on a daily basis, with only 1.9% adhering to dairy intake recommendations [30]. In Qatar, a study investigating snack consumption amongst 9–10 year old students in Doha showed that the most commonly consumed snacks in the study sample included fruit drinks (consumed by 98.8% of students), and a high percentage of children reported the consumption of potato chips (81.5%), candy and chocolates (41.7%), and pizzas and pies (39.8%), while the least consumed snacks were milk (37.1%) and nuts (0.8%) [31].

Studies conducted in Iran reported a relatively high consumption of fruits and vegetables amongst school-aged children, in the range of 400 g/day [20,32], with more than 60% of children being adherent to the WHO recommendations [33]. In contrast, the consumption of milk and dairy products was reported to be low (0.8 servings/day) [34]. A high consumption of sweet snacks (two servings/day) [32], fats and oils (6.2 servings/day) [34], and salty snacks (1.3–1.4 servings/day) [32] was also noted. The average consumption of grains met the recommendations (7.4 servings/day) [34], but approximately 60% of children reported to consume grains in their refined form [35].

3.1.2. Adolescents

The GSHS database provides country-specific information on the consumption of fruits, vegetables, and carbonated beverages amongst adolescents aged 13–17 years [18]. Figure 1 summarizes data available from EMR countries. Amongst 13–15 year old adolescents, the percentage of students who reported the consumption of fruits and vegetables at least five times/day during the month preceding the survey was low, ranging between 12.6% in Libya and 38.1% in Djibouti. In contrast, higher proportions of adolescents reported the consumption of carbonated soft drinks once or more times/day. These proportions ranged between 30.8% and 66.6% amongst 13–15 year old adolescents and between 31.5% and 56.9% in those aged 16 to 17 year old (Figure 2).

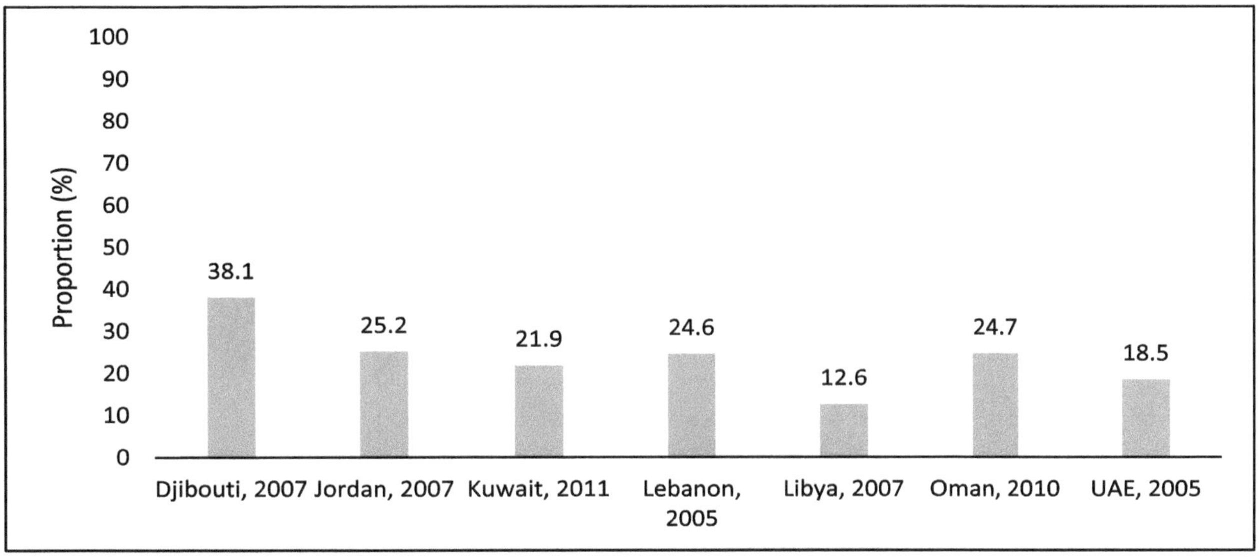

Figure 1. Proportion of students (aged 13–15 years) who had fruits and vegetables at least five times/day during the 30 days preceding the survey, based on the global school-based student health survey (GSHS) database [18].

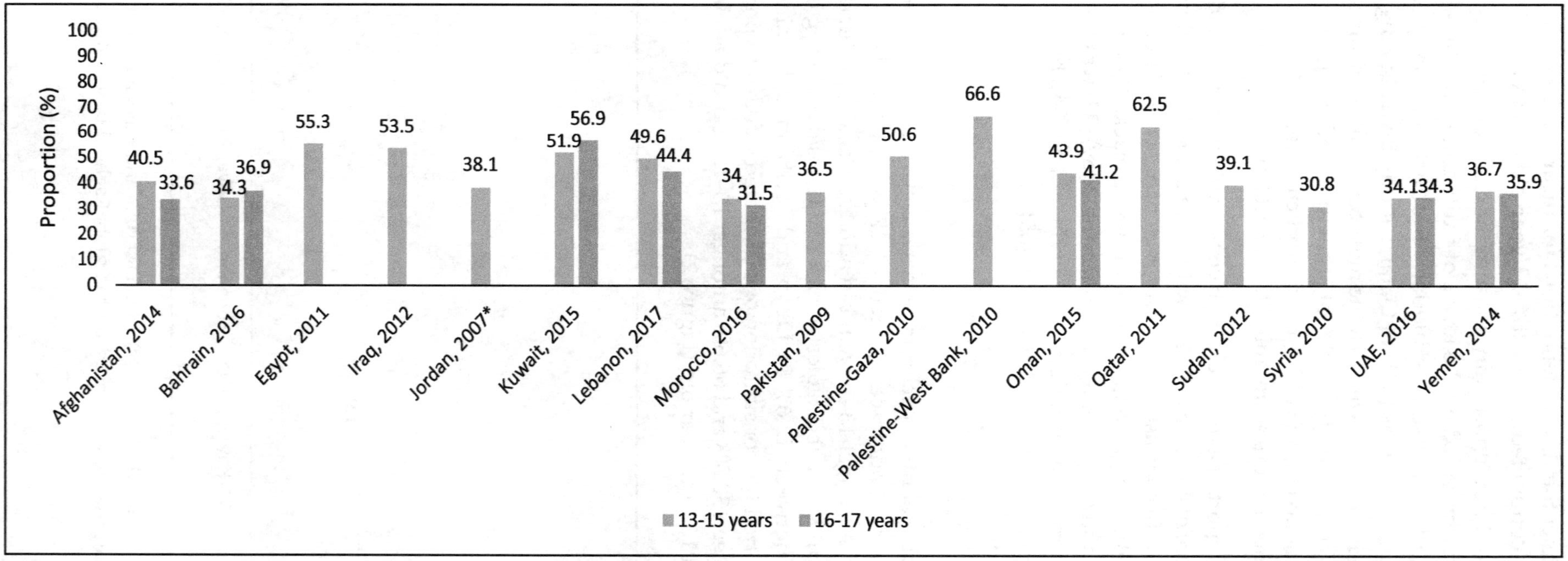

Figure 2. Proportion of students (aged 13–17 years) who drank carbonated soft drinks once or more times per day during the 30 days preceding the survey, based on the global school-based student health survey (GSHS) database [18]. *: This data represents the proportion of students (13–15 years) who drank carbonated soft drinks twice or more times per day during the 30 days preceding the survey in Jordan.

Research studies have also documented suboptimal dietary practices amongst adolescents in the EMR. Table 1, shows that the proportions of adolescents reporting daily intake of fruits ranged between 11% and 33.5% in most countries, except for studies conducted in Iraq [36] and Palestine [37] where higher estimates were reported. The proportions of adolescents reporting daily consumption of vegetables ranged between 20% and 43% in countries like Bahrain, Jordan, Kuwait, Morocco, Qatar, and KSA, while higher estimates were reported from Egypt (78.2%), Iraq (46–62%), Palestine (73%), and Sudan (70%) (Table 1). In Lebanon, a study investigating the diets of adolescents from contrasting socioeconomic backgrounds (n = 209, aged 17–19 years) [38] documented low intakes of vegetables, ranging between 1.4 and 1.9 servings/day, while fruits intake was reported as adequate. Studies conducted in Oman showed that, amongst adolescents, 52–57% consumed less than three servings of vegetables/day [39], and more than a third of adolescents consumed less than two servings of fruits/day [39]. In the UAE, Makansi et al. (2018) indicated that only 28% of adolescents from grades 10–12 (n = 620) met the recommended daily fruit and vegetable intake [40]. In a study conducted amongst 12–16 year old adolescents in Shiraz (Iran), the intake of fruits and vegetables together was estimated at 3.27 servings/day [41].

Food consumption patterns amongst adolescents in the region are also characterized by inadequate intakes of dairy: the proportions reporting daily intake did not exceed a third of adolescents in EMR countries, except for Egypt and Morocco [42–44]. In Muscat, Oman, 76% of adolescent boys and 83% of girls were found to consume less than two servings of dairy/day [39], and in Lebanon, the intake of dairy was estimated to range between 0.5 and 0.7 servings/day [38]. In Iran, Shokrvash et al. (2015) reported that only 14.2% of adolescents met the recommended daily dairy serving consumption, with the average being estimated at 1.64 servings/day [45].

Few studies have assessed the intake of grains and pulses amongst adolescents. In Lebanon and Syria, grains (breads and cereals) were the highest contributor to daily EI, being estimated at 32.7% [24] and 18.4–22% EI [46], respectively. In KSA, the most frequently consumed food items amongst adolescents were grains (rice and breads), with more than 50.5% of adolescents reporting to consume rice at least once daily [47]. Studies conducted in Egypt [42], Iran [48], KSA [49], and Sudan [50], showed that 87–96% of adolescents reported daily consumption of grains (bread, rice, and other cereals). In Muscat, Oman, Waly et al. showed that the proportion of boys and girls consuming less than six servings of grains/day did not exceed one fourth of adolescents [39]. Evidence on the consumption of pulses is scarce. The proportions of adolescents reporting daily consumption of pulses were high in some countries such as Iran (53.8%) [48] and Sudan (64.9%) [51], while estimates from Bahrain [52], Palestine [53], and Jordan [54] ranged between 4% and 19%.

Evidence on the intake of meat, poultry, and fish is also scarce in the region. In Oman, the proportions of adolescents reporting to consume more than three servings of meat, poultry, and fish/day was high, ranging between 68–78% [39]. In Syria, the meat, poultry, and fish group was the second largest contributor to EI (18–21%) [46], while in Lebanon this food group provided 10.2% EI [24]. Despite the fact that the consumption of meat and poultry is frequent in this population group (Table 1), available studies suggest that the intake of fish is suboptimal. Studies conducted in KSA [47,55] reported that half of adolescents did not consume any fish or seafood during the week preceding the survey. In Syria, fish was reported to be rarely consumed by adolescents in Damascus [56], with only 6% consuming it for two times or more/week.

The consumption of high fat, high sugar, high salt foods (HFSS) is common amongst adolescents in the EMR. Table 1 shows that the proportions of adolescents reporting daily intake of SSBs ranged between 37.5% and 80%, except for Palestine and Egypt where these proportions were lower than 20%. A national study in Kuwait [57] has even reported that 43% of adolescents consumed SSBs more than once/day. Country-specific disparities were observed in the proportions of adolescents reporting daily consumption of fast foods, which ranged between 9% and 64% (Table 1). For salty and fried snacks such as potato chips and fries, the proportions of adolescents reporting daily consumption reached as high as 84% in some countries such as Iran (Table 1). Sweet snacks (Cakes/pastries and sweets/chocolates) were also found to be frequently consumed, with the proportions of adolescents reporting daily consumption ranging between 21% and 49% for sweets/chocolates, and exceeding 40% for cakes/pastries in some countries such as Sudan. In Kuwait, Honkola et al. (2006) reported that large proportions of 11–13 years adolescents consumed sweets (42%), SSBs (43%), and cakes (42.5%) several times a day, and that almost every fourth child reported consuming all of these sugary products more than once a day [58]. The frequent consumption of these HFSS suggests that these foods may have significant contributions to EI in adolescents. In Lebanon, fast foods alone were found to contribute 17% EI amongst adolescents [24], and the caloric contribution of sweets and SSBs was estimated at 10% EI and 6.5% EI, respectively [24]. In Syrian adolescents, potato chips alone provided 5% EI and the same was observed for chocolates (5% EI), while sweets and SSBs together provided close to 8% EI [46].

Studies examining water intake amongst adolescents showed that in KSA, close to 60% of 12–15 year old adolescents consumed less than 6 cups of water per day [59] and that water provided only 37% of mean daily fluid intake in 12–13 year old adolescents [60]. Similarly, in Jordan, 74% of 6–18 year olds had fewer than four cups of water daily [61]. A study conducted in Lebanon estimated mean total water intake (TWI) at 1698 mL/day amongst 9–13 years old, and showed that, compared to the adequate intake (AI) level proposed by the Institute of Medicine (IOM) [62], only 5% met the recommendations for daily TWI [63]. In the UAE, mean total daily water intake was estimated at 1116.9 mL amongst 14–18 year old adolescents compared to 922.2 mL amongst 9–13 year olds [64]. The proportion of participants who met the IOM recommendations ranged between 23% and 24% for 9–13 year olds and between 1% and 21% for 14–18 year olds [64].

3.2. *Macronutrient Intakes Amongst School-Aged Children and Adolescents in the EMR*

3.2.1. School-Aged Children

Studies reporting on macronutrient intakes amongst school-aged children in the EMR are scarce. Close to 88% of 6–12 year old children in Cairo met the Recommended Dietary Allowances (RDA) for protein and [71], in Jordan, mean intake of protein ranged between 73% and 85% of the RDA amongst 5–10 year old children from Bedouin or underprivileged communities [27,72]. Another study conducted amongst five year old children from two cities in Jordan reported a high intake of total fat (34.3% EI in boys and 33.8% EI in girls) as well as a high intake of SFA (13.7–14.2% EI) [73]. Fat intake was also found to be high in Lebanese school-aged children, ranging between 35.8% and 39.7% EI, with more than half of the children exceeding the upper level for SFA intake [24,74,75]. In contrast, more than 90% of Lebanese school-aged children did not meet the recommended intakes of alpha-linolenic acid [24,74,76]. In Sudan, Alredaisy and Ibrahim (2011) showed that carbohydrates contributed 58.2% EI amongst rural school-aged children, while noting a high intake level of total fat (32.3% EI) [77]. As for countries of the GCC, a study conducted amongst 6–12 year old girls in KSA [25] showed that protein intake contributed 20.5% EI, while carbohydrates and fat provided 55% and 25.9% EI, repsectively. In the UAE, carbohydrates were reported as the main source of energy in 6–10 year old children (60% of EI) [78]. This level of carbohydrate intake was confirmed by another national study amongst children aged 6 to 13 years in the UAE, where carbohydrates provided 57.4–60.4% of daily EI [29]. It was also reported that 75–92% of participating children had fiber intakes below the requirements [74], 3.7–23% did not meet the protein requirements [74], while 28–46% exceeded the upper level for SFA [29,74].

3.2.2. Adolescents

Macronutrient intakes amongst adolescents in the EMR are displayed, by country, in Table 2.

Average protein intakes reported by the various studies were within the 10–15% range suggested by the WHO. Few countries exceeded this range, and this was particularly true for Oman [79]. In many countries of the region, the intake of total fat exceeded the upper limit of 30% EI, and this was at the expense of carbohydrates.

Table 1. Proportions of adolescents reporting daily consumption (unless otherwise indicated) of various food groups * in countries of the Eastern Mediterranean Region.

Country	Fruits	Vegetables	Dairy	Meat, Poultry, and Fish	Fast Foods	SSBs	Sweet Snacks (Including Confectionary)		Salty and Fried Snacks
							Cakes/Pastries	Sweets/Chocolates	
Bahrain [52] (National)	25.3%	26.3%	37.1%	Meat: 20% Fish: 6.9% Poultry: 18.2%	14.4%	42.2%	–	Sweets: 31.4% Chocolates: 32%	–
Egypt [42]	29%	78.2%	58.9%	–	64.6%	19.7%	–	–	–
Iran [48]	16.2%		16.3%	Meat: 31.9%	–	75.4%	45.5%		84.7%
Iraq [36]	M: 24.3% F: 46.3%	M: 46.1% F: 62.3%	Milk: M: 37.2% F: 35.2%	–	>3 days/w: M: 37.1% F: 24.9%	>3 days/w: M: 66.9% F: 60.4%	>3 days/w: M: 46.1% F: 55%	>3 days/w: M: 43.5% F: 52.2%	>3 days/w: M: 51% F: 64.6%
Jordan [54]	20%	43%	–	1–3 times/w: Meat: 47% Fish: 54% 4–6 times/w: Poultry: 40%	1–3 times/w: 57%	–	–	Chocolates: 40%	–
Kuwait [57]	M: 17.5% F: 11.8%	M: 26% F: 22.1%	M: 36.3% F: 25.3%	–	M: 9.4% F: 10.4%	M: 42.2% F: 37.5%	M: 7% F: 14.7%	M: 21.1% F: 35.6%	Potato fries/chips: M: 9.4%; F: 12.4%
Kuwait [58] (National)	–	–	–	–	–	>1 time/d: 43%	>1 time/d: 42.5%	>1 time/d: 42%	–
Morocco [43,44]	M: 18.7% F: 20.4%	M: 33.1% F: 42.5%	M: 78.1% F: 76.9%	–	>3 times/w: M: 15% F: 12.9%	>3 times/w: M: 37.5% F: 41.9%	>3 times/w: M: 66.9% F: 79%	3 times/w: M: 66.9% F: 72%	>3 times/w: Potato fries/chips: M: 18.8%; F: 29%
Palestine [53]	M: 11.6% F: 16.2%	M: 27.6% F: 34.1%	Milk: M: 33.7% F: 29.9% Yogurt: M: 19.8% F: 20.8%	>3 times/w: Meat: M: 7.3% F: 7.9% Poultry: M: 3.4% F: 3.8%	–	M: 6.2% F: 9.3%	Cookies: M: 14.6% F: 19.6%	Chocolates: M: 10.7% F: 17%	–

Table 1. *Cont.*

Country	Fruits	Vegetables	Dairy	Meat, Poultry, and Fish	Fast Foods	SSBs	Sweet Snacks (Including Confectionary)		Salty and Fried Snacks
							Cakes/Pastries	Sweets/Chocolates	
Palestine [65] (National)	31%	45%	Milk: 22%	Meat and poultry: 16%	–	24%	35%		–
Palestine [37]	M: 58.9% F: 55.2%	M: 72.8% F:73.8%	Milk: M: 32.9% F: 18.3% Yogurt: M: 31.8% F: 28.3%	Meat: M: 11.4% F: 10.7% Poultry: M: 11.9% F: 12.2%	–	M: 39.6% F: 28.4%	M: 42.3% F: 49.2%		Salty snacks: M: 50.3% F: 61.5% Fried potatoes: M: 20.5% F: 23.8%
Qatar [66]	13.9%	20.3%	24.1%	–	≥4 days/w: 27.3%	≥4 days/w: 48.8%	≥4 days/w: 24.5%	≥4 days/w: 49.4%	≥4 days/w: 28.7%
Saudi [67]	M: 16% F: 9.6%	M: 23.3% F: 22.3%	Milk: M: 33.2% F: 25.1%	–	>3 days/w: M: 30.2% F: 24.9%	>3 days/w: M: 67.3% F: 57.4%	>3 days/w: M: 24.8% F: 28.8%	>3 days/w: M: 37.3% F: 52.6%	>3 days/w: M: 25% F: 30.7%
Sudan [50]	M: 33.5% F: 31.9%	M: 70.1% F: 69.7%	–	Meat: M: 55.7% F: 60.7%	–	M: 43.9% F: 44.8%	Sweets: M: 55.4% F: 60.6%	–	Crisps: M: 38.7% F: 39.2% Other salty snacks: M: 42.9% F: 32%
Sudan [51]	>4 times/w: 30.1%	>4 times/w: 63.9%	>4 times/w: 58.1%	>4 times/w: Meat: 59.1% Fish: 11.4% Poultry: 27.8%	>4 times/w: 26.6%	>4 times/w: 43.4%	>4 times/w: 37.1%	>4 times/w: Chocolates: 30.1%	–
Sudan [68]	–	–	–	–	–	80.6%	Dessert: 69.3% Sweet biscuits: 65.3%	Chocolates: 80% Popsicles: 61.4% Sweets: 48.7%	–
UAE [40]	–	–	–	–	≥1 time/w: M: 77.3% F: 81.4%	≥1 time/d: M: 41.1% F: 34%	–	–	–

Abbreviations: SSBs: sugar-sweetened beverages; M: males; F: females; w: week; d: day; UAE: United Arab Emirates. Salty snacks may include potato chips, French fries, popcorn, crackers. *: Food items categorization was adopted and modified based on a review by Keats et al., 2018 [19,69,70]. The following categories were not included in the table due to limited data: Grains, white roots, tubers and plantains; Pulses (beans, peas, lentils); Nuts and seeds; Eggs; Oils and fats.

Adequacy of macronutrient intake was investigated in some of the reviewed studies. In Iran, average protein intake was found to represent 165.4% of the RDA for protein and 154.7% of the WHO recommendations, highlighting an adequate dietary protein intake [80]. In KSA, mean nutrient adequacy ratio (NAR) of protein was estimated at 1.84, which indicates that protein intake met the dietary requirement in the majority of subjects [81]. Another study in KSA showed that mean protein intake (70.8 ± 40.6 g/day) amongst 13–18 year adolescents in Jeddah, was around 1.6 times higher than that recommended by the Academy of Nutrition and Dietetics (44 and 59 g/day for males and females respectively) [82]. In Bahrain, adolescent boys and girls consumed 1.5 times the United Kingdom's (UK's) Reference Nutrient intake (RNI) for protein [28,83], and in Kuwait, 86–92% of adolescents met the Acceptable Macronutrient Distribution range (AMDR) of 10–35% EI for protein [74,84]. In contrast, in Palestine, inadequate protein intake (<80% RDA) was observed amongst 15.1% of boys and 43.1% of girls aged 11–16 years [85], and in Northern Sudan, 50% of adolescents aged 13–18 years had inadequate protein intake (<80% of RDA) [86].

As for the adequacy of intake for the various subtypes of fat intake, a study conducted amongst 10–19 year old adolescents in Iran [87], showed that the average intake of SFA (10.3% EI) was close to the upper limit set by the WHO (10%) [88]. Another study in Iran reported that only a third of 6–18 year old participants, adhered to the WHO recommendations on SFA and half adhered to the recommendations related to PUFAs intakes [33]. Mirmiran et al. (2019) also reported on TFA, estimating its average intake at 2.2% EI, with only 6% of the study participants adhering to the TFA WHO recommendations of less than 1% EI [20,33]. In Lebanon, the average intake of SFA (10.7%) exceeded the WHO upper limit, while the intakes of Linoleic acid (4.8% EI) and Linolenic acid (0.13% EI) were short of the respective AMDRs of 5–10% and 0.6–1.2% EI [74,88,89]. In Palestine, the average intake of SFA amongst 11–16 year old adolescents (10.3% EI) exceeded the WHO maximal intake recommendations particularly amongst boys (12% EI) [85], while the intake of MUFAs (12.2% EI) was below the WHO recommendations of 15–20% EI [85,90]. In the UAE, Ali et al. (2013) showed that amongst 14–18 year old subjects, 12–13% of adolescents exceeded the AMDR for total fat, while 40% of girls and 60% of boys exceeded the 10% upper limit for SFA [29,74]. Similarly, in KSA, the average intake of SFA was high (11.3% EI), while that of MUFAs (10.5% EI) and PUFAs (5.8% EI) were suboptimal [82]. In Kuwait, 31–40% of adolescents exceeded the AMDR for total fat (i.e., 20–35% EI), but only 2–6% of adolescents met the AMDR for n-3 fatty acids, and 16–29% met the AMDR for n-6 fatty acids [74,84]. In Bahrain, the intakes of MUFAs and PUFAs were found to be inadequate, estimated at approximately 9–9.2% EI and 5.2–6.2% EI, respectively [28]. The PUFAs to SFA ratio of 0.6 for both girls and boys in Bahrain, was lower than the usually recommended value of 1, suggesting higher consumption of SFA compared to PUFA sources [28]. In contrast to the previous studies, the intakes of dietary fat subtypes in Tunisia were not far from recommendations, with SFA representing 9% EI, MUFAs 14% EI, and PUFAs 11% EI [91].

The majority of available studies have reported inadequate intake of dietary fiber amongst adolescents. Average dietary fiber intake was estimated at 7.5 g/day in Lebanon [89], 9 g/day in Libya [92], 11.6 g/day in Iran [41], 12.6 g/day in KSA [82], and 12.4–13.5 g/day in Bahrain, which are all considerably lower than the recommendation of the Food and Agriculture (FAO)/WHO of more than 25 g/day [90]. In countries of the GCC, average dietary fiber intake was estimated to range between 16 and 20 g/day amongst adolescents in Kuwait and between 13.6 and 20.7 g/day in the UAE [29,74,84]. The majority of adolescents (81–91% in Kuwait and 95% in UAE) did not meet the AI for fiber. Higher estimates were reported from Northern African countries in the EMR. In Morocco, fiber intake was estimated at 39.6 g/day in adolescent boys and 33.5 g/day in girls, which represented 18.8 g/1000 kcal in boys and 17.7 g/1000 kcal in girls [93,94]. These estimates are considered adequate when compared with the recommendation of 14 g fiber/1000 kcal for optimal cardiovascular health [95]. Similarly, in Tunisia, the average intake of dietary fiber intake was estimated at 36 g/day, thus exceeding the recommended level of >25 g/day [90,91].

Evidence on sugar intake amongst adolescents is very limited. A study conducted in Libya [92] reported that total sugars and FS contributed 20.4% and 12.6% of the daily EI, the latter being above the upper limit set by the WHO (10% EI) [90]. In Bahrain, the mean daily intake of total sugars was estimated to range between 98–114.6 g/day for boys and 85.5–93.8 g/day for girls, which were reported as high when compared with the maximum recommended intake of 60 g/day by the Dietary Reference Values of UK [28,83]. Adolescents aged 10–13 years from KSA were reported to consume high levels of total sugar, providing 26% EI [96]. In Iran, FS intake was estimated at close to 7% EI amongst 6–18 year old children and adolescents, with 81% of boys and 84% of girls adhering to the FS WHO recommendations [20,33].

3.3. Micronutrient Intakes Amongst School-Aged Children and Adolescents in the EMR

3.3.1. School-Aged Children

In Jordan, a study conducted amongst 5–6 year old children [73] showed that mean intakes of several vitamins were below their respective Dietary Reference Intakes (DRIs). More specifically, vitamins A and B12 represented 60–70% of the respective DRIs and similar values were observed for folate (73–75% DRI) and vitamin C (57–60% DRI). Inadequate intakes of calcium (64–68% DRI), iron (66–73% DRI), and zinc (56–60% DRI) were also reported [73]. Other studies conducted in Jordan, especially amongst Bedouins and children from underprivileged areas, reported that mean intakes of iron, calcium, and vitamin A represented 50%, 70%, and 65–80% of their respective RDAs [27,72,102,103]. Similarly, in school-aged children in Lebanon, 84–95%, 73–88%, and 35% did not meet two-thirds of the RDA for vitamin D, calcium, and iron, respectively [76,102,104]. In KSA, mean calcium intakes in children aged 7–12 years old did not exceed 60% of the RDA, and mean vitamin D intake represented only 23% of RDA [102,105]. In the UAE, a national study showed that more than 76% of 6–8 year old children did not meet the respective Estimated Average Requirement (EAR) level for vitamin A, while for vitamin D and vitamin E, more than 93% of 6–8 year old children did not meet the EAR value [29]. In addition, 26% of boys and 43% of girls did not meet the EAR intake level for folate [29]. In Lebanon, a study conducted amongst 5–12 year olds showed that 23% and 95% did not meet 2/3rd of the RDA for vitamin E and D, respectively [76]. In Egypt, 44–76% of 6–12 years old children did not meet 50% RDA for vitamin A [71], and close to a third did not meet 50% RDA for iron and calcium.

High intakes of sodium (Na) coupled with low intakes of potassium (K) were reported by studies in the region. In Iran, mean intakes of Na and K amongst 3–10 year old children were 2017 mg/day and 1119 mg/day, respectively [26], while the recommended intakes in this age group ranged from <1500 to <1900 mg/day and 3000–3800 mg/day, respectively [9]. In Kuwait, 64% of girls and 71% of boys aged 4–8 years, exceeded the Tolerable Upper Intake Level for Na (1900 mg/day) of the IOM [84]. In Morocco, average intake of Na was estimated at 1800 mg/day amongst 6–8 year old children, with 46.7% exceeding the IOM upper limit [106].

3.3.2. Adolescents

Figure 3 illustrates the proportions of adolescents not meeting the recommended intake levels of vitamins A, C, E, D and folate [29,48,85,99]. It is important to note that the data reported by the various studies is not readily comparable given that different studies have used different benchmarks to define nutrient adequacy. Taken together, the data underline suboptimal intakes for the micronutrients in Iran, Pakistan, Palestine and the UAE, with high proportions of adolescents not meeting the recommended nutrient intake levels. Similarly, in KSA, 63% and 87% of adolescents (9–18 year olds) had intakes below EAR for vitamin A and E, respectively [107]. In Lebanon 55.3% of Lebanese children and adolescents (6–19 year olds) did not meet 2/3rd the RDA for vitamin A, with 23–26% also not meeting 2/3rd the RDA for vitamins C and E [89]. Inadequate intakes for thiamin, riboflavin, pyridoxine, vitamin B12 were also reported by some studies in the region [29,48,85].

Table 2. Macronutrients intakes amongst adolescents in countries of the Eastern Mediterranean region.

Country	Study Area	Study Population	Dietary Assessment	CHO (%EI)	Protein (%EI)	Fat (%EI)
Bahrain [28]	11 regions of Bahrain	11–18 year old children and adolescents; $n = 496$	24-HR	M: 45–52.5; F: 52–53	M: 15.5–15.9; F: 15–15.4	M: 31.1–32.5; F: 32.7–33.9
Egypt [97]	Sohag	12–18 year old adolescents; $n = 300$	24-HR	59.1–61.3	15.7–15.9	26.9–28.5
Iran [80]	Lahijan, Northern Iran	14–17 year old girls; $n = 400$	24-HR	59.3	11.9	28.8
Iran [87]	Tehan	10–19 year old girls; $n = 717$	FFQ	–	–	30.6
Iran [48]	Sistan and Baluchistan	14–18 year old girls; $n = 753$	2-day 24-HR	54	14	31.9
Iran [33]	Tehan	6–18 year old; $n = 424$	FFQ	M: 57.2; F: 56.8	M: 12.9; F: 13.2	M: 32.1; F: 32.4
Iran [34]	Isfahan	Primary school and junior high school pupils; $n = 4700$	FFQ	64.1	12	23.8
Kuwait [98]	Different regions in Kuwait	8, 13 and 17 year old students; $n = 588$	Questionnaire	60.6	13	32.2
Kuwait [84]	National	9–18 year old children and adolescents; $n = 614$	24-HR	M: 53–54; F: 53	M: 15; F: 14–15	M: 31–32; F: 32–33
Lebanon [24]	National	12–19 year old adolescents; $n = 498$	24-HR	51.1	13.5	36.2
Lebanon [89]	National	12–19 year old children and adolescents; $n = 3394$	24-HR	51.4	13.4	36
Libya [92]	Benghazi	12 year old adolescents; $n = 180$	3-day food record	54	15.7	30.2
Morocco [93,94]	Ouarzazate	15–18 year old adolescents; $n = 327$	3-day food record	M: 58.8; F: 56.6	M: 12.9; F: 12.1	M: 28.3; F: 31.3
Oman [79]	Muscat	15–18 year old adolescents; $n = 802$	FFQ	M: 55.5; F: 51.1	M: 22.5; F: 18.7	M: 30.4; F: 22.6
Pakistan [99]	Sialkot	Mean age: 14.3 years; $n = 328$	3-day food record	51.5	12.5	36.3
Pakistan [100]	National	6–16 year old children and adolescents; $n = 237$	24-HR	60–74	10–12	18–32
Palestine [85]	East Jerusalem	11–16 year old adolescents; $n = 313$	24-HR	54	12.7	34.7
Saudi-Arabia [101]	Riyadh and Dawadami	17–19 year old adolescents; $n = 600$	24-HR	R: 54.4; U: 54.3	R: 16.9; U: 15.1	R: 29.5; U: 32.8

Table 2. *Cont.*

Country	Study Area	Study Population	Dietary Assessment	CHO (%EI)	Protein (%EI)	Fat (%EI)
Saudi-Arabia [82]	Jeddah	13–18 year old adolescents; $n = 239$	3-day 24-HR	56.6	13	30.5
Sudan [86]	Northern State	10–19 year old adolescents; $n = 401$	24-HR	77.4	12.6	9.9
Tunisia [91]	3 regions in Tunisia	15–19 year old adolescents; $n = 1019$	FFQ	52	12	36
UAE [78]	National	11–18 year old adolescents; $n = 276$	24-HR	M: 59.1; F: 58.2	M: 16; F: 14.9	M: 25.8; F: 27.8
UAE [29]	National	11–18 year old adolescents; $n = 276$	24-HR	–	M: 15–16; F: 14.7–15.3	M: 25.2–26.7; F: 27.6–27.9

Abbreviations: CHO: carbohydrates; EI: energy intake; M: males; F: females; R: rural; U: urban; 24-HR: 24-hr dietary recall; FFQ: food frequency questionnaire.

Figure 4 displays the proportions of adolescents not meeting the recommended intake levels of iron, calcium and zinc. The data suggest that high proportions of adolescents do not meet the recommendations for these nutrients in Iran, Pakistan, Palestine and KSA [48,85,99,107]. A study conducted in Lebanon of 6–19 year old children and adolescents showed that 27% and 36% do not meet 2/3rd the RDA for zinc and iron, respectively, while 77% do not meet two-thirds of the RDA for calcium [89].

Available evidence suggests that sodium (Na) intakes are high in this age group. In Kuwait, 46–61% of females and 73–80% of males aged 9–18 years exceeded the Tolerable Upper Intake Level for Na (2200–2300 mg/day) set by the IOM [84]. Mean Na intakes amongst adolescents in KSA ranged between 2209 and 2250 mg/day, exceeding the AI level (1700 mg/day) and the WHO Upper limit (2000 mg/day) [82,107]. In Morocco, Na intake was estimated at 2193.4 mg/day and 2138.0 mg/day in those aged 9–13 years and 14–18 years, respectively with 26.7–49.3% exceeding the upper intake level set by the IOM [106]. In parallel, low potassium intakes (K) were reported. In Pakistan, 45% of boys and 51% of girls had intakes below the EAR for potassium [99]. In KSA, mean intakes of K ranged between 1530 mg and 1961 mg/day, thus being inferior to the AI of 4500–4700 mg/day [82,107], and 87% of adolescents had intakes less than the AI level for K [107]. In Tunisia, mean K intake was estimated at 1044.5–1053.8 mg/day amongst 15–19 year adolescents [91], and in Morocco, 75% of children and adolescents aged 6–18 year old children and adolescents [106] consumed less than the AI of K [106]. Low intakes of phosphorous, magnesium, manganese, copper and selenium have also been reported by some studies in the region [76,85,99,107].

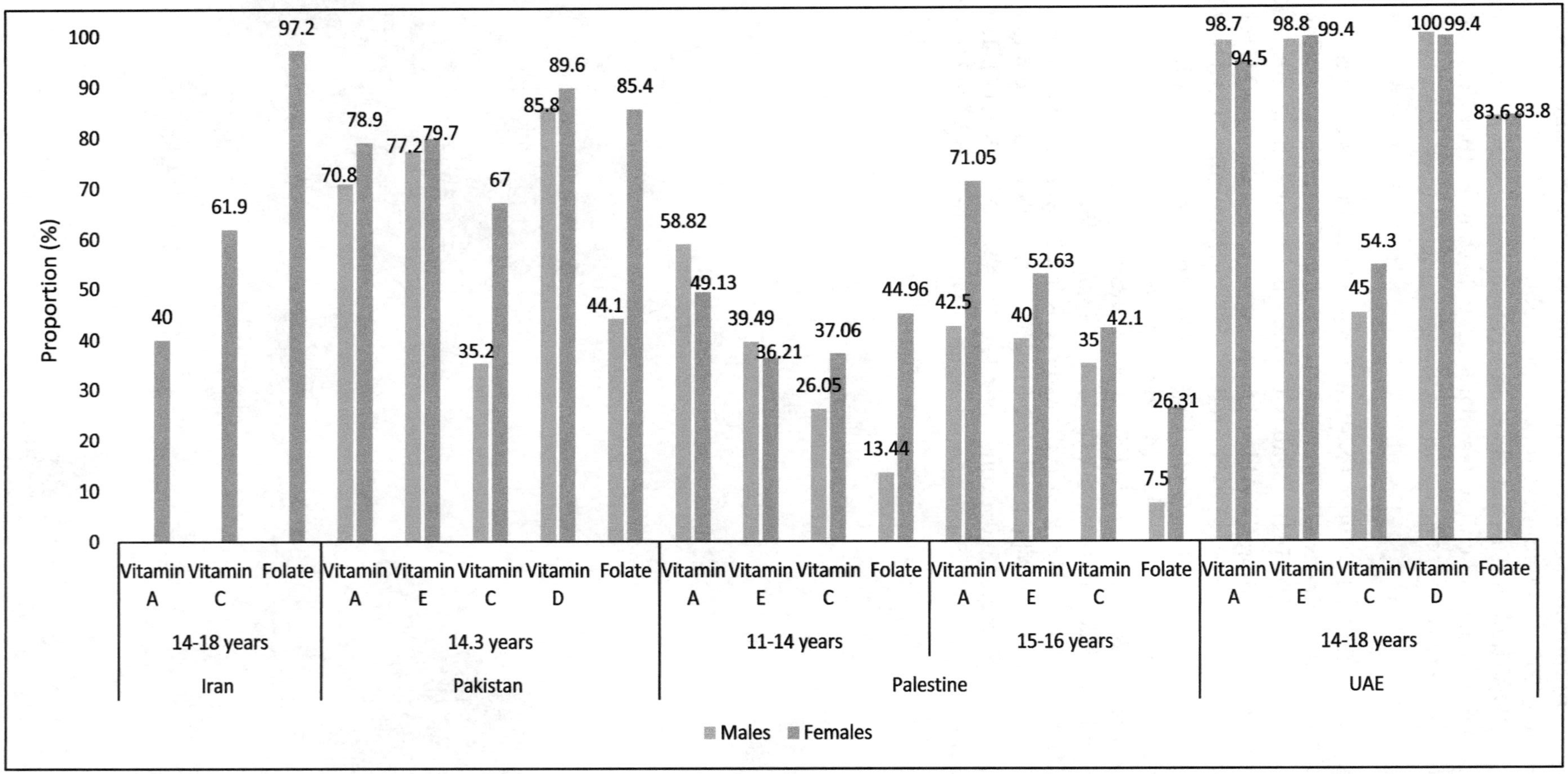

Figure 3. Proportion of adolescents not meeting the recommendations for vitamins A, E, C, D and folate. The criteria used to assess the proportion of adolescents not meeting the recommendation, are as follows: Iran, Recommended Dietary Allowances (RDAs); Pakistan, Estimated Average Requirement (EAR)/Average Intake (AI); Palestine, <80% RDA; United Arab Emirates (UAE), <EAR.

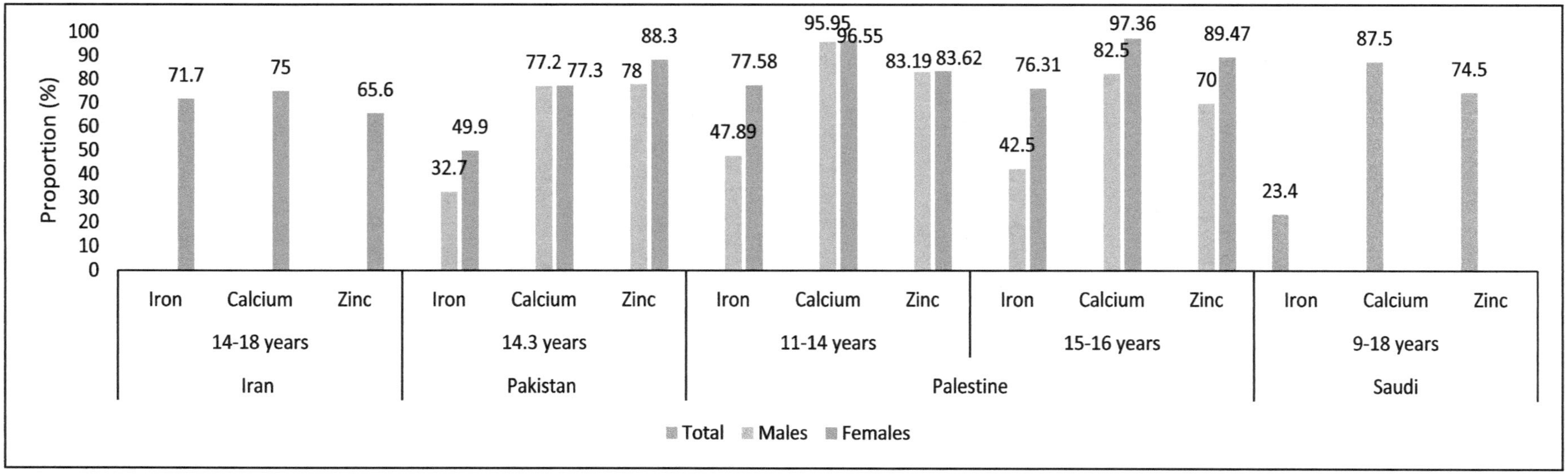

Figure 4. Proportion of adolescents not meeting the recommendation for iron, calcium and zinc. The criteria used to assess the proportion of adolescents not meeting the recommendations, are as follows: Iran, Recommended Dietary Allowances (RDAs); Pakistan, Estimated Average Requirement (EAR)/Average Intake (AI); Palestine, <80% RDA; United Arab Emirates (UAE), <EAR.

4. Discussion

The majority of available studies amongst children and adolescents in the EMR have documented a low intake of fruits, vegetables and fiber, inadequate consumption of water, milk and dairy products, coupled with a high intake of SSBs, and a frequent consumption of energy-dense, nutrient poor foods such as sweet and savory snacks. High intakes of fat and SFA were also observed in several studies conducted in the region, coupled with a number of micronutrient inadequacies, particularly low intakes of calcium, iron, and zinc and vitamins A, D, C and folate.

These food consumption and dietary intake patterns may be linked with suboptimal nutritional status and increased risk for obesity and cardiometabolic risk factors. This is of concern to the EMR given that the region harbors a "triple" burden of malnutrition in children and adolescents, characterized by the persistence of undernutrition, an alarming escalating burden of overweight and obesity, and a high prevalence of micronutrient deficiencies [108,109]. A recent review showed that the estimated weighted regional averages for stunting, wasting and underweight were 28%, 8.69% and 18%, respectively [109]. The prevalence of anemia was found to range between 16% and 81% amongst school-aged children and adolescents in countries of the region, while that of vitamin D deficiency ranged between 21% and 83% [109]. Several countries in the EMR reported an increasing trend in the prevalence of overweight and obesity amongst school-aged children and adolescents, the highest increases being reported from Iran [110,111], Lebanon [112], Qatar [113,114], Saudi Arabia [115–117], Tunisia [118] and Bahrain [119,120]. The prevalence of obesity amongst school-aged children and adolescents reached as high as 29.6% in Kuwait [121] and 21.7% in Bahrain [122]. The escalating and high prevalence of child and adolescent obesity raises questions about its implications for disease burden in the region, given its association with metabolic syndrome, insulin resistance, hypertension, dyslipidemia and hyperglycemia [121,123]. Studies conducted in various EMR countries reported a high prevalence of metabolic syndrome in obese children and adolescents, ranging between 15% and 30% in countries of the Levant and reaching as high as 44% in countries of the GCC, such as the UAE [7,8,124–126]. With those younger than 14 years representing approximately 30% of the population of the EMR, these estimates do not bode well for the future health and well-being of the population, and the development and building of productive societies [108].

The faulty dietary practices documented in this review, and which are in many instances similar to those reported by Keats et al. in low and middle income countries [19], may at least partially explain the increase in pediatric and adolescent adiposity and the persistence of undernutrition in the EMR. For instance, low intakes of fruit and vegetables may be a risk factor for obesity. In fact, available evidence suggests that adequate consumption of fruits and vegetables is usually associated with lower EI and higher intakes of dietary fiber which, through colonic, intrinsic, and/or hormonal effects may be associated with increased satiety, increased fat oxidation, and increased insulin sensitivity, all of which may contribute to the prevention of obesity and metabolic abnormalities [95,127–129]. In addition, high intake of SSBs can promote weight gain through their low satiety, incomplete compensatory reduction in EI at subsequent meals and high content of added sugar [130]. On average, SSBs provide approximately 140–150 calories and 35.0–37.5 g of sugar per 12-oz serving [131]. In addition, fructose from sucrose or from high corn fructose syrup has been linked with the development of visceral adiposity and ectopic fat deposition [132–135]. Several societies and organizations including the American Academy of Pediatrics and the WHO have advocated for reductions in the intake of SSBs to help prevent obesity and enhance overall health [136]. The observed high intakes of fat and SFA may also be linked with the burden of obesity in the region, given their high energy density and the promotion of adipogenesis [137]. The overall food consumption pattern that is low in fruit and vegetables, while being high in high fat, high sugar foods and beverages, is a hallmark of the western dietary pattern, which has been repetitively shown to be associated with increased adiposity risk [138]. At the same time, such food consumption and dietary patterns are associated with low dietary diversity, insufficient consumption of nutrient dense foods and suboptimal micronutrient intakes, which may at least partially explain the persistent burden of undernutrition and micronutrient deficiencies in countries of the EMR. The observed high intake of sodium, coupled with low intakes of potassium, is recognized as a risk factor for raised blood pressure in childhood and adolescents, and may increase the risk for hypertension and cardiovascular disease later in life [139].

Numerous factors may influence the diets of children and adolescents. These comprise both individual and socio-cultural factors as well as economic and environmental factors [140]. At the individual level, poor nutritional knowledge may be associated with unhealthy dietary practices. Studies conducted in countries of the region have documented significant nutrition knowledge gaps in children and adolescents, especially in what relates to nutrient sources, the identification of healthy snacks and diet-disease relationships [38,141,142]. Other factors such as personal likings, taste preferences, self-efficacy, and body image [143–146] may also play an important role in shaping the dietary practices in this age group [140]. Children and adolescents are also highly affected by the food environment, including the affordability, availability, and access to foods [140,147–151]. Marketing and advertising of ultra-processed foods with a high content of fat, sugar and/or salt to children and adolescents was also recognized as a factor that promotes suboptimal diets amongst children and adolescents [140,152]. Studies conducted in countries of the region have shown that the marketing of ultra-processed, nutrient-depleted foods is highly common on television, during children's programs and/or children's viewing time [153,154].

The WHO developed several standards and guidelines for health policies, strategies and interventions aimed at improving the nutrition status of children and adolescents. Aligned with the SDGs, and guided by the Global Strategy for Women's Children's and Adolescent's Health (2016–2030), the WHO Child and Adolescent Health and Nutrition program aims to translate global nutrition guidelines into actions to address the double burden of malnutrition in various countries of the world, build capacity for the monitoring of health and nutrition status, and develop evidence-based policies that contribute to the improvement of health and nutrition of children and adolescents [2]. The WHO has also established the nutrition-friendly school initiative that provides a framework for ensuring integrated school-based programs that address the double-burden of nutrition-related ill health [155], and has further articulated priorities related to adolescent nutrition in the Global Accelerated Action for the Health of Adolescents [156]. In line with its mandate, the regional office of the WHO has been active in shaping the policy environment in Member States, emphasizing the need for policies and initiatives that promote a healthier food environment for the population, with a focus on children and adolescents. The WHO EMR published, in 2018, a set of recommendations on the marketing of food and non-alcoholic beverages to children in the region [157]. The recommendations aim to guide Member States on the promotion of responsible marketing and the regulation of the marketing of foods and beverages that are high in saturated fat, trans fat, free sugar or salt to children [157]. Countries that have adopted legislation that contributes to the implementation of these recommendations include Egypt, Iran and Saudi Arabia. The WHO Regional Strategy (2020–2030) [158] also provides a comprehensive framework for regional and national efforts to reach the various targets on nutrition, including the promotion of healthier diets amongst children and adolescents. It has mapped existent nutrition policies in the region and showed that the main action areas included in nutrition policies across the region are infant and young child nutrition (84%), school health and nutrition programs (84%), healthy diet awareness (84%), vitamin and mineral nutrition (79%), acute malnutrition (53%) and nutrition and infectious diseases (37%). In addition, the Regional framework for action on obesity prevention 2019–2023 [159] provides a set of strategic interventions and progress indicators related to fiscal measures, public procurement, food supply and trade, food labeling, physical activity promotion, mass media campaigns, and product reformulation, coupled with continuous assessment and monitoring to help Member states in their obesity prevention efforts. Moreover, the WHO EMR office has issued several policy statements related to lowering sugar, fat and salt intakes in countries of the EMR [160–162], providing a road map for countries of the region for the progressive and sustainable reduction in national intakes of sugar, fat and salt. Despite the active policy response in several countries of the EMR, recent reports [140,163] are highlighting the need for a broader food system approach in order to improve the diets of children and adolescents. To better address the nutritional needs of children and adolescents, the food system should be leveraged and aligned along its four determinants (food supply chains, external food environments, personal food environments, and behaviors of caregivers, children and adolescents) to improve the quality of the diet in this age group [140].

5. Missing Knowledge and Future Research

Although this review has provided valuable insight into food consumption patterns and dietary intakes amongst school-aged children and adolescents in the EMR, it has identified several challenges and gaps in the existing dietary assessment studies. In particular, findings on food consumption patterns were often limited by the scarcity of data, particularly in school-aged children. This knowledge gap has been reported by the United Nations Children's Fund (UNICEF) [140], stating that the age group of school-aged children is often missing from health and nutrition surveys. The fact that most of the available studies have reported on daily or weekly frequency of intake, rather than quantifying consumption, has also often limited the interpretability of the data. Another challenge stemmed from the fact that most of the available studies were conducted at a small or regional scale, with only few countries having conducted national surveys on food consumption in children and adolescents. Political instabilities and turmoil, coupled with limited research funding, are amongst the challenges that some countries of the region are facing and that may contribute to the scarcity of nationally representative data. It is also important to mention that dietary assessment in many countries of the region may be limited by the availability of complete and up-to-date food composition tables, particularly for traditional foods and composite dishes, highlighting the crucial need for concerted efforts in this domain. The findings of this review may also be limited by the fact that different dietary assessment methods (food frequency questionnaires, FFQ; 24-hr recalls, 24-HR; dietary records) were used by the various countries/studies, which may impact the comparability of the generated food consumption data [108].

Based on the work undertaken in this paper, opportunities for future research include regional collaborations to: (1) consolidate and update food composition tables, with a focus on culture-specific foods and composite dishes; (2) conduct nationwide dietary surveys on children and adolescents using validated and standardized approaches and methodologies; (3) contribute to a better characterization of food consumption patterns and dietary intakes in under-represented age groups, such as school-aged children; (4) assess the intake and sources of free sugar; (5) assess the intake and sources of trans fat; and (6) gain a better understanding of factors that may be associated with unhealthy food consumption patterns in the EMR. These priorities may guide policy makers, researchers, funding agencies, and non-governmental organizations in tackling the identified knowledge gaps and developing culture specific and evidence-based intervention strategies aimed at improving the nutritional status of children in the EMR.

6. Conclusions

This review contributes toward the characterization of food consumption patterns and dietary intakes amongst children and adolescents in the EMR. The findings highlighted poor dietary habits in these age groups characterized by low intakes of fruit, vegetables, and dairy coupled with high intakes of SSBs and frequent consumption of sweets and savory snacks. High intakes of fat and saturated fat were observed, while the intakes of several micronutrients were inadequate. These suboptimal food consumption and dietary intake patterns represent a public health concern, given that the triple burden of malnutrition continues to plague most countries of the region. The findings of this review have therefore broad implications for developing public health strategies and policies to improve the diet of children and adolescents in the EMR. Acknowledging the impact that nutrition may have on building societies and transforming the lives of children, adolescents and their families, there is a crucial need for a food system approach in developing and implementing national and regional policies and interventions aimed at improving the diet of children and adolescents. Such interventions will not only enhance the diet and nutritional status of young people, but will also pave the way towards the achievement of many sustainable development goal targets, including ensuring healthy lives, promoting life-long learning, improving economic growth and building inclusive societies [164].

Author Contributions: Conceptualization, A.A.-J. and L.N.; methodology, L.N.; investigation, A.A.-J. and L.N.; resources, A.A.-J. and L.N.; data curation, M.T.; writing—original draft preparation, L.N.; writing—review and editing, M.T. and A.A.-J.; supervision, A.A.-J. and L.N.; project administration, A.A.-J.; funding acquisition, A.A.-J. All authors have read and agreed to the published version of the manuscript.

References

1. World Health Organization Regional Office for Europe. *Fact Sheets on Sustainable Development Goals: Health Targets: Child and Adolescent Health*; WHO: Copenhagen, Denmark, 2017.
2. World Health Organization Regional Office for Africa. Child and Adolescent Health and Nutrition (CAN) Program. Available online: https://www.afro.who.int/about-us/programmes-clusters/CAN (accessed on 8 October 2020).
3. Institute of Medicine. Nutrition-Related Health Concerns, Dietary Intakes, and Eating Behaviors of Children and Adolescents. In *Nutrition Standards for Foods in Schools: Leading the Way Toward Healthier Youth*; The National Academies Press: Washington, DC, USA, 2007. [CrossRef]
4. Story, M.; Holt, K.; Sofka, D. *Bright Futures in Practice*, 2nd ed.; National Center for Education in Maternal and Child Health: Arlington, VA, USA, 2002.
5. Daniels, S.R. The consequences of childhood overweight and obesity. *Future Child* **2006**, *16*, 47–67. [CrossRef]
6. Institute of Medicine. *Preventing Childhood Obesity: Health in the Balance*; The National Academies Press: Washington, DC, USA, 2005.
7. Nasreddine, L.; Naja, F.; Tabet, M.; Habbal, M.-Z.; El-Aily, A.; Haikal, C.; Sidani, S.; Adra, N.; Hwalla, N. Obesity is associated with insulin resistance and components of the metabolic syndrome in Lebanese adolescents. *Ann. Hum. Biol.* **2012**, *39*, 122–128. [CrossRef]
8. Nasreddine, L.; Ouaijan, K.; Mansour, M.; Adra, N.; Sinno, D.; Hwalla, N. Metabolic syndrome and insulin resistance in obese prepubertal children in Lebanon: A primary health concern. *Ann. Nutr. Metab.* **2010**, *57*, 135–142. [CrossRef]
9. Gidding, S.S.; Dennison, B.A.; Birch, L.L.; Daniels, S.R.; Gilman, M.W.; Lichtenstein, A.H.; Rattay, K.T.; Steinberger, J.; Stettler, N.; Van Horn, L. Dietary recommendations for children and adolescents: A guide for practitioners: Consensus statement from the American Heart Association. *Circulation* **2005**, *112*, 2061–2075. [CrossRef]
10. World Health Organization. *Technical paper. Regional strategy on nutrition 2010–2019. Regional Committee for the Eastern Mediterranean. Fifty-Seventh Session. Agenda Item 4 (b)*; WHO: Geneva, Switzerland, 2010.
11. Nasreddine, L.; Naja, F.; Sibai, A.-M.; Helou, K.; Adra, N.; Hwalla, N. Trends in nutritional intakes and nutrition-related cardiovascular disease risk factors in Lebanon: The need for immediate action. *Leb. Med. J.* **2014**, *103*, 1–9. [CrossRef]
12. Popkin, B.M.; Adair, L.S.; Ng, S.W. Global nutrition transition and the pandemic of obesity in developing countries. *Nutr. Rev.* **2012**, *70*, 3–21. [CrossRef]
13. World Health Organization Regional Office for the Eastern Mediterranean. Nutrition. Available online: http://www.emro.who.int/health-topics/nutrition/index.html (accessed on 26 August 2020).
14. Rahim, H.F.A.; Sibai, A.; Khader, Y.; Hwalla, N.; Fadhil, I.; Alsiyabi, H.; Mataria, A.; Mendis, S.; Mokdad, A.H.; Husseini, A. Non-communicable diseases in the Arab world. *Lancet* **2014**, *383*, 356–367. [CrossRef]
15. Moghames, P.; Hammami, N.; Hwalla, N.; Yazbeck, N.; Shoaib, H.; Nasreddine, L.; Naja, F. Validity and reliability of a food frequency questionnaire to estimate dietary intake among Lebanese children. *Nutr. J.* **2015**, *15*, 4. [CrossRef]
16. Bagchi, K. Nutrition in the eastern Mediterranean region of the World Health Organization. *East. Mediterr. Health J.* **2008**, *14*, S107–S113.

17. World Health Organization Regional Office for the Eastern Mediterranean. Countries in the Eastern Mediterranean Region. Available online: http://www.emro.who.int/countries.html (accessed on 15 July 2020).
18. World Health Organization. Global School-Based Student Health Survey (GSHS). Available online: https://www.who.int/ncds/surveillance/gshs/factsheets/en/ (accessed on 11 August 2020).
19. Keats, E.C.; Rappaport, A.I.; Shah, S.; Oh, C.; Jain, R.; Bhutta, Z.A. The dietary intake and practices of adolescent girls in low-and middle-income countries: A systematic review. *Nutrients* **2018**, *10*, 1978. [CrossRef]
20. World Health Organization. *Healthy Diet FACT SHEET N°394*; WHO: Geneva, Switzerland, 2015.
21. Abbass, M.M.; Mahmoud, S.A.; El Moshy, S.; Rady, D.; AbuBakr, N.; Radwan, I.A.; Ahmed, A.; Abdou, A.; Al Jawaldeh, A. The prevalence of dental caries among Egyptian children and adolescences and its association with age, socioeconomic status, dietary habits and other risk factors. A cross-sectional study. *F1000Research* **2019**, *8*, 1–19. [CrossRef] [PubMed]
22. Hashim, R.; Williams, S.M.; Murray Thomson, W. Diet and caries experience among preschool children in Ajman, United Arab Emirates. *Eur. J. Oral. Sci.* **2009**, *117*, 734–740. [CrossRef] [PubMed]
23. Jaghasi, I.; Hatahet, W.; Dashash, M. Dietary patterns and oral health in schoolchildren from Damascus, Syrian Arab Republic. *East. Mediterr. Health J.* **2012**, *18*, 358–364. [CrossRef]
24. Nasreddine, L.; Naja, F.; Akl, C.; Chamieh, M.C.; Karam, S.; Sibai, A.-M.; Hwalla, N. Dietary, lifestyle, and socio-economic correlates of overweight, obesity and central obesity in Lebanese children and adolescents. *Nutrients* **2014**, *6*, 1038–1062. [CrossRef]
25. Hasanein, M.A.; Jawad, S.H.A. Prevalence of obesity and risk factors among female school-aged children in primary school in Madinah Munawarah. *Life Sci. J.* **2014**, *11*.
26. Kelishadi, R.; Gheisari, A.; Zare, N.; Farajian, S.; Shariatinejad, K. Salt intake and the association with blood pressure in young Iranian children: First report from the middle East and north Africa. *Int. J. Prev. Med.* **2013**, *4*, 475.
27. Khatib, I.; Elmadfa, I. High prevalence rates of anemia, vitamin A deficiency and stunting imperil the health status of Bedouin schoolchildren in North Badia, Jordan. *Ann. Nutr. Metab.* **2009**, *55*, 358–367. [CrossRef]
28. Gharib, N.; Rasheed, P. Energy and macronutrient intake and dietary pattern among school children in Bahrain: A cross-sectional study. *Nutr. J.* **2011**, *10*, 62. [CrossRef]
29. Ali, H.I.; Ng, S.W.; Zaghloul, S.; Harrison, G.G.; Qazaq, H.S.; El Sadig, M.; Yeatts, K. High proportion of 6 to 18-year-old children and adolescents in the United Arab Emirates are not meeting dietary recommendations. *Nutr. Res.* **2013**, *33*, 447–456. [CrossRef]
30. Alsubaie, A.S.R. Intake of fruit, vegetables and milk products and correlates among school boys in Saudi Arabia. *Int. J. Adolesc. Med. Health* **2018**, *1*. [CrossRef]
31. Hassan, A.S.; Al-Dosari, S.N. Breakfast habits and snacks consumed at school among Qatari schoolchildren aged 9–10 years. *Nutr. Food Sci.* **2008**, *38*, 264–270. [CrossRef]
32. Amini, M.; Dadkhah-Piraghaj, M.; Abtahi, M.; Abdollahi, M.; Houshiarrad, A.; Kimiagar, M. Nutritional assessment for primary school children in Tehran: An evaluation of dietary pattern with emphasis on snacks and meals consumption. *Int. J. Prev. Med.* **2014**, *5*, 611. [PubMed]
33. Mirmiran, P.; Ziadlou, M.; Karimi, S.; Hosseini-Esfahani, F.; Azizi, F. The association of dietary patterns and adherence to WHO healthy diet with metabolic syndrome in children and adolescents: Tehran lipid and glucose study. *BMC Public Health* **2019**, *19*, 1457. [CrossRef]
34. Naeeni, M.M.; Jafari, S.; Fouladgar, M.; Heidari, K.; Farajzadegan, Z.; Fakhri, M.; Karami, P.; Omidi, R. Nutritional knowledge, practice, and dietary habits among school children and adolescents. *Int. J. Prev. Med.* **2014**, *5*, S171. [CrossRef]
35. Kelishadi, R.; Ardalan, G.; Gheiratmand, R.; Gouya, M.M.; Razaghi, E.M.; Delavari, A.; Majdzadeh, R.; Heshmat, R.; Motaghian, M.; Barekati, H. Association of physical activity and dietary behaviours in relation to the body mass index in a national sample of Iranian children and adolescents: CASPIAN Study. *Bull. World Health Organ.* **2007**, *85*, 19–26. [CrossRef]
36. Musaiger, A.O.; Al-Mufty, B.A.; Al-Hazzaa, H.M. Eating habits, inactivity, and sedentary behavior among adolescents in Iraq: Sex differences in the hidden risks of noncommunicable diseases. *Food Nutr. Bull.* **2014**, *35*, 12–19. [CrossRef] [PubMed]

37. Mikki, N.; Abdul-Rahim, H.F.; Shi, Z.; Holmboe-Ottesen, G. Dietary habits of Palestinian adolescents and associated sociodemographic characteristics in Ramallah, Nablus and Hebron governorates. *Public Health Nutr.* **2010**, *13*, 1419–1429. [CrossRef]
38. Nabhani-Zeidan, M.; Naja, F.; Nasreddine, L. Dietary intake and nutrition-related knowledge in a sample of Lebanese adolescents of contrasting socioeconomic status. *Food Nutr. Bull.* **2011**, *32*, 75–83. [CrossRef]
39. Waly, I.; Zayed, K.; Al Haddabi, B. Obesity, eating habits and sedentary behaviour of Omani young adolescents: A cross-sectional study. *EC Nutr.* **2017**, *7*, 3–10.
40. Makansi, N.; Allison, P.; Awad, M.; Bedos, C. Fruit and vegetable intake among Emirati adolescents: A mixed methods study. *East. Mediterr. Health J.* **2018**, *24*. [CrossRef]
41. Hejazi, N.; Mazloom, Z. Socioeconomic status, youth's eating patterns and meals consumed away from home. *Pak. J. Biol. Sci.* **2009**, *12*, 730. [PubMed]
42. Abdel-Hady, D.; El-Gilany, A.-H.; Sarraf, B. Dietary habits of adolescent students in Mansoura, Egypt. *Int. J. Collab. Res. Intern. Med. Public Health* **2014**, *6*, 132.
43. El Achhab, Y.; Marfa, A.; Echarbaoui, I.; Chater, R.; El-Haidani, A.; Filali-Zegzouti, Y. Physical inactivity, sedentary behaviors and dietary habits among Moroccan adolescents in secondary school. *Sci. Sport* **2018**, *33*, 58–62. [CrossRef]
44. Hamrani, A.; Mehdad, S.; El Kari, K.; El Hamdouchi, A.; El Menchawy, I.; Belghiti, H.; El Mzibri, M.; Musaiger, A.O.; Al-Hazzaa, H.M.; Hills, A.P. Physical activity and dietary habits among Moroccan adolescents. *Public Health Nutr.* **2015**, *18*, 1793–1800. [CrossRef] [PubMed]
45. Shokrvash, B.; Salehi, L.; Akbari, M.H.; Mamagani, M.E.; Nedjat, S.; Asghari, M.; Majlessi, F.; Montazeri, A. Social support and dairy products intake among adolescents: A study from Iran. *BMC Public Health* **2015**, *15*, 1078. [CrossRef]
46. Nasreddine, L.; Mehio-Sibai, A.; Mrayati, M.; Adra, N.; Hwalla, N. Adolescent obesity in Syria: Prevalence and associated factors. *Child Care Health Dev.* **2010**, *36*, 404–413. [CrossRef]
47. Mahfouz, A.A.; Shatoor, A.S.; Hassanein, M.A.; Mohamed, A.; Farheen, A. Gender differences in cardiovascular risk factors among adolescents in Aseer Region, southwestern Saudi Arabia. *J. Saudi Heart Assoc.* **2012**, *24*, 61–67. [CrossRef]
48. Montazerifar, F.; Karajibani, M.; Dashipour, A.R. Evaluation of dietary intake and food patterns of adolescent girls in Sistan and Baluchistan Province, Iran. *Funct. Foods Health Dis.* **2012**, *2*, 62–71. [CrossRef]
49. Sachithananthan, V.; Gad, N. A Study on the Frequency of Food Consumption and Its Relationship to BMI in School Children and Adolescents in Abha City, KSA. *Cur. Res. Nutr. Food Sci.* **2016**, *4*, 203. [CrossRef]
50. Moukhyer, M.E.; van Eijk, J.T.; De Vries, N.K.; Bosma, H. Health-related behaviors of Sudanese adolescents. *Educ. Health* **2008**, *21*, 184.
51. Musaiger, A.O.; Nabag, F.O.; Al-Mannai, M. Obesity, dietary habits, and sedentary behaviors among adolescents in Sudan: Alarming risk factors for chronic diseases in a poor country. *Food Nutr. Bull.* **2016**, *37*, 65–72. [CrossRef] [PubMed]
52. Musaiger, A.; Bader, Z.; Al-Roomi, K.; D'Souza, R. Dietary and lifestyle habits amongst adolescents in Bahrain. *Food Nutr. Res.* **2011**, *55*, 7122. [CrossRef]
53. Abudayya, A.H.; Stigum, H.; Shi, Z.; Abed, Y.; Holmboe-Ottesen, G. Sociodemographic correlates of food habits among school adolescents (12–15 year) in North Gaza Strip. *BMC Public Health* **2009**, *9*, 185. [CrossRef]
54. Dalky, H.F.; Al Momani, M.H.; Al-Drabaah, T.K.; Jarrah, S. Eating habits and associated factors among adolescent students in Jordan. *Clin. Nurs. Res.* **2017**, *26*, 538–552. [CrossRef]
55. Mahfouz, A.A.; Abdelmoneim, I.; Khan, M.Y.; Daffalla, A.A.; Diab, M.M.; Al-Gelban, K.S.; Moussa, H. Obesity and related behaviors among adolescent school boys in Abha City, Southwestern Saudi Arabia. *J. Trop. Pediatr.* **2008**, *54*, 120–124. [CrossRef] [PubMed]
56. Musaiger, A.O.; Kalam, F. Dietary habits and lifestyle among adolescents in Damascus, Syria. *Ann. Agric. Environ. Med.* **2014**, *21*. [CrossRef] [PubMed]
57. Allafi, A.; Al-Haifi, A.R.; Al-Fayez, M.A.; Al-Athari, B.I.; Al-Ajmi, F.A.; Al-Hazzaa, H.M.; Musaiger, A.O.; Ahmed, F. Physical activity, sedentary behaviours and dietary habits among Kuwaiti adolescents: Gender differences. *Public Health Nutr.* **2014**, *17*, 2045–2052. [CrossRef]
58. Honkala, S.; Honkala, E.; Al-Sahli, N. Consumption of sugar products and associated life-and school-satisfaction and self-esteem factors among schoolchildren in Kuwait. *Acta Odontol. Scand.* **2006**, *64*, 79–88. [CrossRef]

59. Al Muammar, M.; El Shafie, M. Association between dietary habits and body mass index of adolescent females in intermediate schools in Riyadh, Saudi Arabia. *East. Mediterr. Health J.* **2014**, *20*, 39–45. [CrossRef]
60. Bello, L.; Al-Hammad, N. Pattern of fluid consumption in a sample of Saudi Arabian adolescents aged 12–13 years. *Int. J. Paediatr. Dent.* **2006**, *16*, 168–173. [CrossRef]
61. Subih, H.S.; Abu-Shquier, Y.; Bawadi, H.; Al-Bayyari, N. Assessment of body weight, maternal dietary knowledge and lifestyle practices among children and adolescents in north Jordan. *Public Health Nutr.* **2018**, *21*, 2803–2810. [CrossRef]
62. Institute of Medicine; Food and Nutrition Board. Dietary Reference Intakes for Water, Potassium, Sodium, Chloride, and Sulfate. Available online: https://www.nal.usda.gov/sites/default/files/fnic_uploads/water_full_report.pdf (accessed on 10 September 2020).
63. Jomaa, L.; Hwalla, N.; Constant, F.; Naja, F.; Nasreddine, L. Water and beverage consumption among children aged 4–13 years in Lebanon: Findings from a National Cross-Sectional Study. *Nutrients* **2016**, *8*, 554. [CrossRef]
64. Ali, H.I.; Al Dhaheri, A.S.; Elmi, F.; Ng, S.W.; Zaghloul, S.; Ohuma, E.O.; Qazaq, H.S. Water and Beverage Consumption among a Nationally Representative Sample of Children and Adolescents in the United Arab Emirates. *Nutrients* **2019**, *11*, 2110. [CrossRef] [PubMed]
65. Al Sabbah, H.; Vereecken, C.; Kolsteren, P.; Abdeen, Z.; Maes, L. Food habits and physical activity patterns among Palestinian adolescents: Findings from the national study of Palestinian schoolchildren (HBSC-WBG2004). *Public Health Nutr.* **2007**, *10*, 739–746. [CrossRef]
66. Kerkadi, A.; Sadig, A.H.; Bawadi, H.; Al Thani, A.A.M.; Al Chetachi, W.; Akram, H.; Al-Hazzaa, H.M.; Musaiger, A.O. The relationship between lifestyle factors and obesity indices among adolescents in Qatar. *Int. J. Environ. Res. Public Health* **2019**, *16*, 4428. [CrossRef]
67. Al-Hazzaa, H.M.; Abahussain, N.A.; Al-Sobayel, H.I.; Qahwaji, D.M.; Musaiger, A.O. Physical activity, sedentary behaviors and dietary habits among Saudi adolescents relative to age, gender and region. *Int. J. Behav. Nutr. Phys. Act.* **2011**, *8*, 140. [CrossRef]
68. Nazik, M.; Malde, M.; Ahmed, M.; Trovik, T. Correlation between caries experience in Sudanese school children and dietary habits, according to a food frequency questionnaire and a modified 24-hr recall method. *Afr. J. Food Agric. Nutr. Dev.* **2013**, *13*.
69. FAO and FHI 360. *Minimum Dietary Diversity for Women: A Guide for Measurement*; Food and Agriculture Organization of the United Nations: Rome, Italy, 2016.
70. Friel, S.; Hattersley, L.; Snowdon, W.; Thow, A.M.; Lobstein, T.; Sanders, D.; Barquera, S.; Mohan, S.; Hawkes, C.; Kelly, B. Monitoring the impacts of trade agreements on food environments. *Obes. Rev.* **2013**, *14*, 120–134. [CrossRef] [PubMed]
71. El-Gazzar, H.H.; Saleh, S.M.; Khairy, S.A.; Marei, A.S.; ElKelany, K.; Al Soda, M.F. Relationship between dietary intake and obesity among a group of primary school-aged children in Cairo Governorate. *J. Med. Sci. Res.* **2019**, 2, 42.
72. Khatib, I.; Hijazi, S.S. Micronutrient deficiencies among children may be endemic in underprivileged areas in Jordan. *Jordan Med. J.* **2009**, *43*, 324–332.
73. Al-Rewashdeh, A. Assessment of the nutritional status for preschool children in Jordan. *Bull. Fac. Agric. Cairo Univ.* **2009**, *60*, 423–432.
74. Institute of Medicine; Food and Nutrition Board. Dietary Reference Intakes for Energy, Carbohydrate, Fiber, Fat, Fatty Acids, Cholesterol, Protein and Amino Acids. Available online: https://www.nap.edu/catalog/10490/dietary-reference-intakes-for-energy-carbohydrate-fiber-fat-fatty-acids-cholesterol-protein-and-amino-acids-macronutrients (accessed on 30 April 2017).
75. Jabre, P.; Sikias, P.; Khater-Menassa, B.; Baddoura, R.; Awada, H. Overweight children in Beirut: Prevalence estimates and characteristics. *Child Care Health Dev.* **2005**, *31*, 159–165. [CrossRef]
76. Akl, C. *Prevalence and Determinants of Overweight and Obesity in a Nationally Representative Sample of Lebanese Children 5 to 12 Years Old*; American University of Beirut: Beirut, Lebanon, 2012.
77. Alredaisy, M.; Ibrahim, S. Assessment of nutritional status of children less than 10 years old in rural western Kordafan. *IIOABJ* **2011**, *2*, 40–49.
78. Ng, S.W.; Zaghloul, S.; Ali, H.; Harrison, G.; Yeatts, K.; El Sadig, M.; Popkin, B.M. Nutrition transition in the United Arab Emirates. *Eur. J. Clin. Nutr.* **2011**, *65*, 1328–1337. [CrossRef] [PubMed]

79. Kilani, H.; Al-Hazzaa, H.; Waly, M.I.; Musaiger, A. Lifestyle Habits: Diet, physical activity and sleep duration among Omani adolescents. *Sultan Qaboos Univ. Med. J.* **2013**, *13*, 510. [CrossRef] [PubMed]
80. Bazhan, M.; Kalantari, N.; Houhiar-Rad, A.; Alavi-Majd, H.; Kalantari, S. Dietary habits and nutrient intake in adolescent girls living in Northern Iran. *Arch. Adv. Biosci.* **2013**, *4*.
81. ALFaris, N.A.; Al-Tamimi, J.Z.; Al-Jobair, M.O.; Al-Shwaiyat, N.M. Trends of fast food consumption among adolescent and young adult Saudi girls living in Riyadh. *Food Nutr. Res.* **2015**, *59*, 26488. [CrossRef] [PubMed]
82. Washi, S.A.; Ageib, M.B. Poor diet quality and food habits are related to impaired nutritional status in 13-to 18-year-old adolescents in Jeddah. *Nutr. Res.* **2010**, *30*, 527–534. [CrossRef]
83. Department of Health. Dietary Reference Values for Food Energy, Nutrients for the United Kingdom. In *Report of the Panel on Dietary Values of the Committee on Medical Aspects of Food Policy*, 8th ed.; HMSO: London, UK, 1996.
84. Zaghloul, S.; Al-Hooti, S.N.; Al-Hamad, N.; Al-Zenki, S.; Alomirah, H.; Alayan, I.; Al-Attar, H.; Al-Othman, A.; Al-Shami, E.; Al-Somaie, M. Evidence for nutrition transition in Kuwait: Over-consumption of macronutrients and obesity. *Public Health Nutr.* **2013**, *16*, 596–607. [CrossRef]
85. Jildeh, C.; Papandreou, C.; Mourad, T.A.; Hatzis, C.; Kafatos, A.; Qasrawi, R.; Philalithis, A.; Abdeen, Z. Assessing the nutritional status of Palestinian adolescents from East Jerusalem: A school-based study 2002–03. *J. Trop. Pediatr.* **2011**, *57*, 51–58. [CrossRef]
86. Ahmed, N.M.K.; Onsa, Z.O. Nutritional Assessment of the Adolescents in the Northern State of Sudan. *Pak. J. Nutr.* **2014**, *13*, 79. [CrossRef]
87. Mohseni-Takalloo, S.; Mirmiran, P.; Hosseini-Esfahani, F.; Azizi, F. Dietary fat intake and its relationship with serum lipid profiles in tehranian adolescents. *J. Food Nutr. Res.* **2014**, *2*, 330–334. [CrossRef]
88. World Health Organization. Interim summary of conclusions and dietary recommendations on total fat & fatty acids. In *From the Joint FAO/WHO Expert Consultation on Fats and Fatty Acids in Human Nutrition*; World Health Organization: Geneva, Switzerland, 2008.
89. Nasreddine, L.; Chamieh, M.C.; Ayoub, J.; Hwalla, N.; Sibai, A.-M.; Naja, F. Sex disparities in dietary intake across the lifespan: The case of Lebanon. *Nutr. J.* **2020**, *19*, 1–18. [CrossRef] [PubMed]
90. World Health Organization. Diet, Nutrition and the Prevention of Chronic Diseases. Joint WHO/FAO Expert Consultation. WHO Technical Report Series no. 916. Available online: https://apps.who.int/iris/bitstream/handle/10665/42665/WHO_TRS_916.pdf?sequence=1 (accessed on 1 September 2020).
91. Aounallah-Skhiri, H.; Traissac, P.; El Ati, J.; Eymard-Duvernay, S.; Landais, E.; Achour, N.; Delpeuch, F.; Romdhane, H.B.; Maire, B. Nutrition transition among adolescents of a south-Mediterranean country: Dietary patterns, association with socio-economic factors, overweight and blood pressure. A cross-sectional study in Tunisia. *Nutr. J.* **2011**, *10*, 38. [CrossRef]
92. Huew, R.; Maguire, A.; Waterhouse, P.; Moynihan, P. Nutrient intake and dietary patterns of relevance to dental health of 12-year-old Libyan children. *Public Health Nutr.* **2014**, *17*, 1107–1113. [CrossRef]
93. Montero, P.; Mora Urda, A.; Cherkaoui, M.; Anzid, K. Transition nutritionnelle au Maroc: Étude comparative de l'état nutritionnel des adolescents entre 1991 et 2007. *Bull Séances.* **2009**, *60*, 433–450.
94. Montero, M.D.P.; Mora-Urda, A.I.; Anzid, K.; Cherkaoui, M.; Marrodan, M.D. Diet quality of Moroccan adolescents living in Morocco and in Spain. *J. Biosoc. Sci.* **2017**, *49*, 173. [CrossRef] [PubMed]
95. Anderson, J.W.; Baird, P.; Davis, R.H.; Ferreri, S.; Knudtson, M.; Koraym, A.; Waters, V.; Williams, C.L. Health benefits of dietary fiber. *Nutr. Rev.* **2009**, *67*, 188–205. [CrossRef]
96. Collison, K.S.; Zaidi, M.Z.; Subhani, S.N.; Al-Rubeaan, K.; Shoukri, M.; Al-Mohanna, F.A. Sugar-sweetened carbonated beverage consumption correlates with BMI, waist circumference, and poor dietary choices in school children. *BMC Public Health* **2010**, *10*, 234. [CrossRef]
97. Tayel, D.I.; El-Sayed, N.A.; El-Sayed, N.A. Dietary pattern and blood pressure levels of adolescents in Sohag, Egypt. *J. Egypt Public Health Assoc.* **2013**, *88*, 97–103. [CrossRef]
98. Al-Ansari, J.M.; Al-Jairan, L.Y.; Gillespie, G.M. Dietary habits of the primary to secondary school population and implications for oral health. *J. Allied Health* **2006**, *35*, 75–80. [PubMed]
99. Rifat-uz-Zaman, Z.I.; Ali, U. Dietary Intakes of Urban Adolescents of Sialkot, Pakistan Do Not Meet the Standards of Adequacy. *Pak. J. Nutr.* **2013**, *12*, 460–467. [CrossRef]
100. Aziz, S.; Hosain, K. Carbohydrate (CHO), protein and fat intake of healthy Pakistani school children in a 24 hour period. *J. Pak. Med. Assoc.* **2014**, *64*, 1255–1259.

101. Abuzaid, O.I. *Eating Patterns and Physical Activity Characteristics among Urban and Rural Students in Saudi Arabia*; Nutrition and Health Sciences Department, University of Nebraska-Lincoln: Lincoln, NE, USA, 2012.
102. Institute of Medicine; Food and Nutrition Board. Dietary Reference Intakes: RDA and AI for Vitamins and Elements. Available online: http://www.nationalacademies.org/hmd/~{}/media/Files/Activity%20Files/Nutrition/DRI-Tables/2_%20RDA%20and%20AI%20Values_Vitamin%20and%20Elements.pdf?la=en (accessed on 30 April 2017).
103. Khatib, I. High prevalence of subclinical vitamin A deficiency in Jordan: A forgotten risk. *Food Nutr. Bull.* **2002**, *23*, 228–236. [CrossRef] [PubMed]
104. Salamoun, M.; Kizirian, A.; Tannous, R.; Nabulsi, M.; Choucair, M.; Deeb, M.; Fuleihan, G.E.-H. Low calcium and vitamin D intake in healthy children and adolescents and their correlates. *Eur. J. Clin. Nutr.* **2005**, *59*, 177–184. [CrossRef] [PubMed]
105. Al-Musharaf, S.; Al-Othman, A.; Al-Daghri, N.M.; Krishnaswamy, S.; Yusuf, D.S.; Alkharfy, K.M.; Al-Saleh, Y.; Al-Attas, O.S.; Alokail, M.S.; Moharram, O. Vitamin D deficiency and calcium intake in reference to increased body mass index in children and adolescents. *Eur. J. Pediatr.* **2012**, *171*, 1081–1086. [CrossRef]
106. Saeid, N.; Elmzibri, M.; Hamrani, A.; Latifa, Q.; Belghiti, H.; El Berri, H.; Benjeddou, K.; Bouziani, A.; Benkirane, H.; Taboz, Y. Assessment of sodium and potassium intakes in children aged 6 to 18 years by 24 h urinary excretion in city of rabat, Morocco. *J. Nutr. Metab.* **2018**, *2018*. [CrossRef]
107. Al-Daghri, N.M.; Al-Othman, A.; Alkharfy, K.M.; Alokail, M.S.; Khan, N.; Alfawaz, H.A.; Aiswaidan, I.A.; Chrousos, G.P. Assessment of selected nutrients intake and adipocytokines profile among Saudi children and adults. *Endocrine J.* **2012**, EJ12-0167. [CrossRef]
108. Nasreddine, L.M.; Kassis, A.N.; Ayoub, J.J.; Naja, F.A.; Hwalla, N.C. Nutritional status and dietary intakes of children amid the nutrition transition: The case of the Eastern Mediterranean Region. *Nutr. Res.* **2018**, *57*, 12–27. [CrossRef]
109. Nasreddine, L.; Ayoub, J.J.; Al Jawaldeh, A. Review of the nutrition situation in the Eastern Mediterranean Region. *East. Mediterr. Health J.* **2018**, *24*, 77–91. [CrossRef]
110. Kelishadi, R.; Ardalan, G.; Gheiratmand, R.; Majdzadeh, R.; Hosseini, M.; Gouya, M.; Razaghi, E.; Delavari, A.; Motaghian, M.; Barekati, H. Thinness, overweight and obesity in a national sample of Iranian children and adolescents: CASPIAN Study. *Child Care Health Dev.* **2008**, *34*, 44–54. [CrossRef] [PubMed]
111. Mirmohammadi, S.-J.; Hafezi, R.; Mehrparvar, A.H.; Rezaeian, B.; Akbari, H. Prevalence of overweight and obesity among Iranian school children in different ethnicities. *Iran J. Pediatr.* **2011**, *21*, 514. [PubMed]
112. Nasreddine, L.; Naja, F.; Chamieh, M.C.; Adra, N.; Sibai, A.-M.; Hwalla, N. Trends in overweight and obesity in Lebanon: Evidence from two national cross-sectional surveys (1997 and 2009). *BMC Public Health* **2012**, *12*, 798. [CrossRef] [PubMed]
113. Bener, A.; Kamal, A.A. Growth patterns of Qatari school children and adolescents aged 6–18 years. *J. Health Popul. Nutr.* **2005**, *23*, 250–258.
114. Rootwelt, C.; Fosse, K.B.; Tuffaha, A.; Said, H.; Sandridge, A.; Janahi, I.; Greer, W.; Hedin, L. Qatar s Youth Is Putting on Weight: The Increase in Obesity Between 2003 and 2009. In Proceedings of the Qatar Foundation Annual Research Conference Proceedings, Doha, Qatar, November 2014; Volume 2014, p. HBSP1130.
115. El-Hazmi, M.A.; Warsy, A.S. A comparative study of prevalence of overweight and obesity in children in different provinces of Saudi Arabia. *J. Trop. Pediatr.* **2002**, *48*, 172–177. [CrossRef]
116. Al-Almaie, S.M. Prevalence of obesity and overweight among Saudi adolescents in Eastern Saudi Arabia. *Saudi Med. J.* **2005**, *26*, 607.
117. Al-Nuaim, A.A.; Al-Nakeeb, Y.; Lyons, M.; Al-Hazzaa, H.M.; Nevill, A.; Collins, P.; Duncan, M.J. The prevalence of physical activity and sedentary behaviours relative to obesity among adolescents from Al-Ahsa, Saudi Arabia: Rural versus urban variations. *J. Nutr. Metab.* **2012**, *2012*. [CrossRef]
118. Aounallah-Skhiri, H.; El Ati, J.; Traissac, P.; Romdhane, H.B.; Eymard-Duvernay, S.; Delpeuch, F.; Achour, N.; Maire, B. Blood pressure and associated factors in a North African adolescent population. a national cross-sectional study in Tunisia. *BMC Public Health* **2012**, *12*, 98. [CrossRef]
119. Musaiger, A.O. The state of nutrition in Bahrain. *Nutr. Health* **2000**, *14*, 63–74. [CrossRef]
120. Musaiger, A.O. Overweight and obesity in eastern mediterranean region: Prevalence and possible causes. *J. Obes.* **2011**, *2011*. [CrossRef]

121. Black, R.E.; Victora, C.G.; Walker, S.P.; Bhutta, Z.A.; Christian, P.; De Onis, M.; Ezzati, M.; Grantham-McGregor, S.; Katz, J.; Martorell, R. Maternal and child undernutrition and overweight in low-income and middle-income countries. *Lancet* **2013**, *382*, 427–451. [CrossRef]
122. Itoh, H.; Kanayama, N. Nutritional conditions in early life and risk of non-communicable diseases (NCDs) from the perspective of preemptive medicine in perinatal care. *Hypertens. Res. Pregnancy* **2015**, *3*, 1–12. [CrossRef]
123. Weiss, R.; Dziura, J.; Burgert, T.S.; Tamborlane, W.V.; Taksali, S.E.; Yeckel, C.W.; Allen, K.; Lopes, M.; Savoye, M.; Morrison, J. Obesity and the metabolic syndrome in children and adolescents. *N. Engl. J. Med.* **2004**, *350*, 2362–2374. [CrossRef] [PubMed]
124. Khader, Y.; Batieha, A.; Jaddou, H.; El-Khateeb, M.; Ajlouni, K. Metabolic syndrome and its individual components among Jordanian children and adolescents. *Int. J. Pediatr. Endocrinol.* **2010**, *2010*, 316170. [CrossRef] [PubMed]
125. Taha, D.; Ahmed, O.; Sadiq, B.B. The prevalence of metabolic syndrome and cardiovascular risk factors in a group of obese Saudi children and adolescents: A hospital-based study. *Ann. Saudi Med.* **2009**, *29*, 357–360. [CrossRef] [PubMed]
126. Eapen, V.; Mabrouk, A.; Yousef, S. Metabolic syndrome among the young obese in the United Arab Emirates. *J. Trop. Pediatr.* **2010**, *56*, 325–328. [CrossRef]
127. Ho, K.K.; Ferruzzi, M.G.; Wightman, J.D. Potential health benefits of (poly) phenols derived from fruit and 100% fruit juice. *Nutr. Rev.* **2020**, *78*, 145–174. [CrossRef]
128. Tetens, I.; Alinia, S. The role of fruit consumption in the prevention of obesity. *J. Hortic. Sci. Biotech.* **2009**, *84*, 47–51. [CrossRef]
129. Ello-Martin, J.A.; Roe, L.S.; Ledikwe, J.H.; Beach, A.M.; Rolls, B.J. Dietary energy density in the treatment of obesity: A year-long trial comparing 2 weight-loss diets. *Am. J. Clin. Nutr.* **2007**, *85*, 1465–1477. [CrossRef]
130. Malik, V.S.; Schulze, M.B.; Hu, F.B. Intake of sugar-sweetened beverages and weight gain: A systematic review¯. *Am. J. Clin. Nutr.* **2006**, *84*, 274–288. [CrossRef]
131. Malik, V.S.; Pan, A.; Willett, W.C.; Hu, F.B. Sugar-sweetened beverages and weight gain in children and adults: A systematic review and meta-analysis. *Am. J. Clin. Nutr.* **2013**, *98*, 1084–1102. [CrossRef] [PubMed]
132. Teff, K.L.; Grudziak, J.; Townsend, R.R.; Dunn, T.N.; Grant, R.W.; Adams, S.H.; Keim, N.L.; Cummings, B.P.; Stanhope, K.L.; Havel, P.J. Endocrine and metabolic effects of consuming fructose-and glucose-sweetened beverages with meals in obese men and women: Influence of insulin resistance on plasma triglyceride responses. *J. Clin. Endocrinol. Metab.* **2009**, *94*, 1562–1569. [CrossRef]
133. Stanhope, K.L.; Schwarz, J.M.; Keim, N.L.; Griffen, S.C.; Bremer, A.A.; Graham, J.L.; Hatcher, B.; Cox, C.L.; Dyachenko, A.; Zhang, W. Consuming fructose-sweetened, not glucose-sweetened, beverages increases visceral adiposity and lipids and decreases insulin sensitivity in overweight/obese humans. *J. Clin. Investig.* **2009**, *119*, 1322–1334. [CrossRef]
134. Stanhope, K.L.; Griffen, S.C.; Bair, B.R.; Swarbrick, M.M.; Keim, N.L.; Havel, P.J. Twenty-four-hour endocrine and metabolic profiles following consumption of high-fructose corn syrup-, sucrose-, fructose-, and glucose-sweetened beverages with meals. *Am. J. Clin. Nutr.* **2008**, *87*, 1194–1203. [CrossRef] [PubMed]
135. Stanhope, K.L.; Havel, P.J. Endocrine and metabolic effects of consuming beverages sweetened with fructose, glucose, sucrose, or high-fructose corn syrup. *Am. J. Clin. Nutr.* **2008**, *88*, 1733S–1737S. [CrossRef]
136. Muth, N.D.; Dietz, W.H.; Magge, S.N.; Johnson, R.K.; Pediatrics, A.A.O.; Association, A.H. Public policies to reduce sugary drink consumption in children and adolescents. *Pediatrics* **2019**, *143*. [CrossRef]
137. Engin, A. Fat cell and fatty acid turnover in obesity. In *Obes Lipotoxicity*; Springer: Berlin/Heidelberg, Germany, 2017; pp. 135–160.
138. Liberali, R.; Kupek, E.; Assis, M.A.A.d. Dietary Patterns and Childhood Obesity Risk: A Systematic Review. *Child Obes.* **2020**, *16*, 70–85. [CrossRef] [PubMed]
139. Eyles, H.; Bhana, N.; Lee, S.E.; Grimes, C.; McLean, R.; Nowson, C.; Wall, C. Measuring Children's Sodium and Potassium Intakes in NZ: A Pilot Study. *Nutrients* **2018**, *10*, 1198. [CrossRef]
140. UNICEF-GAIN. Food Systems for Children and Adolescents. In *Working Together to Secure Nutritious Diets*; UNICEF Office of Research: Rome, Italy, 2018.
141. Al-Isa, A. Nutritional Knowledge among High School Male Students in Kuwait. *J. Community Med. Health Educ.* **2018**, *8*. [CrossRef]

142. Al-Yateem, N.; Rossiter, R. Nutritional knowledge and habits of adolescents aged 9 to 13 years in Sharjah, United Arab Emirates: A crosssectional study. *East. Mediterr. Health J.* **2017**, *23*, 551–558. [CrossRef]
143. McClain, A.D.; Chappuis, C.; Nguyen-Rodriguez, S.T.; Yaroch, A.L.; Spruijt-Metz, D. Psychosocial correlates of eating behavior in children and adolescents: A review. *Int. J. Behav. Nutr. Phys. Act.* **2009**, *6*, 54. [CrossRef] [PubMed]
144. Banna, J.C.; Buchthal, O.V.; Delormier, T.; Creed-Kanashiro, H.M.; Penny, M.E. Influences on eating: A qualitative study of adolescents in a periurban area in Lima, Peru. *BMC Public Health* **2015**, *16*, 40. [CrossRef] [PubMed]
145. Becker, A.E.; Burwell, R.A.; Herzog, D.B.; Hamburg, P.; Gilman, S.E. Eating behaviours and attitudes following prolonged exposure to television among ethnic Fijian adolescent girls. *Br. J. Psychiatry* **2002**, *180*, 509–514. [CrossRef]
146. Karimi-Shahanjarini, A.; Omidvar, N.; Bazargan, M.; Rashidian, A.; Majdzadeh, R.; Shojaeizadeh, D. Iranian female adolescent's views on unhealthy snacks consumption: A qualitative study. *Iran J. Public Health* **2010**, *39*, 92. [PubMed]
147. Anthrologica-World Food Programme (WFP). *Bridging the Gap: Engaging Adolescents for Nutrition, Health and Sustainable Development*; World Food Programme: Rome, Italy, 2018.
148. Pachón, H.; Simondon, K.B.; Fall, S.T.; Menon, P.; Ruel, M.T.; Hotz, C.; Creed-Kanashiro, H.; Arce, B.; Domínguez, M.R.L.; Frongillo, E.A. Constraints on the delivery of animal-source foods to infants and young children: Case studies from five countries. *Food Nutr. Bull.* **2007**, *28*, 215–229. [CrossRef]
149. Armar-Klemesu, M.; Osei-Menya, S.; Zakariah-Akoto, S.; Tumilowicz, A.; Lee, J.; Hotz, C. Using ethnography to identify barriers and facilitators to optimal Infant and Young Child Feeding in rural Ghana: Implications for programs. *Food Nutr. Bull.* **2018**, *39*, 231–245. [CrossRef]
150. Burns, J.; Emerson, J.A.; Amundson, K.; Doocy, S.; Caulfield, L.E.; Klemm, R.D. A qualitative analysis of barriers and facilitators to optimal breastfeeding and complementary feeding practices in South Kivu, Democratic Republic of Congo. *Food Nutr. Bull.* **2016**, *37*, 119–131. [CrossRef]
151. Darmon, N.; Drewnowski, A. Contribution of food prices and diet cost to socioeconomic disparities in diet quality and health: A systematic review and analysis. *Nutr. Rev.* **2015**, *73*, 643–660. [CrossRef]
152. Kelly, B.; Halford, J.C.; Boyland, E.J.; Chapman, K.; Bautista-Castaño, I.; Berg, C.; Caroli, M.; Cook, B.; Coutinho, J.G.; Effertz, T. Television food advertising to children: A global perspective. *Am. J. Public Health* **2010**, *100*, 1730–1736. [CrossRef]
153. Nasreddine, L.; Taktouk, M.; Dabbous, M.; Melki, J. The extent, nature, and nutritional quality of foods advertised to children in Lebanon: The first study to use the WHO nutrient profile model for the Eastern Mediterranean Region. *Food Nutr. Res.* **2019**, *63*. [CrossRef]
154. Amini, M.; Omidvar, N.; Yeatman, H.; Shariat-Jafari, S.; Eslami-Amirabadi, M.; Zahedirad, M. Content analysis of food advertising in Iranian children's television programs. *Int. J. Prev. Med.* **2014**, *5*, 1337. [PubMed]
155. World Health Organization. Nutrition-Friendly Schools Initiative (NFSI). Available online: https://www.who.int/nutrition/topics/nutrition_friendly_schools_initiative/en/ (accessed on 8 October 2020).
156. World Health Organization. *Global Accelerated Action for the Health of Adolescents (AA-HA!): Guidance to Support Country Implementation*; World Health Organization: Geneva, Switzerland, 2017.
157. World Health Organization Regional Office for the Eastern Mediterranean. *Implementing the WHO Recommendations on the Marketing of Food and Nonalcoholic Beverages to Children in the Eastern Mediterranean Region*; 9290222247; World Health Organization: Cairo, Egypt, 2018.
158. World Health Organization Regional Office for the Eastern Mediterranean. *Strategy on Nutrition for the Eastern Mediterranean Region 2020–2030*; World Health Organization: Cairo, Egypt, 2019.
159. World Health Organization Regional Office for the Eastern Mediterranean. *Regional Framework for Action on Obesity Prevention 2019–2023*; World Health Organization: Cairo, Egypt, 2019.
160. World Health Organization. *Policy Statement and Recommended Actions for Lowering Sugar Intake and Reducing Prevalence of Type 2 Diabetes and Obesity in the Eastern Mediterranean Region*; World Health Organization: Cairo, Egypt, 2016.
161. World Health Organization. *Policy Statement and Recommended Actions for Reducing Fat Intake and Lowering Heart Attack Rates in the Eastern Mediterranean Region*; World Health Organization: Cairo, Egypt, 2014.

162. World Health Organization. *Policy Statement and Recommended Actions to Lower National Salt Intakes and Lower Death Rates from High Blood Pressure and Strokes in the Eastern Mediterranean Region*; World Health Organization: Cairo, Egypt, 2014.
163. HLPE. Nutrition and food systems. In *A Report by the High Level Panel of Experts on Food Security and Nutrition of the Committee on World Food Security*; High Level Panel of Experts: Rome, Italy, 2017.
164. UNICEF. The Faces of Malnutrition. Available online: https://www.unicef.org/nutrition/index_faces-of-malnutrition.html (accessed on 30 September 2020).

Permissions

All chapters in this book were first published by MDPI; hereby published with permission under the Creative Commons Attribution License or equivalent. Every chapter published in this book has been scrutinized by our experts. Their significance has been extensively debated. The topics covered herein carry significant findings which will fuel the growth of the discipline. They may even be implemented as practical applications or may be referred to as a beginning point for another development.

The contributors of this book come from diverse backgrounds, making this book a truly international effort. This book will bring forth new frontiers with its revolutionizing research information and detailed analysis of the nascent developments around the world.

We would like to thank all the contributing authors for lending their expertise to make the book truly unique. They have played a crucial role in the development of this book. Without their invaluable contributions this book wouldn't have been possible. They have made vital efforts to compile up to date information on the varied aspects of this subject to make this book a valuable addition to the collection of many professionals and students.

This book was conceptualized with the vision of imparting up-to-date information and advanced data in this field. To ensure the same, a matchless editorial board was set up. Every individual on the board went through rigorous rounds of assessment to prove their worth. After which they invested a large part of their time researching and compiling the most relevant data for our readers.

The editorial board has been involved in producing this book since its inception. They have spent rigorous hours researching and exploring the diverse topics which have resulted in the successful publishing of this book. They have passed on their knowledge of decades through this book. To expedite this challenging task, the publisher supported the team at every step. A small team of assistant editors was also appointed to further simplify the editing procedure and attain best results for the readers.

Apart from the editorial board, the designing team has also invested a significant amount of their time in understanding the subject and creating the most relevant covers. They scrutinized every image to scout for the most suitable representation of the subject and create an appropriate cover for the book.

The publishing team has been an ardent support to the editorial, designing and production team. Their endless efforts to recruit the best for this project, has resulted in the accomplishment of this book. They are a veteran in the field of academics and their pool of knowledge is as vast as their experience in printing. Their expertise and guidance has proved useful at every step. Their uncompromising quality standards have made this book an exceptional effort. Their encouragement from time to time has been an inspiration for everyone.

The publisher and the editorial board hope that this book will prove to be a valuable piece of knowledge for researchers, students, practitioners and scholars across the globe.

List of Contributors

Lucinda K. Bell, Celeste Schammer and Rebecca K. Golley
Caring Futures Institute, College of Nursing and Health Sciences, Flinders University, Adelaide 5001, Australia

Gemma Devenish and Jane A. Scott
School of Public Health, Curtin University, Perth 6102, Australia

Diep Ha, John A. Spencer and Loc G. Do
Australian Research Centre for Population Oral Health, School of Dentistry, The University of Adelaide, Adelaide 5000, Australia

Murray W. Thomson
Division of Health Sciences, University of Otago, Dunedin 9016, New Zealand

Rehana A. Salam, Zahra A. Padhani, Jai K. Das, Amina Y. Shaikh and Zahra Hoodbhoy
Division ofWomen and Child Health, Aga Khan University Hospital, Karachi 74800, Pakistan

Sarah Masroor Jeelani
Department of Trauma & Orthopaedics, Macclesfield District General Hospital, East Cheshire NHS Trust Victoria Rd, Macclesfield SK10 3BL, UK

Zohra S. Lassi
Robinson Research Institute, University of Adelaide, Adelaide, SA 5005, Australia

Zulfiqar A. Bhutta
Centre for Global Child Health, the Hospital for Sick Children, Toronto, ON M5G 1X8, Canada

Rachael T. Leon Guerrero, L. Robert Barber, Tanisha F. Aflague, Yvette C. Paulino, Margaret P. Hattori-Uchima and Mark Acosta
Office of Research & Sponsored Programs, University of Guam, Mangilao, Guam 96923, USA

Lynne R. Wilkens
University of Hawaii Cancer Center, Honolulu, HI 96813, USA

Rachel Novotny
College of Tropical Agriculture and Human Resources, University of Hawaii At Manoa, Honolulu, HI 96822, USA

Rute Borrego
Escola Superior de Tecnologia da Saúde de Lisboa, Instituto Politécnico de Lisboa, 1990-096 Lisboa, Portugal

Ana Catarina Moreira
Escola Superior de Tecnologia da Saúde de Lisboa, Instituto Politécnico de Lisboa, 1990-096 Lisboa, Portugal
H &TRC—Health & Technology Research Center, 1990-096 Lisboa, Portugal

Patrícia Almeida Oliveira
Escola Superior de Tecnologia da Saúde de Lisboa, Instituto Politécnico de Lisboa, 1990-096 Lisboa, Portugal
Faculdade de Medicina, Universidade de Lisboa, 1649-004 Lisboa, Portugal

Telma Nogueira
Laboratório de Nutrição, Faculdade de Medicina, Universidade de Lisboa, 1649-028 Lisboa, Portugal
Instituto de Saúde Ambiental, Faculdade de Medicina, Universidade de Lisboa, 1649-028 Lisboa, Portugal

Raquel Ferreira
Escola Superior de Tecnologia da Saúde de Lisboa, Instituto Politécnico de Lisboa, 1990-096 Lisboa, Portugal
Núcleo de Educação e Qualidade Alimentar, Câmara Municipal de Sintra, 2710-307 Sintra, Portugal

Daniel Virella
Research Unit, Centro Hospitalar Universitário Lisboa Central, 1150-199 Lisboa, Portugal

Abina Chaudhary
Independent Researcher, Kastrupvej 79, 2300 Copenhagen, Denmark

František Sudzina
Department of Materials and Production, Faculty of Engineering and Science, Aalborg University, A. C. Meyers Vænge 15, 2450 Copenhagen, Denmark
Department of Systems Analysis, Faculty of Informatics and Statistics, University of Economics, nám. W. Churchilla 1938/4, 130 67 Prague, Czech Republic

Bent Egberg Mikkelsen
Department of Geosciences and Natural ResourceManagement, Faculty of Science, University of Copenhagen, Rolighedsvej 23, 1958 Frederiksberg C, Denmark

Chishinga Callender, Denisse Velazquez, Meheret Adera, Jayna M. Dave and Debbe Thompson
USDA/ARS Children's Nutrition Research Center, Department of Pediatrics, Baylor College of Medicine, 1100 Bates Street, Houston, TX 77030, USA

Norma Olvera
Psychological, Health, and Learning Sciences Department, University of Houston, 3657 Cullen Boulevard Room 491, Houston, TX 77204, USA

Tzu-An Chen
HEALTH Research Institute, University of Houston, 4849 Calhoun Road, Houston, TX 77204, USA

Shana Alford
Common Threads, 222W. Merchandise Mart Plaza, Suite 1212, Chicago, IL 60654, USA

Gonzalo Colmenarejo
Biostatistics and Bioinformatics Unit, IMDEA Food, CEI UAM+CSIC, E28049 Madrid, Spain

Julianne Williams, Marta Buoncristiano, Giulia Rathmes, Anne Charlotte Bunge and Ivo Rakovac
WHO European Office for the Prevention and Control of Noncommunicable Diseases, 125009 Moscow, Russian Federation

Paola Nardone and Angela Spinelli
Italian National Institute of Health (Istituto Superiore Di Sanità), 00161 Rome, Italy

Tatjana Hejgaard
Danish Health Authority, 2300 Copenhagen S, Denmark

Lene Kierkegaard
National Institute of Public Health, University of Southern Denmark, 1455 Copenhagen K, Denmark

Eha Nurk
Department of Nutrition Research, National Institute for Health Development, 11619 Tallinn, Estonia

Marie Kunešová
Institute of Endocrinology, Obesity Unit, 116 94 Prague, Czechia

Sanja Musić Milanović
Croatian Institute of Public Health, University of Zagreb, School of Medicine, 10000 Zagreb, Croatia

Marta García-Solano and Enrique Gutiérrez-González
Spanish Agency for Food Safety and Nutrition, 28014 Madrid, Spain

Lacramioara Aurelia Brinduse and Alexandra Cucu
Department of Public Health and Management, University of Medicine and Pharmacy Carol Davila, 030167 Bucharest, Romania

Anna Fijałkowska
Department of Cardiology, Institute of Mother and Child, 01-211 Warsaw, Poland

Victoria Farrugia Sant'Angelo
Primary Health Care, Ministry for Health, 1940 Floriana, Malta

Shynar Abdrakhmanova
National Center of Public health, Ministry of Health of the Republic of Kazakhstan, 010000 Nur-Sultan City, Kazakhstan

Iveta Pudule
Centre for Disease Prevention and Control, LV-1005 Latvia, Riga

Vesselka Duleva
National Center of Public Health and Analyses, 1431 Sofia, Bulgaria

Nazan Yardim
Turkish Ministry of Health, Public Health General Directorate, 34400 Istanbul, Turkey

Andrea Gualtieri
Health Authority, Department of Health and Social Security, 47893 San Marino, San Marino

Mirjam Heinen and Silvia Bel-Serrat
National Nutrition Surveillance Centre, University College Dublin, Dublin, Ireland

Zhamyla Usupova
Republican Center for Health Promotion and Mass Communication, 720040 Bishkek, Kyrgyzstan

Valentina Peterkova
Institute of Paediatric Endocrinology, National Medical Research Centre for Endocrinology of the Ministry of Health of the Russian Federation, 117036 Moscow, Russian Federation

Lela Shengelia
National Center for Disease Control and Public Health of Georgia, 0198 Tbilisi, Georgia

Jolanda Hyska
Institute of Public Health, 1007 Tirana, Albania

Maya Tanrygulyyeva
Internal Diseases Department of the Scientific Clinical Centre of Mother and Child Health, 744036 Ashgabat, Turkmenistan

Ausra Petrauskiene
Department of Preventive Medicine, Lithuanian University of Health Sciences, 44307 Kaunas, Lithuania

Sanavbar Rakhmatullaeva
Department for Organization of Health Services to Children, Mothers, Adolescents and Family Planning, Ministry of Health and Social Protection of Population, 734025 Dushanbe, Tajikistan

Enisa Kujundzic
Institute of Public Health of Montenegro, Podgorica, Montenegro

Sergej M. Ostojic
Applied Bioenergetics Lab, University of Novi Sad, 21000 Novi Sad, Serbia

Daniel Weghuber
Department of Pediatrics, Paracelsus Medical University, 5020 Salzburg, Austria

Marina Melkumova
Arabkir Medical Centre-Institute of Child and Adolescent Health, 0014 Yerevan, Armenia

Igor Spiroski
Institute of Public Health, Faculty of Medicine, Ss. Cyril and Methodius University, 1000 Skopje, North Macedonia

Gregor Starc
Faculty of Sport, University of Ljubljana, 1000 Ljubljana, Slovenia

Harry Rutter
Department of Social and Policy Sciences, University of Bath, Bath BA2 7AY, UK

Khadichamo Boymatova
WHO Country Office for Tajikistan, 734019 Dushanbe, Tajikistan

Martin Weber
WHO Child and Adolescent Health and Development, WHO Regional Office for Europe, 2100 Copenhagen, Denmark

Narae Yang and Kirang Kim
Department of Food Science and Nutrition, College of Natural Sciences, Dankook University, Dandae-ro, Dongnam-gu, Cheonan-si, Chungnam 31116, Korea

Reetta Lehto, Riikka Pajulahti, Essi Skaffari, Pauliina Hiltunen and Carola Ray
Folkhälsan Research Center, Topeliuksenkatu 20, FI-00250 Helsinki, Finland
Department of Food and Nutrition, University of Helsinki, FI-00014 Helsinki, Finland

Henna Vepsäläinen, Liisa Korkalo and Maijaliisa Erkkola
Department of Food and Nutrition, University of Helsinki, FI-00014 Helsinki, Finland

Rejane Figuereido
Folkhälsan Research Center, Topeliuksenkatu 20, FI-00250 Helsinki, Finland
Clinicum, Faculty of Medicine, University of Helsinki, FI-00014 Helsinki, Finland

Katri Sääksjärvi
Department of Teacher Education, University of Helsinki, FI-00100 Helsinki, Finland

Taina Sainio and Elviira Lehto
Folkhälsan Research Center, Topeliuksenkatu 20, FI-00250 Helsinki, Finland
Department of Teacher Education, University of Helsinki, FI-00100 Helsinki, Finland

Nina Sajaniemi
Department of Teacher Education, University of Helsinki, FI-00100 Helsinki, Finland
School of Applied Educational Science and Teacher Education, Philosophical Faculty, University of Eastern Finland, FI-80101 Joensuu, Finland

Eva Roos
Folkhälsan Research Center, Topeliuksenkatu 20, FI-00250 Helsinki, Finland
Department of Food and Nutrition, University of Helsinki, FI-00014 Helsinki, Finland
Department of Public Health, Clinicum, University of Helsinki, FI-00014 Helsinki, Finland

Isabel Castanheira
WHO Collaborating Centre on Nutrition and Childhood Obesity—National Institute of Health Dr. Ricardo Jorge (INSA, IP), 1649-016 Lisbon, Portugal

Ana Isabel Rito
WHO Collaborating Centre on Nutrition and Childhood Obesity—National Institute of Health Dr. Ricardo Jorge (INSA, IP), 1649-016 Lisbon, Portugal
Centre for Studies and Research in Social Dynamics and Health (CEIDSS), 1649-016 Lisbon, Portugal
National Institute of Health Dr. Ricardo Jorge, 1600 560 Lisbon, Portugal

Mariana Santos
WHO Collaborating Centre on Nutrition and Childhood Obesity—National Institute of Health Dr. Ricardo Jorge (INSA, IP), 1649-016 Lisbon, Portugal
National School of Public Health, NOVA University of Lisbon, 1600-560 Lisbon, Portugal

Sofia Mendes
Centre for Studies and Research in Social Dynamics and Health (CEIDSS), 1649-016 Lisbon, Portugal
National School of Public Health, NOVA University of Lisbon, 1600-560 Lisbon, Portugal

Francisco Goiana-da-Silva and Ara Darzi
Centre for Health Policy, Institute of Global Health Innovation, Imperial College London, London SW7 2AZ, UK

Francesco Paolo Cappuccio
University ofWarwick, WHO Collaborating Centre for Nutrition, Warwick Medical School, Coventry CV2 2DX, UK

Stephen Whiting and João Breda
WHO European Office for the Prevention and Control of Noncommunicable Diseases, 125009 Moscow, Russia

Ana Dinis and Carla Rascôa
Regional Health Administration of Lisbon and Tagus Valley (ARSLVT), 1700-179 Lisbon, Portugal

Ayoub Al-Jawaldeh
World Health Organization (WHO), Regional Office for the Eastern Mediterranean (EMRO), Cairo 7608, Egypt

Mandy Taktouk and Lara Nasreddine
Nutrition and Food Sciences Department, Faculty of Agriculture and Food Sciences, American University of Beirut, Beirut 11-0236, Lebanon

Index

Printed in the USA
CPSIA information can be obtained
at www.ICGtesting.com
JSHW052343050224
56675JS00008B/80

9 781639 877782